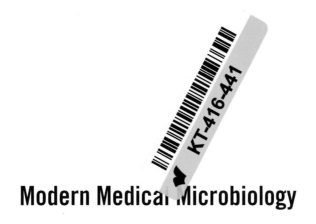

Modern Medical Microbiology

Modern Medical Microbiology
the fundamentals

Stuart C. Clarke MSc PhD FIBMS

Director, Scottish Meningococcus and Pneumococcus
Reference Laboratory, Glasgow, UK

Honorary Senior Research Fellow, Faculty of Biomedical and Life Sciences,
University of Glasgow, Glasgow, UK

Honorary Research Fellow, Faculty of Medicine,
University of Glasgow, Glasgow, UK

ARNOLD

A member of the Hodder Headline Group
LONDON

First published in Great Britain in 2004 by
Arnold, a member of the Hodder Headline Group,
338 Euston Road, London NW1 3BH

http://www.arnoldpublishers.com

Distributed in the United States of America by
Oxford University Press Inc.,
198 Madison Avenue, New York, NY10016
Oxford is a registered trademark of Oxford University Press

© 2004 Arnold

Whilst the advice and information in this book are believed to be true and
accurate at the date of going to press, neither the author nor the publisher
can accept any legal responsibility or liability for any errors or omissions
that may be made. In particular (but without limiting the generality of the
preceding disclaimer) every effort has been made to check drug dosages;
however, it is still possible that errors have been missed. Furthermore,
dosage schedules are constantly being revised and new side effects
recognized. For these reasons the reader is strongly urged to consult the
drug companies' printed instructions before administering any of the drugs
recommended in this book.

British Library Cataloguing in Publication Data
A catalogue record for this book is available from the British Library

Library of Congress Cataloging-in-Publication Data
A catalog record for this book is available from the Library of Congress

ISBN   0 340 81044 0

1 2 3 4 5 6 7 8 9 10

Commissioning Editor: Serena Bureau
Development Editor: Layla Vandenbergh
Project Editor: Wendy Rooke
Production Controller: Deborah Smith
Cover Design: Stewart Larking

Typeset in 10 on 13 Sabon by Phoenix Photosetting, Chatham, Kent
Printed and bound in Spain

What do you think about this book? Or any other Arnold title?
Please send your comments to **feedback.arnold@hodder.co.uk**

Contents

Author biography

Stuart C. Clarke trained as a biomedical scientist at Wexham Park Hospital, Slough between 1988 and 1995 before undertaking a PhD in the Faculty of Medicine at Leicester University. There he specialized in the molecular virulence of enteropathogenic *Escherichia coli*. He then took up the post of Senior Clinical Scientist at the Scottish Meningococcus and Pneumococcus Reference Laboratory (SMPRL) in Glasgow in 1998. He has been the Director of the SMPRL since 2000. He holds two honorary positions at Glasgow University, as a Research Fellow in the Faculty of Medicine and as a Senior Research Fellow in the Faculty of Biomedical and Life Sciences. Dr Clarke's main interests lie in the fields of bacterial virulence, bacterial typing and molecular epidemiology. He has published over 50 research papers and more than 90 other articles.

Preface

Writing a book requires a lot of effort from the author and an equal amount of support from family, friends and colleagues. This book is the result of almost 10 years of writing articles for *Biomedical Scientist*, formerly *The Gazette*, for the Institute of Biomedical Science. While training as a biomedical scientist (MLSO), and just before starting my postgraduate education, I realized that there was little to read in *The Gazette* if you were a student of the profession. So I set about starting this long series of articles, which still continues today, albeit in a more irregular fashion. The aim of this book is to bring together many of these articles in a single format. My worry was that the articles, which are used widely by students, would get lost on bookshelves over time and that the aim of starting them in the first place would fail. This book, consisting of 72 chapters, provides an introduction to the fascinating world of medical microbiology by describing most of the main diseases and the micro-organisms that cause them. The first major section provides a background to medical microbiology in broad terms, including subjects such as health and safety, antibiotics and molecular biology. This is followed by four major sections on bacteriology, virology, parasitology and mycology. As such, the book will appeal to students of microbiology and biomedical science, clinical microbiologists and academic researchers. It will also help those undertaking reading towards their continuous professional development. In the modern world, medical microbiology has an impact on everyone, from our general health, to hospital-acquired infections, to the serious repercussions of bioterrorism; the book will also therefore appeal to a general readership.

Acknowledgements

There are obviously many people to acknowledge along the way, the first of whom are my parents and other immediate family. They helped me get into the profession and have supported me throughout my career. During recent years, my wife has given me much support, including proof-reading the final manuscript. Colleagues and friends have also been paramount, of whom there are too many to mention. However, my mentors deserve much more than a big thanks because they provided opportunities. Dr Mike McIntyre (Wexham Park Hospital) supported me throughout my Master's degree and helped me publish my early peer-reviewed papers. Professor Peter Williams (Leicester University) questioned my knowledge of molecular biology before starting my PhD, and look where that got me! And Dr Tony Girdwood (Stobhill Hospital, now retired) gave me the opportunity to head a national reference laboratory at the age of 27 years and then become director two years later. But mentors are not the only ones who shape careers. My sincere thanks therefore go to everyone in the Department of Microbiology at Wexham Park Hospital, particularly Rosemary and Tom. In Leicester, my gratitude is extended to Richard, Primrose and Rob for making my PhD so enjoyable. Obviously, this book would not exist without the support of the IBMS, particularly Roy Owen, former Editor of *Biomedical Scientist*. Without him, the articles would not have been published and therefore the concept of this book would not have been born. More recently, the support of the current editor, Brian Nation, and my colleagues on the Medical Microbiology Panel of the IBMS has been invaluable. My final thanks to Arnold for believing in my idea.

Abbreviations

ACDP	Advisory Committee on Dangerous Pathogens	EIA	enzyme immunoassay	
ADP	adenosine diphosphate	EIEC	enteroinvasive *Escherichia coli*	
AIDS	acquired immune deficiency syndrome	ELISA	enzyme-linked immunosorbent assay	
AK	adenylate kinase	EPEC	enteropathogenic *Escherichia coli*	
AMP	adenosine monophosphate	EPV	epidermodysplasia verruciformis	
APC	antigen-presenting cell	ETEC	enterotoxigenic *Escherichia coli*	
ARV	AIDS-associated retrovirus	FAS	fluorescent actin-staining	
ATP	adenosine triphosphate	FTA-ABS test	fluorescent treponemal antibody absorbed test	
BCG	bacille Calmette-Guérin	GBS	Guillain–Barré syndrome	
Bfp	bundle-forming pili	GRID	gay-related immune deficiency	
CAP	community-acquired pneumonia	HAI	haemagglutination inhibition	
CCU	Common Cold Unit	HAT	hypoxanthine, aminopterin, thymidine	
CDT-EC	cytolethal distending toxin-producing *Escherichia coli*	HAV	hepatitis A virus	
CFT	complement fixation test	HBcAb	hepatitis B core antibody	
CIE	counter-current immunoelectrophoresis	HBsAg	hepatitis B surface antigen	
		HBV	hepatitis B virus	
CMV	cytomegalovirus	HCV	hepatitis C virus	
CNS	central nervous system	HDV	hepatitis D virus	
COSHH	Control of Substances Hazardous to Health	HEV	hepatitis E virus	
		HHV	human herpes virus	
CRP	C-reactive protein	Hib	*Haemophilus influenzae* type b	
CSF	cerebrospinal fluid	HIV	human immunodeficiency virus	
DAEC	diffuse-adherent *Escherichia coli*	HLA	human leukocyte antigen	
DHF	dengue haemorrhagic fever	HSC	Health and Safety Commission	
DIC	disseminated intravascular coagulation	HSV	herpes simplex virus	
		HTIg	human tetanus immunoglobulin	
DNA	deoxyribonucleic acid	HTLV	human T-cell leukaemia virus	
DoH	Department of Health	HTLV-III	human T-cell leukaemia virus type III	
EAF	enteropathogenic *Escherichia coli* adherence factor	HUS	haemolytic uraemic syndrome	
EAggEC	enteroaggregative *Escherichia coli*	IFA	immunofluorescent antibodies	
EAST1	enteroaggregative heat-stable enterotoxin	IFAT	indirect fluorescent antibody test	
		IgA	immunoglobulin A	
EBV	Epstein–Barr virus	IgG	immunoglobulin G	
EHEC	enterohaemorrhagic *Escherichia coli*	IgE	immunoglobulin E	

IgM	immunoglobulin M
IHAT	indirect haemagglutination test
IL-1	interleukin 1
IL-6	interleukin 6
IVC	intravascular catheter
LAV	lymphadenopathy-associated virus
LCR	ligase chain reaction
LEE	locus of enterocyte effacement
LFTs	liver function tests
LGV	lymphogranuloma venereum
LRT	lower respiratory tract
MAb	monoclonal antibody
MAC	membrane attack complex
MBC	minimum bactericidal concentration
MCA	Medicines Control Agency
MDR-TB	multidrug-resistant tuberculosis
MDT	multidrug therapy
MHC	major histocompatibility complex
MIC	minimum inhibitory concentration
MLST	multi-locus sequence typing
MMR	measles, mumps, rubella
MRSA	methicillin-resistant *Staphylococcus aureus*
NHS	National Health Service
NIH	National Institutes of Health
NK	natural killer
NSAID	non-steroidal anti-inflammatory drug
PCP	*Pneumocystis carinii* pneumonia
PCR	polymerase chain reaction

PHLS	Public Health Laboratory Service
PID	pelvic inflammatory disease
PT	phage types
RIA	radioimmunoassay
RNA	ribonucleic acid
RPR	rapid plasma reagin
RSV	respiratory syncytial virus
RT-PCR	reverse-transcriptase polymerase chain reaction
SIV	simian immunodeficiency virus
SLE	systemic lupus erythematosus
SRH	single radial haemolysis
STD	sexually transmitted disease
TB	tuberculosis
TNF	tumour necrosis factor
TPHA	*Treponema pallidum* haemagglutination assay
TPI test	*Treponema pallidum* immobilization test
URTI	upper respiratory tract infection
UTI	urinary tract infection
UV	ultraviolet
VDRL	Venereal Disease Reference Laboratory
VT	Vero cytotoxin
VTEC	Vero cytotoxin-producing *Escherichia coli*
VZV	varicella zoster virus
WHIF	whole-cell inclusion immunofluorescence test
WHO	World Health Organization

PART I

Introduction

1
Health and safety in the laboratory

The laboratory environment contains many potential hazards, and the safety of every individual is of supreme importance. It is the responsibility of the employer that all health and safety policies are instigated correctly and adhered to at all times, although much of this responsibility may be delegated to departmental health and safety officers. Employees are also responsible for their own actions, and they have a responsibility to be aware of all health and safety codes at local and national levels. All protocols should be adhered to at all times to minimize any risks involved. Any doubt or uncertainty over a procedure should be discussed with a senior member of staff. Associated risks can be identified, perhaps minimized, and the procedure completed safely.

Health and safety covers a wide range of topics involved in the everyday work of a laboratory. These include the use of protective clothing, the provision of good washing facilities, the correct usage and storage of chemicals, the awareness of fire safety and first aid, and the implementation of other safety precautions not covered under these headings.

The general Health and Safety at Work Act was implemented in 1974 and required employers to ensure health, safety and welfare at work for its employees. A number of documents and codes have since been published by the Health and Safety Commission (HSC) and the Department of Health (DoH) so that health and safety issues are updated (Health Services Advisory Committee, 1998; Health and Safety Commission, 1999). Others are published as more specific documents for particular laboratory environments (Health Services Advisory Committee, 1991a; Health Services Advisory Committee, 1991b; Advisory Committee on Dangerous Pathogens, 1995; Health Services Advisory Committee, 1999; Health and Safety Commission, 1995). For example, the Howie Code was first issued by the DoH in response to the Health and Safety Act in 1978 and was directed specifically at clinical laboratories and post-mortem rooms. Since the publication of the early documents in the late 1970s, the general awareness and understanding of health and safety matters has increased dramatically. Over the past decade, changes in health and safety procedures have occurred due to changes in legislation, greater involvement of trade unions, the introduction of laboratory health and safety officers, and a greater knowledge of chemicals and infectious diseases. The changes that have taken place have resulted in safer laboratory environments.

Two documents were published in the 1980s that provided up-to-date guidance on certain health and safety issues. The first, *Categorisation of Pathogens According to Hazard and Categories of Containment*, was issued by the Advisory Committee on Dangerous Pathogens (ACDP) in 1984 and later updated (Advisory Committee on Dangerous Pathogens, 1995). It introduced the terms 'hazard group' and 'containment level'. These are now commonly used phrases in the laboratory and provide the necessary national standard for working safely with infectious agents. The second document, *Control of Substances Hazardous to Health (COSHH) Regulations*, was introduced in October 1989, with documentation being updated in 1999 (Health and Safety Commission, 1999). This requires the employer to assess health risks arising from hazardous substances and processes used in work activities and to introduce controls that are effective in protecting people's health. However, COSHH has also made the employee more responsible for health and safety. COSHH details should be checked on any chemical before its use and any necessary precautions taken.

More recently, the HSC published a revised code on safe working and prevention of infection in clinical laboratories and post-mortem rooms entitled *Safety in health service laboratories*. This is a three-section document that updated and superseded the Howie Code, particularly in the context of risk assessment contained in the COSHH regulations (Health Services Advisory Committee, 1991a; Health Services Advisory Committee, 1991b; Health Services Advisory Committee, 1999). Advice on risk of infection and the necessary precautions was also included, as well as a revised system for the classification of pathogens and corresponding containment requirements recommended by the ACDP.

Laboratories have also introduced their own policies to complement legal requirements and to clarify local requirements. Safe lifting, waste disposal, and fire safety courses have informed staff, while occupational health departments ensure the good health of employees. The introduction of vaccination programmes, most notably hepatitis B, in certain establishments has improved health standards and protection against laboratory pathogens. Major equipment, such as centrifuges and airflow cabinets, are regularly serviced and certified, and logbooks are kept. In the laboratory, general improvements have taken place that have increased safety levels significantly. These include eyewashes, better lighting, fire equipment, safety showers, and first-aid boxes. Access to laboratories has also been reduced so that unauthorized staff cannot enter. Ultimately, the best safety precaution is the educa-tion of staff. Concerns over budgets should never allow compromises in health and safety.

The increased knowledge of the effects of chemicals and infectious diseases has led to changes in health and safety procedures. As we learn even more, the guidelines may change accordingly, so that safer and more effective handling procedures are implemented. There are a number of issues in health and safety, such as laboratory accreditation, which should improve the conditions in the clinical laboratory still further.

REFERENCES

Advisory Committee on Dangerous Pathogens (1995). *Categorisation of Biological Agents According to Hazard and Categories of Containment*, 4th edn. London: HSE Books.

Health and Safety Commission (1995). *A Guide to the Reporting of Injuries, Diseases and Dangerous Occurrences Regulations*. London: HSE Books.

Health and Safety Commission (1999). *COSHH Regulations*. London: HSE Books.

Health Services Advisory Committee (1991a). *Safe Working and the Prevention of Infection in Clinical Laboratories*. London: HMSO.

Health Services Advisory Committee (1991b). *Safe Working and the Prevention of Infection in the Mortuary and Post Mortem Room*. London: HMSO.

Health Services Advisory Committee (1998). *Manual Handling in the Health Services*. London: HSE Books.

Health Services Advisory Committee (1999). *Safe Working and the Prevention of Infection in Clinical Laboratories – Model Rules for Staff and Visitors*. London: HMSO.

2

Emerging and re-emerging diseases

Infectious diseases are known to have affected mankind for thousands of years. This evidence has been gained from literature such as the Bible and from the preserved remains of individuals, such as Egyptian mummies. Today, after all the advances in medicine and public health over the past century, infectious diseases remain a major threat to humans in all areas of the world. New diseases continue to be 'discovered', while others thought to be of little significance or to be easily treatable are re-emerging and creating problems (Chamberland, 2002; Weinstock and Brown, 2002; Williams *et al.*, 2002). Even diseases such as meningococcal meningitis are termed as 'emerging' due to the changing epidemiology of the disease worldwide.

In the past few decades, at least 30 'new' infectious diseases have been described (Table 2.1). The human immunodeficiency virus (HIV), perhaps the most widely known cause of these new diseases, has infected millions of individuals worldwide and continues to spread in the developing world, although the number of cases is levelling out slowly in developed countries. Other diseases such as the Ebola infection are restricted geographically at present but have high mortality rates and are therefore of great concern. *Cryptosporidium* spp., although first described early in the twentieth century, has only recently become regarded as a human pathogen and has been shown to have dramatic public health implications due to waterborne transmission via improperly treated drinking water.

'Old' diseases that were on the decline for various reasons are re-emerging. These diseases are usually treatable through the use of antibiotics or vaccination or are declining due to improved sanitation and changes in human social behaviour.

Table 2.1 Examples of emerging and re-emerging infectious diseases

Bubonic plague
Cholera
Cryptosporidiosis
Cyclosporiasis
Dengue fever
Diphtheria
Ebola infection
Escherichia coli 0157
Hantavirus
HIV infection
Legionnaires' disease
Lyme disease
Tuberculosis

Diphtheria, for example, has been declining in many countries and can be treated with antibiotic therapy. However, cases of diphtheria increased and outbreaks occurred in the former Soviet Union during the 1990s (Skogen *et al.*, 2002). This pattern is also occurring with other diseases. There are a number of reasons for the re-emergence of 'old' diseases. First, antibiotic resistance is on the increase due to overuse or misuse in some countries (Metlay, 2002; Smith *et al.*, 2002). Some organisms were once treatable with commonly available and cheap antibiotics but are now resistant to them. Second, as mentioned earlier, the changes in epidemiology of some diseases may be attributed to the changes in social behaviour of humans.

However, some diseases are actually increasing for the same reason. Over the past two decades, the amount of global travel has increased enormously. Whether travel is by land, sea or air, infectious diseases can spread from one country to another, and diseases that were once limited geographically are now being found in similar climates in areas where they did not exist previously.

Another major contribution to the increasing threat of infectious diseases is population growth. The urban population alone is over 2.6 billion individuals, and this is increasing continually. This inevitably leads to an increase in poverty. Urbanization has increased the possibility for the increase of infectious diseases. Two decades ago it was thought that the advances in medicine and the public health measures that were in place would eventually limit the importance of infectious diseases. Although this is true to an extent, urbanization can lead to overcrowding, and if there is inadequate clean water or sanitation provisions, then diseases or their vectors can emerge. Also, micro-organisms are able to adapt surprisingly well and evolve fairly rapidly to their environment and gain resistance to antibiotics. Malaria, for example, is now becoming a problem in urban areas where the mosquito vector has adapted and found suitable breeding waters. Therefore, any of the following factors can affect the emergence or re-emergence of major infectious diseases:

- changes in human social behaviour;
- population growth;
- population dynamics;
- inadequate public health systems in many developing countries;
- misuse and overuse of antibiotics;
- human invasion and destruction of tropical forests;
- adaptation and evolution of micro-organisms.

Localized outbreaks are now more likely to spread to become major epidemics than ever before. This worry has been seen on a number of occasions due to outbreaks in the developing world. For example, in recent years outbreaks of plague have occurred in India (Deodhar *et al.*, 1998; Shivaji *et al.*, 2000), and outbreaks of Ebola haemorrhagic fever have occurred in Africa (Tukei, 1996). During such outbreaks, there is the worry in developed countries of the possibility of an infected but asymptomatic individual travelling widely within the same country or, worse, travelling abroad. In either case, there is the potential for this individual to infect others. This has not occurred yet, but rapid public health measures were taken on both occasions to prepare for such an eventuality.

One of the most important infectious diseases to re-emerge in both the developing and developed world in recent years is tuberculosis (Alexander *et al.*, 2002; Murray, 1991). Although the disease can usually be treated with combination antibiotic therapy, this has always been a problem in the developing world due to antibiotic availability, cost, and patient compliance. Bacille Calmette-Guérin (BCG) vaccination has proved to be very useful since its introduction in the developing world; however, there was an approximate 28% increase in global case notifications between 1990 and 1993 compared with between 1984–86, and in some countries it continues to emerge (Brennan, 1997; Inoue and Matoba, 2001). Some strains of tuberculosis are now resistant to a number of drugs that were previously useful in treating the disease, and the HIV pandemic has not helped. Tuberculosis has been declared a global emergency by the World Health Organization (WHO).

It is now hoped that a global alert system, involving a number of agencies worldwide, can provide rapid and effective action when outbreaks of infectious diseases that are of major significance occur. It is also hoped that improved global infectious disease surveillance will take place, so that disease trends can be followed to enable the necessary short- or long-term action to be put in place. Although such alerting or surveillance systems are very costly, more lives and money are saved in the long term. For example, it is hoped that polio will soon be eradicated globally (Hull and Aylward, 2001). If this becomes the case, WHO predicts that there will be global savings of $3 billion/year by 2015.

Infectious diseases therefore remain a major threat to mankind even though many important advances have been made in medicine and public health. Global surveillance systems are required to enable rapid action during major outbreaks. Eradication of those micro-organisms for which there are safe vaccines may be required to lessen the global burden of infectious diseases as a whole.

REFERENCES

Alexander, K A., Pleydell, E., Williams, M.C., Lane, E.P., Nyange, J.F. and Michel, A.L. (2002). *Mycobacterium* tuberculosis: an emerging disease of free-ranging wildlife. *Emerg Infect Dis* **8**, 598–601.

Brennan, P.J. (1997). Tuberculosis in the context of emerging and reemerging diseases. *FEMS Immunol Med Microbiol* **18**, 263–9.

Chamberland, M.E. (2002). Emerging infectious agents: do they pose a risk to the safety of transfused blood and blood products? *Clin Infect Dis* **34**, 797–805.

Deodhar, N.S., Yemul, V.L. and Banerjee, K. (1998). Plague that never was: a review of the alleged plague outbreaks in India in 1994. *J Public Health Policy* **19**, 184–99.

Hull, H.F. and Aylward, R.B. (2001). Progress towards global polio eradication. *Vaccine* **19**, 4378–84.

Inoue, K. and Matoba, S. (2001). Counterattack of re-emerging tuberculosis after 38 years. *Int J Tuberc Lung Dis* **5**, 873–5.

Metlay, J.P. (2002). Update on community-acquired pneumonia: impact of antibiotic resistance on clinical outcomes. *Curr Opin Infect Dis* **15**, 163–7.

Murray, J.F. (1991). An emerging global programme against tuberculosis: agenda for research, including the impact of HIV infection. *Bull Int Union Tuberc Lung Dis* **66**, 207–9.

Shivaji, S., Bhanu, N.V. and Aggarwal, R.K. (2000). Identification of *Yersinia pestis* as the causative organism of plague in India as determined by 16S rDNA sequencing and RAPD-based genomic fingerprinting. *FEMS Microbiol Lett* **189**, 247–52.

Skogen, V., Cherkasova, V.V., Maksimova, N., *et al.* (2002). Molecular characterization of *Corynebacterium diphtheriae* isolates, Russia, 1957–1987. *Emerg Infect Dis* **8**, 516–18.

Smith, D.L., Harris, A.D., Johnson, J.A., Silbergeld, E.K. and Morris, J.G., Jr (2002). Animal antibiotic use has an early but important impact on the emergence of antibiotic resistance in human commensal bacteria. *Proc Natl Acad Sci USA* **99**, 6434–9.

Tukei, P.M. (1996). Threat of Marburg and Ebola viral haemorrhagic fevers in Africa. *East Afr Med J* **73**, 27–31.

Weinstock, D.M. and Brown, A.E. (2002). *Rhodococcus equi*: an emerging pathogen. *Clin Infect Dis* **34**, 1379–85.

Williams, E.S., Yuill, T., Artois, M., Fischer, J. and Haigh, S.A. (2002). Emerging infectious diseases in wildlife. *Rev Sci Tech* **21**, 139–57.

3

Disease in the developing world

GLOBAL HEALTH PROBLEMS

Approximately two-thirds of the world's population live in areas regarded as underdeveloped. Over 10 million children die each year before their fifth birthday, despite most children now being immunized against all of the major childhood infectious diseases. Although the figures were once higher, they remain high despite continuing research and vaccine development and have not changed significantly. A large proportion of these deaths are due to diarrhoeal diseases, and it is therefore crucial to global health that basic research into diarrhoeal and other diseases continues.

This chapter provides a background to diarrhoeal disease in the developing world as an example of the major challenges facing the future public health of these countries.

THE GLOBAL PROBLEM OF DIARRHOEAL ILLNESS

Diarrhoeal disease has been recognized since the beginning of civilization, perhaps as early as 3300 BC, and remains one of the most important health problems of today. In developing countries, it is estimated that over 1.3 billion cases of diarrhoeal illness occur each year, resulting in over 5 million deaths. Of these, over 2.7 million deaths occur in children under five years of age. Underdeveloped areas do not have adequate sanitary provisions, housing is poor and overcrowded, and personal hygiene is of a low standard. Disease is therefore transmitted readily between people, and the mor-

tality rate is much higher than in developed countries due to the lack of supportive medicine. Diarrhoeal disease is largely a problem in children, and it is the second most common illness in this age group after respiratory disease; it therefore remains a problem in both developed and developing countries, although it is a greater problem in the latter. The rates of diarrhoeal disease range from an average of 1.7 episodes per person per year in the USA to an average of 17 episodes per person per year in some developing countries. Diarrhoeal disease may be caused by a number of bacterial, parasitic and viral aetiologies, which are discussed below. Certain species within each group are very important causes of diarrhoea, resulting in millions of deaths worldwide each year. The final outcome of diarrhoeal illness depends on numerous factors, including age, breastfeeding, the pathogen involved, complications such as dehydration and renal failure, and the availability of medical treatment.

GASTROINTESTINAL PATHOGENS

There are numerous causes of gastrointestinal illness in humans. These include various genera and species of viruses, protozoa and bacteria. The search for aetiological agents of diarrhoea began in 1875, with the discovery of *Entamoeba histolytica* by Lösch in Russia. Since then, new species of organisms have been continually discovered as 'new' aetiological agents of diarrhoeal disease. Even so, in some developing countries the known causes of diarrhoea account for only 60% of all episodes, with the remaining 40% being due to unknown aetiologies. Additionally, the costs associated with the diagnosis of gastrointestinal pathogens are high, being estimated to be between $900 and $1000 for a positive case in the USA (Guerrant *et al.*, 1985). There have been clear advances in recent years in the fields of research related to gastrointestinal infectious disease. Newly identified pathogens have been described, such as *Helicobacter pylori* and various pathovars of *Escherichia coli* (Clarke, 2001; Suerbaum & Michetti, 2002). However, much more is to be learnt before effective therapies or vaccines can be produced.

Viral gastrointestinal pathogens

Viruses are an important cause of diarrhoeal disease worldwide and account for approximately 10% of cases of traveller's diarrhoea. Rotavirus and Norwalk virus are the most common causes of viral diarrhoea, although other viruses such as the small round structured viruses, adenoviruses and astroviruses are also important (Jiang *et al.*, 2002; Subekti *et al.*, 2002). Symptoms of viral diarrhoea are usually of abrupt onset and short-lived; they include diarrhoea, vomiting and sometimes mild fever. Diarrhoeal viruses are spread primarily via contaminated water, particularly during rainy season in developing countries.

Protozoan and nematode gastrointestinal pathogens

Diarrhoeal diseases due to protozoan and nematode infections are numerous. Pathogens include organisms as diverse as the flagellates, amoebae, coccidia and helminths (worms). Not all genera within these groups are pathogenic, but those that are are responsible for a whole range of acute and chronic diseases in humans. Many of the pathogens that cause diarrhoeal disease are waterborne and are responsible for either sporadic cases or outbreaks. Two important protozoan diseases are caused by *Giardia* and *Cryptosporidium*, and and these two organisms are estimated to infect more than 600 million people worldwide (Lima, 2001; Walker-Smith, 2001). Another pathogen, *Entamoeba histolytica* (now known as *Entamoeba dispar*), is also common, accounting for 500 million infections and an estimated 100 000 deaths each year. In addition, nematode infections account for a further 3.5 billion infections, the majority of which are due to only four organisms: *Ascaris lumbricoides* (roundworm), *Trichuris trichiuria* (whipworm), *Necator americanus* and *Ancylostoma duodenale* (hookworm).

Bacterial gastrointestinal pathogens

There are three types of bacterial gastrointestinal infection according to the site of pathogenesis and, therefore, to the causative organism. Most gastrointestinal infections are non-inflammatory, occur in the small bowel, and are caused by the action of an enterotoxin, such as cholera toxin, or by a pathogenic process such as that of enteropathogenic *E. coli*. Inflammatory infection occurs in the colon and is caused by an invasive pathogen such as *Shigella*. The third type of infection, characterized by enteric fever, is caused by pathogens such as *Salmonella typhi*, which enter the Peyer's patches and regional lymph nodes. Such pathogens cause systemic infection before returning to the gastrointestinal tract via the biliary tract.

Throughout the world, the species of bacterial agents of diarrhoeal illness are very similar. In developing countries, the most common bacterial causes of diarrhoea are enterotoxigenic *E. coli*, *Vibrio cholerae*, *Salmonella typhi*, *Shigella flexneri*, *Shigella dysenteriae* and enteropathogenic *E. coli*. In developed countries, *Campylobacter*, nontyphoid salmonellae and *Shigella sonnei* are most common. *Campylobacter* spp., *Yersinia* spp., noncholera vibrios, *Staphylococcus aureus* and *Clostridium perfringens* occur in both developing and developed countries (Lima, 2001).

CONTROL OF DIARRHOEAL DISEASE

The control of diarrhoeal disease is a global challenge for people of all ages. Diarrhoeal disease can be controlled largely by the introduction of basic sanitary measures. However, clean water is only a vision in many developing countries, and the vast areas of undeveloped land mean that the provision of such a basic amenity is almost impossible. The level of funding required to develop these countries is beyond the scope of most charities and supporting agencies from developed nations. Whilst the introduction of basic sanitation to such countries is therefore a slow and ongoing process, there are more immediate measures that can be taken to aid the control of diarrhoeal disease.

Many disease-specific control programmes have taken place during the past few decades, and a lot has been learnt from these. The aim is to apply this knowledge to new, coordinated programmes that are not disease-specific and to integrate the action of different agencies so that childhood diseases such as diarrhoea can be prevented and managed. Cheap drugs, including oral antibiotics, antiparasitic drugs, oral rehydration salts and vitamins, may be made available so that they cover all types of diarrhoea. Such programmes also aim to prevent many of these illnesses in the first place by improving the uptake of immunization and improving general nutritional and hygiene levels by methods such as breastfeeding. Education is also an important facet of these programmes.

The correct management of diarrhoea, particularly that occurring during childhood, could save around 2 million lives each year. Most cases of diarrhoeal illness can be prevented or treated. The cause of diarrhoea may be determined by healthcare workers by assessing the duration of illness, the level of dehydration, and the presence of blood in stools. This approach saves lives and is cost-effective because the correct treatment and the right dose is then given, whether for acute diarrhoea or dysentery. Treatment of a child with diarrhoea also provides the healthcare worker with the opportunity of assessing the child's general health status. If health is generally poor, then appropriate action can be taken in the form of treatment, support and education. As malnutrition is an important cause of subsequent disease, such opportunities for health assessment are important.

DISEASE ERADICATION

It is very easy in today's world to wish for the global eradication of many infectious diseases. Smallpox was eradicated over 20 years ago and polio is approaching eradication, while other diseases are under control. In the developed world, infectious disease is not the problem it was 50 years ago, but the same cannot be said for developing countries. Most of the improvements seen in infectious disease control are due to a few changes that have occurred as countries have developed. These include the establishment of an infrastructure, the availability of good sanitation, and the introduction of antibiotics and vaccines. As such, the rates of infectious disease in developed countries are very small compared with those in developing countries, although the emergence or re-emergence of some diseases may cause problems in the future. Many readers may wonder why antibiotics and vaccines cannot be introduced into developing countries so that infectious diseases are controlled better in such areas. And surely improvements in infrastructure and sanitation would reduce the burden of infectious disease? If stagnant waters could be removed, then malaria would be much less of a problem; prophylaxis and vaccination efforts may then be reduced. The simple answer is that all these improvements could be made, but the politics of governments and international pharmaceutical companies often hinder any advances. Media attention has been given to the problems of third-world debt; this debt is owed to various banks in developed countries, and the amount being paid in interest on these loans each year is equivalent to the amount donated by charity each year.

THE FUTURE OF INFECTIOUS DISEASE IN DEVELOPING COUNTRIES

The WHO and many other organizations are doing much to reduce the burden of infectious disease in developing countries. Third-world debt will remain a problem and hinder such efforts if governments in developed countries continue to ignore the consequences felt by developing countries. In the meantime, charitable organizations will continue to provide improvements in health within their capabilities so that the morbidity and mortality are reduced.

REFERENCES

Clarke, S.C. (2001). Diarrhoeagenic *Escherichia coli* – an emerging problem? *Diagn Microbiol Infect Dis* **41**, 93–8.

Guerrant, R.L., Shields, D.S., Thorson, S.M., Schorling, J.B. and Groschel, D.H. (1985). Evaluation and diagnosis of acute infectious diarrhea. *Am J Med* **78**, 91–8.

Jiang, Z.D., Lowe, B., Verenkar, M.P., *et al.* (2002). Prevalence of enteric pathogens among international travelers with diarrhea acquired in Kenya (Mombasa), India (Goa), or Jamaica (Montego Bay). *J Infect Dis* **185**, 497–502.

Lima, A.A. (2001). Tropical diarrhoea: new developments in traveller's diarrhoea. *Curr Opin Infect Dis* **14**, 547–52.

Subekti, D., Lesmana, M., Tjaniadi, P., *et al.* (2002). Incidence of Norwalk-like viruses, rotavirus and adenovirus infection in patients with acute gastroenteritis in Jakarta, Indonesia. *FEMS Immunol Med Microbiol* **33**, 27–33.

Suerbaum, S. and Michetti, P. (2002). *Helicobacter pylori* infection. *N Engl J Med* **347**, 1175–86.

Walker-Smith, J.A. (2001). Post-infective diarrhoea. *Curr Opin Infect Dis* **14**, 567–71.

4

Food poisoning

Foodborne illness, or food poisoning, is an extremely important problem in both developed and developing countries (Tauxe, 2002). Reports of foodborne illness continue to increase worldwide for a number of reasons. Although many control measures have been implemented, especially in developed countries, there remain a number of methods by which foodborne illness can still occur. Furthermore, there are also reasons in developed countries why food poisoning reports have increased.

Food poisoning is defined as any disease of an infectious or toxic nature caused by, or thought to be caused by, the consumption of food or water. An outbreak of food poisoning may be defined as two or more linked cases of the same illness. Some food poisoning outbreaks result in high-profile media attention because of their importance or their location, such as in hospitals or schools, or because they are caused by well-known branded foods. In the developed world, food poisoning is an unpleasant experience resulting in an uneventful recovery for most people. However, the costs resulting from such illnesses may be high, and therefore food poisoning is important economically in terms of lost working hours, public health and diagnostic investigation costs, and treatment costs (Todd, 1989). Greater costs may also be borne by the food manufacturer, as has been seen after salmonella outbreaks during the 1980s in the UK (Roberts *et al.*, 1989), which cost one company more than £20 million. Such an economic burden would be largely avoidable through education and prevention strategies, although such measures are difficult to implement and then retain.

Although most cases of food poisoning are caused by bacteria, it must not be forgotten that foodborne illness may be caused by other microbes such as viruses or parasites, by a product of microbes such as a toxin, or by a chemical agent such as a pesticide (Table 4.1) (Bishai and Sears, 1993; Granum, 1990; Granum and Lund, 1997; Koopmans *et al.*, 2002). However, the risk of microbial contamination is estimated to be 100 000 times greater than the risk of chemical contamination. The principal bacteria associated with food poisoning in the UK are campylobacter and salmonella. These organisms are considered to be zoonoses. They have attracted media attention in recent years; campylobacter has attracted the least attention, even though it is the most common cause of foodborne illness. Cases of food poisoning are required to be reported; these data are then used for epidemiological purposes in both the short and long term. Outbreaks that have been reported may require national notification, which is essential for providing early warnings. Statistics can also be used for recognizing infectious disease trends.

Changes in eating habits are a major contributory factor to the increase in foodborne illness in recent years, and there are many social factors responsible for the shift in habits. People tend to eat out more often today, but when they do eat at home they often prepare convenience foods. Foods are also stored in the home for longer, and food preparation times have shortened, mostly due to the introduction of microwave ovens. Growing public and governmental concern during the 1980s led to the introduction of the Food Safety Act in 1990, which replaced seven previous Acts. This Act and two Government committee reports, known as the Richmond Reports, followed by other reports

Table 4.1 Examples of microbial causative agents of foodborne illness[a,b]

Organism	Associated foods
Bacteria	
Aeromonas	Cooked rice, vegetables
Campylobacter	Milk, poultry
Enterotoxigenic E. coli	Salads, vegetables
Enterohaemorrhagic E. coli	Meats, milk
Listeria monocytogenes	Soft cheeses, milk
Non-typhoid salmonellae	Meat, poultry
Shigella spp.	Milk, vegetables
Yersinia enterocolitica	Milk, pork, poultry
Parasites	
Cryptosporidium	Water, milk
Entamoeba histolytica	Fruit, vegetables
Ascaris lumbricoides	Soil-contaminated foods
Taenia saginata	Meats
Viruses	
Hepatitis A	Shellfish, vegetables
Norwalk virus	Shellfish

[a]Many foodborne pathogens may also be transmitted by water.
[b]This is not a comprehensive list.

in response to outbreaks, have had a significant impact on the food industry. One of the main aims of the Act was to make it illegal to sell for human consumption food that is contaminated beyond the accepted level. Obviously, this is open to some interpretation, but the Act gives more power for criminal prosecution. In 1994, the DoH also published an informal guide, *Management of Outbreaks of Foodborne Illness*, providing a framework for the management of food-poisoning outbreaks. Such documents are important for providing the necessary guidance during food-poisoning outbreaks, and their need was noted by the Committee on the Microbiological Safety of Food (the Richmond Report) in 1990 (Anon, 1990; Anon, 1991) and by the Advisory Committee on the Microbiological State of Food (*Salmonella in Eggs Report*) in 1993.

Although prevention is better than cure, food poisoning appears to be a disease that is easier to cure than prevent. Due to the large range of different organisms that may be responsible for food poisoning, and the fact that many of the causative organisms may be waterborne or zoonotic, post-infection treatment is often easier. It would be an impossible task to eradicate these organisms from both water and animals that are used for human consumption. The only preventive measure that is realistically promising is the production of effective vaccines against the causative organisms. However, as food poisoning is caused by so many different organisms, such vaccine availability is probably decades away. Also, mass vaccination with a dozen or so vaccines would seem impractical. It would therefore seem that food poisoning is a fact of life that will remain with us. The best individual prevention is good hygiene and good cooking methods. However, we also rely on manufacturers and restaurants to do the same. For now, cases of food poisoning will continue to increase until better preventive measures become available.

REFERENCES

Advisory Committee on the Microbiological Safety of Food (1993). *Report on* Salmonella *in Eggs*. London: HMSO.

Anon (1990). *The Microbiological Safety of Food. Report of the Committee on the Microbiological Safety of Food*, part I. London: HMSO.

Anon (1991). *The Microbiological Safety of Food. Report of the Committee on the Microbiological Safety of Food*, part II. London: HMSO.

Bishai, W.R. and Sears, C.L. (1993). Food poisoning syndromes. *Gastroenterol Clin North Am* 22, 579–608.

Department of Health (1994). *Management of Outbreaks of Foodborne Illness. Guidance Produced by a Department of Health Working Group*. London: Department of Health.

Granum, P.E. (1990). *Clostridium perfringens* toxins involved in food poisoning. *Int J Food Microbiol* 10, 101–11.

Granum, P.E. and Lund, T. (1997). *Bacillus cereus* and its food poisoning toxins. *FEMS Microbiol Lett* 157, 223–8.

Koopmans, M., von Bonsdorff, C.H., Vinje, J., de Medici, D. and Monroe, S. (2002). Foodborne viruses. *FEMS Microbiol Rev* 26, 187–205.

Roberts, J.A., Sockett, P.N. and Gill, O.N. (1989). Economic impact of a nationwide outbreak of salmonellosis: cost-benefit of early intervention. *BMJ* 298, 1227–30.

Tauxe, R.V. (2002). Emerging foodborne pathogens. *Int J Food Microbiol* 78, 31–41.

Todd, E.C. (1989). Costs of acute bacterial foodborne disease in Canada and the United States. *Int J Food Microbiol* 9, 313–26.

5

Evasion of the immune response by bacteria

The presence of an appropriate immune response provides an individual with protection from pathogens. The resultant mechanisms of the innate or acquired immune responses, however, may cause more damage than the organism itself. The course of an infectious disease is determined by several interactions between the bacteria and the host, such as entry of the bacteria into the host, invasion and colonization of the host tissues, evasion from the host immune responses, and tissue injury or functional impairment.

Attachment to host tissue is the first interaction by bacteria; the bacteria must be able to adhere to host epithelium to avoid the action of ciliated epithelium or the flushing action of the body fluids before attempting to multiply and cause disease. Some bacteria possess adhesins, proteins that aid their adherence to host epithelium. Extracellular determinants involved in adherence include fimbriae, flagella, capsule, lipopolysaccharide (endotoxin), and outer-membrane proteins (Aizawa, 2001; Ernst *et al.*, 2001).

All Gram-negative bacteria possess endotoxins, complex lipopolysaccharide molecules present on their outer membrane. Endotoxins must be released before they are effective, and this occurs mainly when bacterial cells die. Once free, the endotoxins induce interleukin 1 (IL-1) and tumour necrosis factor (TNF) secretion by macrophages and neutrophils, thereby causing fever and vascular collapse. Macrophages and other cells produce several other cytokines that induce migration, local accumulation, and activation of neutrophils and monocytes to phagocytose the bacteria. One of these cytokines, interleukin 6 (IL-6), induces the synthesis of acute-phase proteins such as C-reactive protein (CRP) and complement in the liver. Other cytokines are able to recruit T- and B-lymphocytes to produce a specific immune response.

Bacteria possess cell-associated and intracellular mechanisms that are as diverse as those that are extracellular. They include exotoxins, enterotoxins, enzymes and antibacterial substances. These chemicals are manufactured inside the bacterial cell and released into the local tissue of the host. Exotoxins have specific effects at low concentration and usually have an enzymatic function; they fall into four categories:

- toxins affecting the passage of nerve impulses;
- toxins promoting the survival or spread of bacteria;
- toxins that damage or destroy cells;
- toxins that interfere with cell metabolism.

Many 'classical toxins', such as that produced by *Clostridium tetani*, are usually the only mechanism by which the bacteria are able to evade the host immune response. Their main functions are probably in competing against commensal flora and in weakening the host to ensure survival. Exotoxins of the 'non-classical' type are not the only mechanism produced by some bacteria to evade the immune response. Enterotoxins, a type of exotoxin, are produced by some enteropathogenic Gram-negative bacteria. Again, they probably play a role in the competition against commensal flora of the gut. Toxins may also aid the invasiveness of those bacteria that cross the gut wall into the blood vessels and other organs, e.g. *Salmonella typhi*. Shiga toxin, produced by *Shigella dysenteriae*, may cause cellular destruction, allowing penetration and multiplication of the bacteria within colonic epithelial cells. Immunoglobulin A (IgA) is the major component of immunoglobulin in gastric secretions, and it prevents attachment of bacteria to the gut epithelium. Neutralizing antibodies (immunoglobulin M (IgM) and immunoglobulin G (IgG)) may be produced against bacterial toxins, and these can have two modes of action. They are able to bind to the active site of the toxin, thereby inhibiting its activity, and they are able to enhance the removal of the toxin from the circulation by phagocytosis. Some bacterial toxins acting as superantigens, such as staphylococcal enterotoxins and exotoxins, have been shown to non-specifically activate CD4-positive T-cells (T-helper cells), which results in massive quantities of cytokines being produced; the immunopathology of this is very similar to endotoxic shock. Many bacteria produce a range of extracellular enzymes that aid in the evasion of innate immune mechanisms, competition against commensal bacteria, and resistance against phagocytosis or opsonization. Some bacteria release antibacterial substances such as bacteriocins, organic acids or alcohols that allow them to compete against the commensal flora.

In response to infection, the host may reduce the levels of intracellular and extracellular iron (Wooldridge and Williams, 1993). Bacteria require iron for growth, and successful bacterial pathogens have evolved mechanisms to counteract the host response, such as the reduction of ferric iron to ferrous iron, the utilization of host iron compounds, and the production of siderophores.

IgG produced against surface determinants of the bacteria serve as opsonins, thereby enhancing phagocytosis. Both IgM and IgG are able to activate the classical complement pathway, whereas endotoxin activates the alternative complement pathway. C3a and C5a fragments produced act as chemotactic factors by attracting neutrophils to the site of infection. Individuals with C3 deficiency are prone to recurrent bacterial infections, e.g. pneu-

monia, septicaemia and meningitis. The final product of both the complement pathways is the membrane attack complex (MAC), which causes lysis of bacterial cells, particularly *Neisseria* spp. Patients with complement deficiencies of C5–9 have a unique susceptibility to neisserial infection.

Intracellular bacteria, such as *Mycobacterium* spp. and *Listeria* spp., are able to survive and replicate inside mononuclear phagocytes, and sometimes within other host cells. The survival of these bacteria within cells provides protection from phagocytosis and the action of antibodies. Immunity to these bacteria crucially depends on interactions between T-lymphocytes and macrophages. After activation by interferon-γ from T-lymphocytes, macrophages become major effectors against these bacteria. Natural killer (NK) cells are also important in early defence against intracellular bacterial. NK cells recognize and lyse infected monocytes.

Although the virulent determinants of Gram-negative anaerobes are not understood fully, encapsulation probably protects the bacterium from phagocytosis, while the production of extracellular/cell-bound enzymes results in the degradation of immunoglobulins. The production of endotoxin causes local tissue damage through the destruction of phagocytes.

It can be seen that bacteria possess several mechanisms by which they evade the host immune response. A compromise in the efficiency of the immune system will further predispose an individual to bacterial infection, and this may be brought about by acquired or congenital states.

REFERENCES

Aizawa, S.I. (2001). Bacterial flagella and type III secretion systems. *FEMS Microbiol Lett* **202**, 157–64.

Ernst, R.K., Guina, T. and Miller, S.I. (2001). *Salmonella typhimurium* outer membrane remodeling: role in resistance to host innate immunity. *Microbes Infect* **3**, 1327–34.

Wooldridge, K.G. and Williams, P.H. (1993). Iron uptake mechanisms of pathogenic bacteria. *FEMS Microbiol Rev* **12**, 325–48.

6

DNA vaccination

Immunization programmes are aimed at controlling infectious diseases via safe and effective vaccines. Successful vaccination relies upon the production of an effective immune response that is able to protect the host against the required disease. Not all vaccines meet these requirements, and for many diseases no vaccine is available despite there being a definite need for one. The advent of molecular biology has led to a greater understanding of both infectious disease agents and the host immune response. This understanding has enabled better vaccine design. Even so, it is unlikely that vaccines for a number of diseases will be available in the near future. However, the virulence mechanisms of various pathogens have been elucidated, and the mechanisms by which these interact with the host at the molecular and cellular level have been investigated. Likewise, in the host, mechanisms involved in the immune response have been determined. Traditional methods of vaccination for infectious diseases often rely upon the use of killed or attenuated organisms. However, in recent years DNA has become a focus for vaccination design (Kucerova, 1998; Watts and Kennedy, 1999).

The ideal vaccine would be safe, cheap and heat-stable, would provide protection against multiple pathogens, and would be administered in a single dose. Although no vaccine intended for human use has yet met all these requirements, vaccination has reduced the morbidity and mortality of numerous diseases worldwide. Smallpox has been eradicated due to vaccination, while the eradication of polio is now also realistic (Hull and Aylward, 2001; Raskin, 2001). Due to most vaccines not meeting all of the above requirements, developing countries are largely unable to adopt

vaccination strategies. Most vaccines are not heat-stable and are not cheap, and therefore they cannot be used in such areas.

Antigens derived from pathogens, whether they be bacterial, protozoan or viral, are either processed within the cell and then displayed on the cell surface in association with class I major histocompatibility complex (MHC) molecules or are taken up by antigen-presenting cells (APCs) and displayed on the cell surface with MHC class II molecules (Momburg and Hengel, 2002; Unanue, 2002). In the former mechanism CD8-positive T-cells are activated, which lyse the infected cells, whilst in the latter mechanism CD4-positive T-helper cells are activated, which secrete cytokines that regulate other mechanisms of the immune response. B-cell antibody production is also critical in host defence and, in general, humoral responses are important in protecting against bacterial infections. Cell-mediated immunity is important during viral infections. DNA vaccination must therefore address these aspects of host immunity and provide adequate protection against disease. Over the past decade, intense research has been performed to answer such questions. Animal models have been used to indicate whether DNA vaccination is worthy of human clinical trials. Such research has shown that both humoral and cell-mediated immune responses are induced after DNA vaccination. This is in contrast to killed-cell vaccines, which are unable to activate the MHC class I pathway. A number of micro-organisms have now been used successfully in DNA vaccination (Table 6.1).

A decade ago, it was shown that when plasmid DNA containing a marker gene was injected intramuscularly into mice, persistent expression of the

Table 6.1 Examples of DNA vaccines used successfully in animal models

Cytomegalovirus
HIV
Hepatitis B virus
Mycoplasma pharyngis
Influenza
Mycobacterium tuberculosis
Rabies
Malaria

gene occurred at the site of injection. Subsequent work has shown that this strategy can be used with naked DNA encoding a viral polypeptide. DNA encoding type A influenza nucleocapsid protein linked to the human cytomegalovirus promoter has been injected into mice. This resulted in a serum antibody response to the nucleocapsid protein and subsequent protection against both morbidity and mortality when challenged intranasally with a heterotypic strain of influenza. Such findings have important implications in human vaccination strategies. At the moment, influenza vaccines are based on the most common strain in circulation. Therefore, humans are not protected against other strains and must rely upon their immediate immune defences, which, in some individuals, are not sufficient. The experiment described above suggests that vaccination of DNA encoding conserved antigens may provide heterotypic protection, which would be of great use in humans for vaccination against influenza and other micro-organisms where heterogenicity occurs frequently. Furthermore, such a strategy would be particularly useful where the use of whole cell or whole virus is not recommended. For example, it is undesirable to use whole HIV or hepatitis virus for vaccination; however, if for each virus a conserved antigen could be targeted, which elicited a good humoral response, then DNA vaccination would be feasible.

DNA vaccination relies upon gene expression after injection, and this is influenced by the vector used and the method of administration (Kucerova, 1998; Shedlock and Weiner, 2000). A number of methods have been used to administer DNA. The first involves direct injection of DNA in saline or DNA complexed with lipids. The second involves propelling the DNA as an aerosol or as coated gold beads using pressurized gas or an electrical charge. The most common method has been direct injection of DNA into skeletal muscle. Recently, intradermal immunization has shown promise; it induces long-term protection and requires less DNA than intramuscular injection.

DNA vaccines do not possess many of the disadvantages associated with current vaccination methods (Shedlock and Weiner, 2000). In addition to possessing all the good points associated with live or killed-cell vaccines, they are easy to prepare and purify, and they are heat-stable and inexpensive. Importantly, DNA vaccine efficacy is not reduced by the presence of maternal antibody, and there is no risk of reversion to pathogenicity.

Although DNA vaccination is an attractive proposition, there are a number of safety concerns. First, the long-term effects of in vivo expression are unknown. It is not known whether antigen persistence will lead to inflammation or immune disorders. Second, although DNA was thought to be inert in normal, healthy individuals, there is growing evidence that it is not, and therefore strong immune responses may be provoked against 'carrier' DNA (i.e. the plasmid carrying the vaccine DNA). Further future vaccination with the same carrier DNA would therefore be useless. Finally, injected DNA may integrate into the host genome and disrupt normal gene function. However, the risk of this is thought to be extremely low, and there is no evidence that integration occurs even after long periods in animal models. It is also not known whether anaphylaxis will be induced when DNA is injected into hosts already sensitized to the antigen.

Clinical trials are being performed in humans to test the safety and efficacy of DNA vaccination. These trials should answer many of the safety concerns raised above. If the clinical trials are successful and DNA vaccination is found to be safe, then the first DNA vaccines could be available in the near future. The use of epitope vaccines is also being explored, as these are the smallest immunogenic subunits derived from protein antigens (Smith, 1999). The long-term prospects of producing more vaccines against infectious diseases will then be more realistic and provide protection against diseases for which there are currently no vaccines or antibiotic treatments. Furthermore, these vaccines will be cheap and heat-stable, thereby providing developing countries with vaccination strategies.

REFERENCES

Hull, H.F. and Aylward, R.B. (2001). Progress towards global polio eradication. *Vaccine* **19**, 4378–84.

Kucerova, L. (1998). DNA/genetic vaccination (minireview). *Viral Immunol* **11**, 55–63.

Momburg, F. and Hengel, H. (2002). Corking the bottleneck: the transporter associated with antigen processing as a target for immune subversion by viruses. *Curr Top Microbiol Immunol* **269**, 57–74.

Raskin, S.A. (2001). Smallpox: elimination or possible re-infection? *Md Med* **2**, 36–8.

Shedlock, D.J. and Weiner, D.B. (2000). DNA vaccination: antigen presentation and the induction of immunity. *J Leukoc Biol* **68**, 793–806.

Smith, S.G. (1999). The polyepitope approach to DNA vaccination. *Curr Opin Mol Ther* **1**, 10–15.

Unanue, E.R. (2002). Perspective on antigen processing and presentation. *Immunol Rev* **185**, 86–102.

Watts, A.M. and Kennedy, R.C. (1999). DNA vaccination strategies against infectious diseases. *Int J Parasitol* **29**, 1149–63.

7

Antibiotics

Antibiotic therapy is an interesting and diverse subject that invokes the fields of pharmacy, microbial physiology, microbial biochemistry and general microbiology. Antibiotics aspire to the definition of 'magic bullets', i.e. chemical compounds that, when given to a patient, can travel to a site of infection and kill the causative organism without harming the patient. Most 'magic bullets' target bacterial infection, although other infections, such as those caused by fungi and parasites, also have their antimicrobials. Most viruses, by virtue of their very different nature, cannot be considered susceptible to such treatment, although some antiviral agents are available. After the introduction of the penicillins in the 1940s, large-scale production of a range of antibiotics started during the 1950s, and the use of antibiotics in modern medicine has greatly reduced the morbidity and mortality associated with many diseases.

Antibiotics may be of natural origin, may be derived from compounds of natural origin, or may be wholly synthetic. Fungal moulds were the earliest source of natural antibiotics. Derived forms tend to be chemically modified versions of natural antibiotics. Synthetic antibiotics may be identical to natural forms or may be modified derivatives, sometimes far removed from their origins. One problem with the use of antimicrobial agents is that successive generations of bacteria may become resistant to them. Such evolution in bacteria may be rapid because of the short interval between generations. Susceptibility to any antibiotic varies according to the species, and even the strain, of a given bacterium. Susceptibility patterns for most bacteria have altered enormously since the 1940s and 1950s. For example, staphylococci were the

first previously susceptible bacteria to develop resistance to penicillin. This is because of the use, and often misuse, of antibiotics. Some bacteria are inherently resistant to certain antibiotics, and this is due to their physiological organisation. Resistance may also be acquired and develop in normally susceptible species or strains. Development of resistance may reflect either a mutation, which can occur quite rapidly in a population, or the acquisition of certain genes. However, for resistance to develop to antibiotics, there must be a reason. This is due mainly to the overuse or misuse of antibiotics, whether in humans or animals. There are three genetic reasons for a bacterium developing resistance:

- gene mutation;
- transformation, whereby DNA is taken up from another bacterium;
- plasmid-mediated.

The actual mechanisms for the development of such resistance are threefold. The first is by the production of enzymes that inactivate or modify the antibiotic either before or after it enters the bacterium. Inactivating enzymes include the beta-lactamases, the aminoglycoside-modifying enzymes, and chloramphenicol acetyltransferase. However, other agents have been discovered or synthesized that may counteract such adaptations, meaning that some antimicrobial agents can still be of therapeutic use. The second mechanism is a reduced affinity of the antibiotic for a target molecule or structure within the bacterium due to modification or bypassing of a vital and susceptible target. Such reduced affinity may be mediated by structures such as penicillin-binding proteins. The third mechanism is reduced permeability or total impermeability to the antibiotic. The latter is more common in Gram-negative bacteria than in Gram-positive bacteria due to the differences in structure of the cell walls and cell membranes.

Beta-lactamase production is arguably the most common mechanism of resistance to antibiotics in bacteria. Most Gram-negative bacteria are able to produce beta-lactamase. It is produced within the cell and is not normally excreted extracellularly. The enzyme acts on the beta-lactam ring component of beta-lactam antibiotics, resulting in the destruction of their antimicrobial properties. Beta-lactamase production was first noted in the early 1940s, and since then the understanding and importance of the enzyme has grown. Other mechanisms of resistance play a very important part in bacterial resistance to antibiotics. Resistance caused by variance in cell structure of Gram-negative bacteria is normally inherent. For example, outer-membrane impermeability is common in many Gram-negative bacteria, where it may occur because of mutation.

Antibiotic resistance in many bacterial pathogens is worrying. Streptococci, salmonellae, campylobacter and *Mycobacterium tuberculosis*, amongst many others, have developed resistance in the past decade against one or more antibiotics that were previously used therapeutically (Beall *et al.*, 2002; Bingen *et al.*, 2002; Davis *et al.*, 2002; Herrera *et al.*, 2002; Low *et al.*, 2002; Zampaloni *et al.*, 2002). Methicillin-resistant *Staphylococcus aureus* (MRSA) is increasing in both incidence and antibiotic resistance (Cespedes *et al.*, 2002; Charlebois *et al.*, 2002; Dominguez *et al.*, 2002; Nishijima and Kurokawa, 2002; Rezende *et al.*, 2002). The management of patients is therefore increasingly difficult due to the pressures of existing or emerging antibiotic resistance. The prescribing and dosing of antibiotics requires good management and communication between clinicians and microbiologists in hospitals and the community (Gupta, 2002; Norman, 2002). Therefore, antibiotic susceptibility testing is very important so

that the correct dose of the correct antibiotic can be given to a patient. Dose sizes are important: too little antibiotic may be ineffective and may facilitate the development of resistance mechanisms, whereas too much antibiotic may result in a dose that may be toxic to the patient's own tissues. Susceptibility patterns of bacteria can be determined in order to provide information relating to whether a given bacterium is sensitive, resistant or moderately sensitive to a given antibiotic when compared with a standard control. Breakpoint tests can also be performed: broths of solid or liquid medium at a range of antibiotic concentrations are used and can provide information relating to the minimum inhibitory concentration (MIC) and minimum bactericidal concentration (MBC) for a given antibiotic against a given bacterium. Although not all bacterial isolates are tested for their MIC and MBC, in certain clinical cases, such as subacute bacterial endocarditis, it may be important to find out these data. Methods used for antibiotic susceptibility testing include the Stokes disc diffusion method, the E-test MIC strip method, and the Vitek machine, to name only a few.

REFERENCES

Beall, B., McEllistrem, M.C., Gertz, R E., Jr, *et al.* (2002). Emergence of a novel penicillin-nonsusceptible, invasive serotype 35B clone of *Streptococcus pneumoniae* within the United States. *J Infect Dis* **186**, 118–22.

Bingen, E., Leclercq, R., Fitoussi, F., *et al.* (2002). Emergence of group A streptococcus strains with different mechanisms of macrolide resistance. *Antimicrob Agents Chemother* **46**, 1199–203.

Cespedes, C., Miller, M., Quagliarello, B., Vavagiakis, P., Klein, R.S. and Lowy, F.D. (2002). Differences between *Staphylococcus aureus* isolates from medical and nonmedical hospital personnel. *J Clin Microbiol* **40**, 2594–7.

Charlebois, E.D., Bangsberg, D.R., Moss, N.J., *et al.* (2002). Population-based community prevalence of methicillin-resistant *Staphylococcus aureus* in the urban poor of San Francisco. *Clin Infect Dis* **34**, 425–33.

Davis, M.A., Hancock, D.D. and Besser, T.E. (2002). Multiresistant clones of *Salmonella enterica*: the importance of dissemination. *J Lab Clin Med* **140**, 135–41.

Dominguez, E., Zarazaga, M. and Torres, C. (2002). Antibiotic resistance in *Staphylococcus* isolates obtained from fecal samples of healthy children. *J Clin Microbiol* **40**, 2638–41.

Gupta, K. (2002). Addressing antibiotic resistance. *Am J Med* **113** (suppl 1A), 29–34S.

Herrera, L., Salcedo, C., Orden, B., *et al.* (2002). Rifampin resistance in *Streptococcus pyogenes*. *Eur J Clin Microbiol Infect Dis* **21**, 411–13.

Low, D.E., de Azavedo, J., Weiss, K., *et al.* (2002). Antimicrobial resistance among clinical isolates of *Streptococcus pneumoniae* in Canada during 2000. *Antimicrob Agents Chemother* **46**, 1295–301.

Nishijima, S. and Kurokawa, I. (2002). Antimicrobial resistance of *Staphylococcus aureus* isolated from skin infections. *Int J Antimicrob Agents* **19**, 241–3.

Norman, D.C. (2002). Management of antibiotic-resistant bacteria. *J Am Geriatr Soc* **50**, S242–6.

Rezende, N.A., Blumberg, H.M., Metzger, B.S., Larsen, N.M., Ray, S.M. and McGowan, J.E., Jr (2002). Risk factors for methicillin-resistance among patients with *Staphylococcus aureus* bacteremia at the time of hospital admission. *Am J Med Sci* **323**, 117–23.

Zampaloni, C., Vitali, L.A., Prenna, M., Toscano, M.A., Tempera, G. and Ripa, S. (2002). Erythromycin resistance in Italian isolates of *Streptococcus pyogenes* and correlations with pulsed-field gel electrophoresis analysis. *Microb Drug Resist* **8**, 39–44.

8

Microbiology of catheters

Catheterization is an essential part of medical care. It has a long history, dating back to Roman times or earlier, when reeds and other natural materials were used. Today, catheters are made from one of three base materials – latex, silicone or plastic – and are coated with other materials depending on their specific use. Although catheterization has many merits, it also contributes to significant morbidity, mortality and economic burden because of nosocomial infections.

URETHRAL CATHETERS

In a typical district general hospital, urethral catheterization will occur in over 10% of inpatients in any one year. Many more patients will be catheterized at home with in-dwelling catheters or by intermittent self-catheterization. Urethral catheterization is indicated in patients with acute or chronic urinary retention, urinary incontinence, paralysis and spinal cord injury. It is also used for bladder irrigation and pre- and postoperative drainage. Catheterization may be short-term (one to seven days), intermittent, in-dwelling or long term (28 days or more). Once inserted, care of the catheter is of utmost importance to reduce the possibility of infection. The catheter must remain in place, should not get blocked, and should not irritate the urethra or bladder, and the system should be kept closed and undisturbed. Leakage should not occur, and encrustation, formed by the precipitation of calcium and ammonium salts, should be avoided (Godfrey and Evans, 2000). Any departure from the above will increase the risk of infection.

The urethral catheter has been recognized as a major cause of nosocomial infection for many years. It is estimated that bacteriuria occurs in up to one-third of catheterized patients within five days, but in more than 70% of these patients the bacteriuria is asymptomatic. In many cases, the bacteriuria resolves without treatment while the catheter is still in place or shortly after it has been removed. However, catheter-associated bacteriuria increases the risk of Gram-negative bacteraemia fivefold and lengthens hospital stay by one to five days. The diagnosis of catheter-associated bacteriuria is therefore important. Infection occurs because the catheter is a foreign body and interferes with the normal process of urine excretion. The catheterized bladder may be thought of as a continuous culture apparatus. There is a constant flow of urine, a good growth medium, and a constant drain, which leaves a 20-mL reservoir, enabling bacteria to establish and multiply. The risk of infection is increased in certain groups of patients, such as those with diabetes or severe underlying illness.

Bacteria might be able to enter the catheter and cause infection via the external urethral meatus or the junction of the catheter and the bag tubing. Some bacteria may also be able to migrate up the tubing from the drainage bag. The risk of exogenous infection from the hands of staff or from the environment may be limited by the application of strict aseptic methods. However, the risk of endogenous infection is more difficult to control and may occur with either faecal or urethral bacteria. The Gram-positive cocci are also commonly associated with urethral catheter infections and may subsequently cause septicaemia. The microbiology analysis of urine from catheterized bladders is therefore required for a number of reasons. It is an aid to prognosis and is helpful in indicating the need for prophylactic treatment to prevent septicaemia or endocarditis. However, prophylaxis is not normally indicated for the treatment of bacteriuria. Microscopy of the catheter urine for the presence of white cells is usually unhelpful since white cells may often be present because of underlying illness, transurethral operation or the catheter itself, and not because of bacteriuria.

Once the catheter has remained in situ for some time, a biofilm may start to form on its surface (Morris et al., 1999). This consists of a collection of bacteria and their extracellular products and has been observed on all types of catheter material. Some bacteria have been shown to be able to adhere to catheter material through the possession of haemagglutinins. Antibiotic therapy and antiseptic washouts are largely ineffective against these biofilms and therefore catheter removal is most effective in preventing infection. However, catheters coated with hydrophilic polymer discourage bacterial colonization and therefore the formation of biofilms. The prevention of urethral catheter-associated infection is needed and requires more than the use of antimicrobial therapy. There are several ways by which this can be achieved, but many are impractical or are not fully effective. Changes in the composition and design of catheters might be the way forward.

INTRAVASCULAR CATHETERS

The introduction of intravascular catheters (IVCs) revolutionized treatment and improved the management of patients requiring nutritional or intravenous therapy (Harrison, 1997). IVCs are used in the short term for fluid replacement, drug administration and cardiovascular monitoring, and in the long term for parenteral nutrition, chemotherapy and haemodialysis. Over 200 000 central vascular catheters are used each year in the UK, and more than three million are used annually in the USA. Infection associated with these catheters is therefore a significant cause of morbidity and mortality

(Harrison, 1997). It is estimated that up to 10% of IVCs result in bacteraemia, but it is generally accepted that the advantages of vascular catheterization far outweigh the possible complications and disadvantages. Thousands of IVC-associated bacteraemias are reported each year in the UK, caused by both Gram-positive and Gram-negative bacteria, including coagulase-negative staphylococci, *Staphylococcus aureus*, streptococci and coliforms (Saad, 2001). Candida species are a less common cause of IVC-associated bacteraemia.

There are many ways by which bacteria may gain access to the catheter and cause infection. These may be divided into four main routes:

- extraluminal
- intraluminal
- haematogenous spread
- via contaminated infusates.

The two most common are the extraluminal and intraluminal routes; these often involve the skin-insertion site or the catheter hub. Infection may result from the spread of the patient's own skin flora or by contamination from hospital staff. There are also a number of factors that influence the risk of catheter-associated infection, including the duration of catheterization, the location of the catheter, the catheter design, and the type of dressing used at the catheter entry site. The local bacterial flora of the patient at the catheter insertion site also influence the incidence of IVC-associated bacteraemia. This is because some bacteria are able to adhere to the materials used in catheters. It has been suggested that coagulase-negative staphylococci may be able to adhere to plastic catheters better than other organisms.

IVC-associated infections can be categorized as localized or systemic. The former may be associated with oedema, a purulent exudate, local cellulitis and abscess formation, although signs of local inflammation are present in only about one-half of cases. Systemic infections may be associated with low-grade pyrexia, leukocytosis and bacteraemia, although in some patients infection may be subclinical. Further complications due to bacteraemia may include endocarditis. The diagnosis of IVC-associated infection is obviously important but is sometimes difficult. There are a number of ways in which microbiological investigations can confirm a clinical diagnosis. Many catheter tips are removed, often unnecessarily, when there is a question of IVC-associated infection, and it is often useful to culture these tips. However, most methods of catheter culture provide a diagnosis after removal when it would be useful to know the result before. Other microbiological investigations include semi-quantitative cultures of the catheter, various surveillance culture methods of the catheter, and quantitative blood cultures. Some of these methods are more useful in selected patients. In any case, IVC-associated bacteraemia may be confirmed by isolating the same organism from both the catheter and peripheral blood cultures. In some circumstances, it is useful to have rapid confirmation of IVC-associated infection. Gram-staining of the catheter tip has been shown to correlate well with subsequent culture results, but its sensitivity is questionable.

As with urethral catheterization, the prevention of IVC-associated infection is needed (O'Grady et al., 2002). Although antibiotics are usually given for both local and systemic complications in patients with IVC-associated infection, other methods are needed to prevent, or at least reduce, the incidence of infection. Procedures that can be implemented to reduce the incidence of IVC-associated infection include the implementation of guidelines for the insertion and care of catheters and improvements in control of cross-infection. The use of antimicrobial prophylaxis upon insertion of IVCs is an issue that is still not recommended. Although it may prevent infection in some patients, it has been shown that its use may increase bacterial colonization of some catheters and lead to bacterial antibiotic resistance. Again, there have been developments in the composition and design of catheters to increase their antimicrobial and anti-adherence properties (Elliott and Tebbs, 1998). The use of these catheters has shown a reduction in the incidence of IVC-associated infection. However, more work still needs to be done in this area to provide further improvements.

REFERENCES

Elliott, T.S. and Tebbs, S.E. (1998). Prevention of central venous catheter-related infection. *J Hosp Infect* **40**, 193–201.

Godfrey, H. and Evans, A. (2000). Management of long-term urethral catheters: minimizing complications. *Br J Nurs* **9**, 74-6, 78–81.

Harrison, M. (1997). Central venous catheters: a review of the literature. *Nurs Stand* **11**, 43–5.

Morris, N.S., Stickler, D.J. and McLean, R.J. (1999). The development of bacterial biofilms on indwelling urethral catheters. *World J Urol* **17**, 345–50.

O'Grady, N.P., Alexander, M., Dellinger, E.P., *et al.* (2002). Guidelines for the prevention of intravascular catheter-related infections. *Infect Control Hosp Epidemiol* **23**, 759–69.

Saad, T.F. (2001). Central venous dialysis catheters: catheter-associated infection. *Semin Dial* **14**, 446–51.

9

Monoclonal antibodies in medicine

Monoclonal antibody (MAb) technology is well-recognized as a significant development for the production of specific serological reagents to a wide variety of antigens. Such reagents provide the means for developing a number of highly specific, sensitive and reproducible immunological assays for the rapid and accurate diagnosis of infectious and non-infectious diseases as well as providing the potential for a number of new therapeutic preparations.

MAb technology relies upon the use of B-lymphocytes, which produce antibodies of a single specificity. The process is naturally random, and it is therefore impossible to predict to which antigen the monoclonal tumour (or myeloma) is specific. However, a technique was developed in 1975 by Georges Kohler and Cesar Milstein at the Medical Research Council Laboratory of Molecular Biology (Kohler and Milstein, 1975). The work was published in *Nature*, and the authors later received Nobel Prizes. Their original method involved the repeated immunization of a mouse with the desired antigen, followed by removal of the spleen, which contains proliferating B-cells. Somatic cell hybridization between a normal antibody-producing B-cell and a myeloma line takes place. Selection of the fused cells that secrete antibody of the desired specificity is performed by culture in selective HAT (hypoxanthine, aminopterin, thymidine) medium. Non-hybrid cells are unable to grow in HAT medium. In just over a week, a small amount of cloned hybrid grows, and the secreted antibody is present in the culture supernatant. Such fusion-derived immortalized antibody-producing cell lines are called hybridomas, and the antibodies they produce are called monoclonal antibodies. The antibodies are tested for their activity by use of a screening assay. Hybridomas from which positive antibodies are obtained can then be bulk-cultured in HAT medium or the peritoneal cavity of syngeneic mice. From standard cell culture, the average MAb yield is less than 20 mg/L. A number of large-scale culture methods have therefore been developed for the industrial production of MAbs. Improvements of the original technique have been made, but the basic concept for MAb production still remains. The technique is now so refined that even laboratories with only modest tissue-culture equipment can produce MAbs.

In 1977, due to the development of Kohler and Milstein's technique, it was shown that MAbs could be raised against biologically interesting molecules. This gave hope for the treatment of some human diseases. However, it soon became apparent that rodent MAbs are unsuitable because they are poor at initiating human immune defence systems due to their slightly different structure. The MAbs themselves were also the target of the human immune response. It was therefore attempted to produce MAbs in human hybridomas, but these antibodies were less specific at binding. Genetic manipulation has since enabled the production of chimeric antibodies. These are largely human antibodies, so that a good immune response is initiated, but they possess rodent variable domains for specific binding.

MAbs have many uses in medicine (Waldmann, 1991). Probably the most exploited use of MAbs currently is in the diagnosis and treatment of infectious diseases (Castillo *et al.*, 1995; Gomez *et al.*, 1997; Irmen and Kelleher, 2000; Verhoef and Torensma, 1990). MAbs have been produced against antigens of numerous bacteria, parasites and viruses, and many assays are now available for the diagnosis of a number of infections, ranging from chlamydia to respiratory syncytial virus (RSV). These assays employ latex agglutination, immunofluorescence or enzyme immunoassay (EIA) techniques and provide more rapid methods of diagnosis than other serological assays or culture. Results may be obtained within a few hours from MAb assays, whereas other methods may take days. Obviously, a rapid diagnosis is helpful in enabling prompt and effective chemotherapy for patients. MAbs may also be used in the diagnosis of non-infectious diseases. For example, MAbs are used in immunohistology for the diagnosis of autoimmune disorders and certain cancers (Kuhn and Thomas, 1994; Schulte, 1996).

MAbs have also been produced for the treatment of many infectious and non-infectious diseases and other medical conditions (Waldmann, 1991). MAbs provide an alternative to conventional therapies and are sometimes safer, with fewer or no side effects. The first MAb to be approved for use in human therapy was OKT3, an immunosuppressive murine reagent for the treatment of renal transplant rejection (Parlevliet and Schellekens, 1992). OKT3 is less toxic than other therapies, but it is not without its own side effects. MAbs have also been developed against the lymphocyte antigens CD4, Tac and Cdw52. Other antibody preparations have been used for a number of years in the treatment of several viral diseases. These preparations have often consisted of polyclonal human immunoglobulin. Humanized MAbs are being developed for use against viruses and bacteria. MAbs have also found a use in the treatment of cancers. However, results have been mostly disappointing, probably due to the inability of MAbs to reach target tumour cells. Further research is therefore being carried out to address this problem. MAbs have been developed against endotoxin and tumour necrosis factor (TNF). Endotoxin is a component of bacterial cell walls and is the cause of septic shock, while TNF is produced by the body in response to the presence of endotoxin. MAbs against these two molecules may therefore reduce the rate of mortality seen in patients with bacteraemia and septic shock.

MAbs are also used commercially. They may be used for the identification and purification of microbial products, e.g. in the production of vaccines and in industrial processes. MAbs may also be used in the water industry for the identification of microbes such as cryptosporidia in contaminated water supplies.

It may be concluded, therefore, that in only two decades MAbs have found a major niche in medicine. Many new developments employ MAb technology, and hopefully many more diagnostic and therapeutic tools will result from such technology.

REFERENCES

Castillo, L., Castillo, D., Silva, W., *et al.* (1995). Development of highly specific monoclonal antibodies for the diagnosis of *Vibrio cholerae* 01. *Hybridoma* **14**, 271–8.

Gomez, B.L., Figueroa, J.I., Hamilton, A.J., *et al.* (1997). Use of monoclonal antibodies in diagnosis of paracoccidioidomycosis: new strategies for detection of circulating antigens. *J Clin Microbiol* **35**, 3278–83.

Irmen, K.E. and Kelleher, J.J. (2000). Use of monoclonal antibodies for rapid diagnosis of respiratory viruses in a community hospital. *Clin Diagn Lab Immunol* **7**, 396–403.

Kohler, G. and Milstein, C. (1975). Continuous cultures of fused cells secreting antibody of predefined specificity. *Nature* **256**, 495–7.

Kuhn, J.A. and Thomas, G. (1994). Monoclonal antibodies and colorectal carcinoma: a clinical review of diagnostic applications. *Cancer Invest* **12**, 314–23.

Parlevliet, K.J. and Schellekens, P.T. (1992). Monoclonal antibodies in renal transplantation: a review. *Transpl Int* **5**, 234–46.

Schulte, W.J. (1996). Use of monoclonal antibodies in colorectal cancer: a review. *World J Surg* **20**, 238–40.

Verhoef, J. and Torensma, R. (1990). Prospects for monoclonal antibodies in the diagnosis and treatment of bacterial infections. *Eur J Clin Microbiol Infect Dis* **9**, 247–50.

Waldmann, T.A. (1991). Monoclonal antibodies in diagnosis and therapy. *Science* **252**, 1657–62.

10

Lactic acid bacteria and human health

The lactic acid bacteria are a group of organisms with a number of common properties. The main property is that they all produce lactic acid via the fermentation of sugar. The group includes four main genera, namely *Lactobacillus*, *Leuconostoc*, *Pediococcus* and *Streptococcus*, although these have been reclassified to include several subgenera (Stiles and Holzapfel, 1997):

- *Streptococcus*
- *Lactococcus*
- *Enterococcus*
- *Pediococcus*
- *Tetragenococcus*
- *Lactobacillus*
- *Carnobacterium*
- *Leuconostoc*
- *Weisella*
- *Oenococcus*
- *Vagococcus*
- *Bifidobacterium*

There are a number of major factors associated with lactic acid fermentation that result in the inhibition of other micro-organisms. These include the production of antimicrobial substances, lactic acid, hydrogen peroxide, bacteriocins and bacteriocin-like substances. The metabolism also results in a low pH, low redox potential, and nutrient depletion. Other substances including ethanol, organic acid and diacetyl may also be produced. These factors have been shown throughout history and from recent scientific data to possess a number of health benefits, including nutritional improvement, lac-

tose tolerance, resistance to gastrointestinal infection, hypocholestemic action, and anti-tumour activity.

Lactic acid bacteria have been used by humans throughout history, even before the science of microbiology began. It is thought that humans utilized lactic acid bacteria to produce fermented milk at least 11 000 years ago. Through time, a number of fermentation processes have been developed to produce a range of dairy products, vegetables, meats, fish and cereals. Many of these foods are produced in developing countries under comparatively unhygienic conditions. However, they are still of satisfactory microbiological quality. Today, lactic acid bacteria are present in a whole range of foods, both solid and liquid, either as part of their natural composition or as an additive, including:

- milk products (e.g. cheese, milk, butter, yoghurt);
- fermented vegetables (e.g. pickles, olives);
- sausages;
- sourdough bread.

The properties of lactic acid bacteria have been exploited in the manufacture, preservation and content of foods, and are being investigated for use in medical therapeutics in both animals and humans (Gorbach, 1990). The lactic acid bacteria themselves are rarely implicated in human disease and are therefore considered to be non-pathogenic for humans. However, a number of cases of infection with lactobacilli have been reported, occurring mainly in patients with an underlying disease. We therefore need to be aware of the possibility, although low, of lactobacilli emerging as opportunistic pathogens.

Certain lactic acid bacteria may have the potential to aid nutritional improvement and to restore bacterial flora (Naidu *et al.*, 1999). Bacteria used in this way are known as probiotic bacteria. The term 'probiotic' was first described by Parker in 1974. However, a more suitable definition of probiotic bacteria was suggested by Fuller (1989): 'a live microbial feed supplement which beneficially affects the host animal by improving its microbial balance.' Probiotics may be applied to the upper or lower gastrointestinal tract, the upper respiratory tract, and the urogenital tract.

Lactobacilli have a long history of use in the gastrointestinal tract to prevent or cure a variety of illnesses. Elie Metchnikoff is thought to be the first to propose the use of lactic acid bacteria as probiotics. He used lactobacilli for the restoration of normal gastrointestinal flora in the 1890s. Lactobacilli were also used in the early part of the twentieth century to treat urinary tract infections based on the fact that lactic acid has antibacterial properties. However, the interest in probiotics waned after the introduction of antibiotics in the 1940s, and it was not until relatively recently that an upsurge in interest occurred. In contrast to conventional therapies, probiotic therapy is seen as being natural and without harmful side effects, although the majority of evidence for a beneficial role of probiotics has been gained through experience of their use in livestock. However, studies have shown that when lactic acid bacteria are given in sufficient numbers, they can survive passage through the human gastrointestinal tract and exert effects on the resident intestinal flora (Salminen and Deighton, 1992). These changes disappear when supply of the bacteria is stopped. It is likely that one or more of the properties possessed by lactic acid bacteria, as described already, are responsible for these effects. A future use of lactobacilli may be to protect against travellers' diarrhoea by inhibiting infection with enteropathogens, although the protection would be only short-term. It has been shown in vitro that lactic acid bacteria may hinder the multiplication of foodborne pathogens. However, the use of probiotic therapies can only be speculated upon at present. Lactobacilli have also been exploited for the prevention of urogenital infections, such as bacterial vaginosis, vulvovaginal candidiasis, and recurrent urinary tract infections. It is therefore a possibility that part of the protective role of lactobacilli is due to the induction of a local immune response in both the gastrointestinal tract and the urogenital tract (Perdigon *et al.*, 2001). Certain components of the gastrointestinal flora may also translocate to and survive in the spleen or other organs, resulting in the stimulation of phagocyte and lymphocyte production.

As mentioned already, bacteriocins and bacteriocin-like substances are produced by lactic acid bacteria (Rodriguez *et al.*, 2003). These may play a part in the inhibition of other bacteria. Normally, bacteriocins from one strain act against a closely related strain. Therefore, the actual significance of bacteriocins produced by lactic acid bacteria and their effect on human health is unclear. However, nicin is a bacteriocin produced by *Lactococcus lactis*. Unlike other bacteriocins, it has a broad range of activity and many bacteria and bacterial endospores are sensitive to it. Nicin is currently used for food preservation, but its uses in human medicine have not yet been determined. Whether it provides any benefit when ingested as part of the diet is not known.

Some lactic acid bacteria, such as *Lactobacillus delbrueckii* subspecies *bulgaricus*, have been shown to possess anti-tumour activity (Hirayama and Rafter, 1999; Rafter, 2002). Epidemiological studies in human colon cancer have shown low incidences in areas where consumption of foods fermented by lactic acid bacteria have been consumed. Scientific reports have confirmed this in both animal and human studies. Species or subspecies of *Lactobacillus*, *Lactobacillus lactis*, *Streptococcus salivarius*, *Leuconostoc* and *Bifidobacterium* have so far shown anti-tumour activity. The anti-tumour factors are thought to be glycopeptides and are thought to be intracellular and not produced extracellularly.

There is an increased knowledge of the risk of heart disease due to high serum cholesterol both in animals and in humans. Animal studies have shown that ingestion of selected strains of *Lactobacillus acidophilus* leads to a significant reduction in serum cholesterol. Much of this work has been carried out in pigs because they are thought to simulate the human gastrointestinal and physiological systems to a reasonable degree. However, studies in humans have led to mixed results, with only some reports showing a reduction in human serum cholesterol after ingestion of various fermented milk products.

Lactose intolerance in humans has a worldwide distribution. The condition results in abdominal pain, bloating, cramps, loss of appetite, and diarrhoea due to the inability of the small intestine to digest lactose. This occurs because of the lack of the lactase enzyme in the brush-border epithelial cells. Individuals with lactose intolerance are unable to ingest milk products without experiencing these symptoms. However, it has been shown that lactose-containing yoghurt enhances the lactose tolerance of lactose intolerant individuals. This has been attributed to the presence of live lactic acid bacteria in these products. Lactobacilli possess varying amounts of lactase activity depending on the species or subspecies.

Lactic acid bacteria are therefore used in a number of human processes, such as food preparation. The potential health benefits of these bacteria are wide-ranging and could make a big impact on a number of conditions if the benefits of lactic acid bacteria are harnessed. However, as many of these benefits are currently poorly understood, further research, including genomics, is required, and it will be some time before any real impact is seen on human health (Champomier-Verges *et al.*, 2002; Klaenhammer *et al.*, 2002).

REFERENCES

Champomier-Verges, M.C., Maguin, E., Mistou, M.Y., Anglade, P. and Chich, J.F. (2002). Lactic acid bacteria and proteomics: current knowledge and perspectives. *J Chromatogr B Analyt Technol Biomed Life Sci* **771**, 329–42.

Fuller, R. (1989). Probiotics in man and animals. *J Appl Bacteriol* **66**, 365–78.

Gorbach, S.L. (1990). Lactic acid bacteria and human health. *Ann Med* **22**, 37–41.

Hirayama, K. and Rafter, J. (1999). The role of lactic acid bacteria in colon cancer prevention: mechanistic considerations. *Antonie Van Leeuwenhoek* **76**, 391–4.

Klaenhammer, T., Altermann, E., Arigoni, F., *et al.* (2002). Discovering lactic acid bacteria by genomics. *Antonie Van Leeuwenhoek* **82**, 29–58.

Naidu, A.S., Bidlack, W.R. and Clemens, R.A. (1999). Probiotic spectra of lactic acid bacteria (LAB). *Crit Rev Food Sci Nutr* **39**, 13–126.

Parker, R.B. (1974). Probiotics, the other half of the antibiotics story. *Animal Nutrition and Health* **29**, 4–8.

Perdigon, G., Fuller, R. and Raya, R. (2001). Lactic acid bacteria and their effect on the immune system. *Curr Issues Intest Microbiol* **2**, 27–42.

Rafter, J. (2002). Lactic acid bacteria and cancer: mechanistic perspective. *Br J Nutr* **88** (suppl 1), S89–94.

Rodriguez, J.M., Martinez, M.I., Horn, N. and Dodd, H.M. (2003). Heterologous production of bacteriocins by lactic acid bacteria. *Int J Food Microbiol* **80**, 101–16.

Salminen, S. and Deighton, M. (1992). Lactic acid bacteria in the gut in normal and disordered states. *Dig Dis* **10**, 227–38.

Stiles, M.E. and Holzapfel, W.H. (1997). Lactic acid bacteria of foods and their current taxonomy. *Int J Food Microbiol* **36**, 1–29.

11

Clinical applications of leeches and maggots

Medicine has advanced a long way in the past few decades. Life expectancy is at its longest ever, diseases that were once incurable are either curable or can be put in abeyance, and the idea of cloning has become a reality. Not all these advances are welcomed, of course, due to ethical, political and common-sense reasons, but some are good for human medicine. Some advances have also returned from 'old medicine' due to the failure of modern medicines such as some antibiotics.

LEECHES: UNWELCOME BLOOD SUCKERS?

Leeches have a traditionally bad reputation, along with vampire bats, as being evil creatures that just want to suck blood. However, leeches have been used in medicine for many centuries in treating a number of diseases, probably as far back as 1000 BC in ancient India. Their peak use was during the time of Napoleon. They were still used commonly in the 1950s, but they fell out of fashion in the medical world during the 1960s–80s. In recent years, however, interest in their use has increased again (Valauri, 1991; Wells *et al.*, 1993).

Leeches are segmented, hermaphroditic worms that are distributed widely throughout the world. They are able to ingest ten times their bodyweight of blood (5–15 mL). When leeches attach with their suckers, ready to feed, they secrete a local anaesthetic and an anticoagulant, called hirudin, so that blood flow is not hindered (Markwardt, 2002). It is this method of feeding that has proved useful to

medicine. Leeches are now used widely in Russia for the treatment of a number of conditions in areas such as cardiovascular disease, ophthalmology and dermatology. Leeches are thought to act as anti-inflammatories, anti-thrombolytics and anti-hypertensives. They are even thought by some practitioners to be the saving grace for treating terminal glaucoma. Most leeches used in medicine are of the species *Hirudo medicinalis* (European medicinal leech) (Andrews, 2001), although the species *Hirudinaria manillensis* (Asian medicinal leech) and *Haementeria ghillanii* (Amazon leech) may also be used. The actual benefit in modern medicine is to provide a good blood flow at the required site in cases such as post-surgery (Irish *et al.*, 2000; Weinfeld *et al.*, 2000). Their use is especially useful in plastic and reconstructive surgery, as the leech bite induces blood flow that lasts up to ten hours (Chepeha *et al.*, 2002); this has a tremendous benefit to the surgical site in shortening healing time.

The main problem associated with leech use in medicine is patient acceptability. Some older patients who remember leeches being used when they were young are more accepting of their use. In other patients, however, basic education on the benefits of leeches is needed before they may be used. The actual procedure is painless because of the secretion of local anaesthetic by the leeches.

MAGGOTS: FRIENDLY WORMS?

As with leeches, maggots are not exactly the treatment one expects when visiting the doctor.

However, maggots are well known for their ability to clean wounds, thereby helping them to heal more rapidly (Dossey, 2002). The healing uses of maggots have been known since Ambroise Paré noted them in the sixteenth century. Maggots have been used throughout history since then, especially for treating wounds sustained during battles. William Baer, an American doctor, noticed during the First World War that soldiers with maggot infestations in wounds recovered better than soldiers treated by conventional methods in hospital. After the war, further work was done on the medical use of maggots, and by the 1930s maggot therapy was widespread, being used in over 300 hospitals in the USA alone. However, with the advent of antibiotic therapy in the 1940s, the use of maggot therapy decreased.

The lifecycle of a maggot begins with the parent housefly (or similar species) laying eggs (Figure 11.1). After about a day the eggs hatch and the larval stage of the fly – the maggot – emerges. The maggots feed quickly, moult twice, and after about five to six days turn into pupae. Development takes place within the pupa for about ten days, after which they emerge as flies. It is during the feeding stage that the maggots are most useful for therapy.

In 1982, interest in maggot therapy surged when an orthopaedic surgeon, John Church, observed that wounds infested with maggots healed quicker than those not infested in a car crash victim. Maggot infestation of humans is known as myiasis. In controlled medical situations, where it is also known as maggot debridement therapy, maggot infestation can be beneficial (Jones and Thomas, 2000; Rayner, 1999). The healing properties of maggots are thought to exist for two reasons. First, the maggots used eat dead flesh but not live, healthy flesh. Second, the maggots are thought to excrete substances that are inhibitory to, or even kill, infecting bacteria. Maggot therapy is particularly useful in areas of the body receiving a poor blood supply. In these areas, antibiotic penetration is poor but maggots can help the healing process. Care must be taken, however, when using maggots: not all maggots eat dead flesh; some, such as the maggot of the screw-worm fly, eat live, healthy flesh.

A number of ethical considerations arise with maggot therapy (Sherman *et al.*, 2000). The first question is whether maggots can be classed as a medicine. If they can, then they would come under the control of the Medicines Control Agency (MCA). One ethical problem that has been solved is that of sterility: as living organisms, maggots are not naturally sterile, but scientists have managed to farm sterile maggots for medical use. The cost of maggot therapy provides support for their use: one study indicated that typical maggot therapy costs half as much as conventional therapy (Wayman *et al.*, 2000).

CONCLUSION

Leeches and maggots clearly have a role in modern medicine (Dossey, 2002). Although these uses may be limited, they provide useful remedies in certain situations, particularly where other modern methods in medicine fail to deliver. Also, leeches and maggots, although not entirely acceptable to the general public, provide non-toxic and cost-effective methods when conventional drugs may not be appropriate. No doubt, other 'traditional' forms of medicine will resurface in this modern era of medicine.

REFERENCES

Andrews, S. (2001). *Hirudo medicinalis*: the medicinal leech. *J Audiov Media Med* **24**, 126–7.

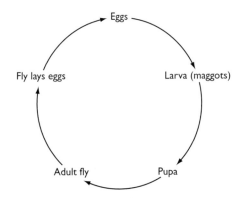

Figure 11.1 Lifecycle of a housefly.

Eggs

Fly lays eggs

Larva (maggots)

Adult fly

Pupa

Chepeha, D.B., Nussenbaum, B., Bradford, C.R. and Teknos, T.N. (2002). Leech therapy for patients with surgically unsalvageable venous obstruction after revascularized free tissue transfer. *Arch Otolaryngol Head Neck Surg* **128**, 960–65.

Dossey, L. (2002). Maggots and leeches: when science and aesthetics collide. *Altern Ther Health Med* **8**, 12–16, 106–7.

Irish, J.C., Gullane, P.J., Mulholland, S. and Neligan, P.C. (2000). Medicinal leech in head and neck reconstruction. *J Otolaryngol* **29**, 327–32.

Jones, M. and Thomas, S. (2000). Larval therapy. *Nurs Stand* **14**, 47–51, quiz 53–4.

Markwardt, F. (2002). Hirudin as alternative anticoagulant – a historical review. *Semin Thromb Hemost* **28**, 405–14.

Rayner, K. (1999). Larval therapy in wound debridement. *Prof Nurse* **14**, 329–33.

Sherman, R.A., Hall, M.J. and Thomas, S. (2000). Medicinal maggots: an ancient remedy for some contemporary afflictions. *Annu Rev Entomol* **45**, 55–81.

Valauri, F.A. (1991). The use of medicinal leeches in microsurgery. *Blood Coagul Fibrinolysis* **2**, 185–7.

Wayman, J., Nirojogi, V., Walker, A., Sowinski, A. and Walker, M.A. (2000), The cost effectiveness of larval therapy in venous ulcers. *J Tissue Viability* **10**, 91–4.

Weinfeld, A.B., Yuksel, E., Boutros, S., Gura, D.H., Akyurek, M. and Friedman, J.D. (2000). Clinical and scientific considerations in leech therapy for the management of acute venous congestion: an updated review. *Ann Plast Surg* **45**, 207–12.

Wells, M.D., Manktelow, R.T., Boyd, J.B. and Bowen, V. (1993). The medical leech: an old treatment revisited. *Microsurgery* **14**, 183–6.

12

Applications of molecular biology

The advent of molecular biology and genetic engineering in the past few decades has resulted in the discovery and application of many techniques and products that have revolutionized medical research. The technology has also recently entered the healthcare industry in a number of areas. Initially, genetic engineering was considered by much of the general public to be a field of science that could be detrimental to mankind because it would be used in ways seen in science-fiction films, such as for the production of weapons or genetically manipulated humans. However, genetic engineering covers a broad range of subjects and industries, including medicine, the pharmaceutical industry, and the brewing industry, and can therefore be of benefit to mankind. It enables the genetic material of cells to be explored and manipulated so that improvements or discoveries may be made. Improvements via such methods enable industries to be more efficient and productive, whilst medical discoveries include new antibiotics and other drugs.

THE BEGINNING OF MOLECULAR BIOLOGY

In 1953, the proposed structure of double-stranded deoxyribonucleic acid (DNA) was reported by Watson and Crick. This ignited the beginning of the molecular revolution and our initial understanding of gene function. Other important events within the molecular revolution included the development of purified restriction enzymes, which allowed further manipulation of DNA. Noteworthy contributions have also been made

with the development of Southern blotting and Northern blotting, gene probe methods for DNA and ribonucleic acid (RNA), respectively. Gene probing is an essential component of molecular biology and is used widely in areas of research involving the detection and manipulation of genes. A gene probe is essentially a DNA sequence that, if specific, can detect its complementary DNA or RNA sequence. It is a powerful tool that can be used to determine the presence or absence of certain genes, and the technology is used so widely in research that a market in the medical field for clinical applications has recently been sought. Gene probes, if designed and used correctly, can be applied to the diagnosis of infectious and non-infectious diseases via the identification of species or specific strains of bacteria, parasites or viruses.

Arguably, it was not until 1986 that the next significant development arose, when a unique DNA amplification method called the polymerase chain reaction (PCR) was developed (Mullis *et al.*, 1986). This has revolutionized molecular biology, enabling the amplification of specific DNA sequences. It is so sensitive that it has been suggested that if 1 mL of DNA from a PCR reaction was distributed evenly in an Olympic swimming pool, then DNA could still be detected if another 1 mL was removed and another PCR reaction performed. The method is therefore of use in diseases where only a few cells may be present and where gene probes may not be sensitive enough. The main potential diagnostic problem with PCR in medicine is that the method detects both 'live' and 'dead' DNA. Therefore, inactive or past infections may also be detected by the method, thus creating problems. Commercial kits for the clinical diagnosis of a number of infectious diseases are now available, including those for mycobacteria, chlamydia and human immunodeficiency virus (HIV). The greatest impact of PCR on clinical diagnosis will probably be on the diagnosis of slow-growing or incultivatable organisms, such as mycobacteria, rickettsia and leptospira, or on the diagnosis of infectious diseases, where a rapid diagnosis is required, or where very small amounts of target DNA are present (Clarke, 2002; Olive and Bean, 1999). Variants of the original PCR method have also been introduced, such as inverse PCR and reverse-transcriptase polymerase chain reaction (RT-PCR).

Another significant technique is the luciferase assay. This is already used widely in the food industry, e.g. in the detection of microbial contamination of work surfaces, and it is being used increasingly for clinical research purposes. The technique makes use of luciferase, an enzyme found in the tails of fireflies, which, in the presence of adenosine triphosphate (ATP), results in the release of visible light. The technique can be used solely as a qualitative assay, or it can be set up to be quantitative, with light emission levels being measured via a photomultiplier. The use of the luciferase assay is probably limited in the healthcare industry, although it may have a few applications.

Currently, a system known as BacLite is being developed. This is based upon technology originally developed by the Defence Science and Technology Laboratory (Dstl) at Porton Down in the UK. It is based not on luciferase activity but on the measurement of bioluminescence produced by adenylate kinase (AK). Studies have shown that AK technology is as sensitive as PCR for the detection of bacteria. Under suitable conditions, a single bacterium can be detected in a matter of a few minutes as a result of the amplification provided by AK. This technique is more than 100-fold more sensitive than ATP bioluminescence and shows significantly better correlation with numbers of bacteria present than conventional ATP measurements. The technology is now being commercialized by Acolyte Biomedica as part of a joint venture with Dstl. If the development of this technology is successful, it could lead to a move away from the traditional methods of bacterial identification and antimicrobial susceptibility testing to a more rapid and sensitive assay that achieves both.

DNA chips, or microarrays, have also changed molecular biology over the past five years and promise to do more so in the future. With genome sequencing, there has been an urgent need for the function of genes to be understood better not only in bacteria but also in viral, animal and plant genes. Microarrays bring together traditional molecular biology techniques, such as PCR and DNA hybridization, with modern electronics and robotics. DNA microarrays have been available for a few years now, and protein arrays are now being produced. The future possibility is that microarrays could be taken to the bedside and a patient diagnosed on the spot. However, microarrays can produce a minefield of information within hours, often on thousands if not hundreds of thousands of genes. This is because each slide, or microarray, is made up of thousands of 'spots' that are essentially made up of single-stranded DNA. These act as probes for fluorescently tagged genes (also single-stranded DNA) that are applied to the microarray. If they match and bind to the probe, they will fluoresce and can then be read with a scanner. If they do not bind, then they are simply washed off the slide. This process allows the identification of certain gene sequences for either mutation detection or expression analysis. Bioinformatics, the marriage of biology and computers, has coped with the analysis of these data quite well, and supercomputers are now able to process genome-scale analyses. The main problem with current microarray systems is their size and cost. To process an appropriate number of samples, liquid-handling robotics are required, as well as the microarray spotter and reader. The cost of this can run into hundreds of thousands of pounds. Therefore, a small laboratory can soon be filled with at least three items of bulky equipment and computer hardware even before any data are gained. The possibility of bedside diagnosis is therefore some distance away.

More recently, genetically modified animals have been produced. This may be a great breakthrough for medicine, although the subject is still rather controversial. Animals have been cloned so that they express some human genes; this enables their organs to be used for transplantation (xeno-transplantation) to humans without rejection by the recipient's immune response. Such animals provide hope for those people who wait a number of years for transplants, some of whom die before they ever receive a transplant. Nevertheless, there is opposition to this, concerning the belief that animals should not be bred and used merely for extending the life of humans.

Molecular biology and genetic engineering have and will continue to have a great impact on a number of industries and, perhaps most importantly, on healthcare. In theory, one-day diagnoses and antimicrobial susceptibility patterns of TB could be achieved, compared with the current situation of four to eight weeks. Detection would be achieved using PCR, identification using gene probes, and antimicrobial susceptibility using the luciferase assay. The next few years will determine how big an impact such technologies will make on our everyday lives.

REFERENCES

Clarke, S.C. (2002). Nucleotide sequence-based typing of bacteria and the impact of automation. *Bioessays* **24**, 858–62.

Mullis, K., Faloona, F., Scharf, S., Saiki, R., Horn, G. and Erlich, H. (1986). Specific enzymatic amplification of DNA in vitro: the polymerase chain reaction. *Cold Spring Harb Symp Quant Biol* **51** (part 1), 263–73.

Olive, D.M. and Bean, P. (1999). Principles and applications of methods for DNA-based typing of microbial organisms. *J Clin Microbiol* **37**, 1661–9.

13

Bioterrorism

All weapons, whether they are traditional, nuclear, biological or chemical, are evaluated on their effectiveness, method of delivery, cost and availability. Biological weapons fulfil all of these criteria very well. Biological weapons provide an amplified effect compared with other weapons due to the lack of counter-defence. Therefore, terrorists and developing nations with such weapons pose a real threat, even though western nations are more powerful in traditional methods of warfare.

There is a long history of chemical and biological warfare, but it remained fairly limited until the start of the twentieth century, when the chemical industry improved (Atlas, 2001). In the twentieth century, there was a bipolar power base – essentially the East and the West – which resulted in the two world wars and the cold war. In the twenty-first century, there is a multipolar power base, which is no longer clearly the East and the West. As has been seen in recent times, there is an increased power base in the Middle and Far East. More countries now possess nuclear capability, and the threat of terrorism is at its greatest due to the power behind terrorist organizations.

Biochemical agents are varied in their composition, method of deployment, and effectiveness. Chemical weapons are designed to kill or incapacitate, whereas traditional methods of warfare, such as bombs and shells, are designed to seriously wound or kill. Sufferers of chemical warfare are often able to continue life shortly after exposure. This was demonstrated clearly during the First World War, when gas was used as a chemical weapon, although there were only small numbers of casualties. The use of gas also led to the introduction of respirators. Blister agents were intro-

duced in 1917 and were better in tactical terms. However, overall effectiveness of chemical agents was low: only 2% of all chemical-exposed casualties actually died, whereas 23% of casualties from other weapons died. With chemical warfare ammunition, the percentage of casualty deaths is increased to 25–50%, although it is still difficult to control in certain weathers and terrain. However, chemical agents remain a good tactic in small areas, where they can cause a high percentage of casualties and deaths. It is in this respect that the Tokyo subway attack in 1995 was successful. The nerve agent, sarin, was applied in a small area with a large number of people and therefore resulted in a large number of casualties. A total of 5500 people were injured and 11 were killed. Moreover, chemical agents can be specifically designed and deployed to create large numbers of casualties but small numbers of fatalities. This has the advantage, in terrorist terms, of producing a large number of hospitalized individuals and therefore increasing the terror and power base of the terrorist.

Unfortunately, terrorists do not abide by the laws of war or conventions. The reduction in military capacity in most western nations in many different ways has resulted in the capacity for terrorist organizations and rogue nations to exist and grow. Therefore, the major players in modern bioterrorism are no longer the main military states but religious cults and groups, rogue nations, and even individuals (Noah *et al.*, 2002). One problem with bioterrorism is the relative ease with which biological weapons can be made. Although without the use of modern technology even the most basic of weapon is not very effective, many bacteria are quite easily available to people with appropriate contacts. Such bacteria include salmonella, shigella and cholera. Even influenza and cryptosporidia could be used as biological weapons, with the main aim of causing disruption and terror in the community. For many biological agents, vaccine research and development started in the 1980s, but it is only now that products are reaching the licensing stage. Therefore, no vaccines are currently available for use in the event of a bioterrorist attack (Simberkoff, 2002), although new stocks of smallpox vaccine are being produced.

The current threat of bioterrorism and the response measures that could be taken are important issues. The first challenge in bioterrorism is to deter an attack in the first place: prevention is better than cure. However, if the attack cannot be deterred, then it must be detected and intercepted before it causes large-scale damage (Klietmann and Ruoff, 2001; Varkey et al., 2002). Response measures and dealing with the consequences of an attack are also important; these will vary according to the type of attack. Chemical attacks, for example, would require a rapid response because it is an instant and short-lived attack, whereas biological attacks require a slower-moving and longer-term response. In the current global climate, the increased concern of bioterrorism is fully justified and, although an attack is of a low probability, an attack would be a high-consequence event. Importantly, no state is fully prepared for a response, and it is probable that no state ever could be. That is why chemical and biological agents are so attractive as weapons. If an attack were to take place, then in the short term there would obviously be casualties and fatalities. However, long-term factors are also important, including the effects on socioeconomics and on traditional western-style living.

A facet of biological warfare that is often not realized is that it does not have to be directed against human beings to have an effect on world economies or human health (Clarke, 2002). For example, animals or crops that represent a high percentage of domestic product can be targeted (Owens, 2002). Outbreaks such as the recent foot and mouth disease epidemic could, potentially, be started by bioterrorism, which would not cause the terror traditionally associated with such acts but nevertheless would cost billions in terms of animal loss, decreased tourism revenues, and compensation.

As mentioned previously, biological agents do not need to be complex to be used in acts of bioterrorism. Therefore, an 'amateur' terrorist could make use of a biological agent and cause a large amount of terror. For example, the anthrax letter attacks that occurred shortly after 11 September 2001 struck even more terror into the US community and had repercussions worldwide (Benjamin, 2002; Blendon et al., 2002). Cutaneous anthrax was confirmed in seven individuals and suspected in five; inhalation anthrax was confirmed in 11 individuals.

The method of delivery plays a major part in the success of a biological weapon. Aerobiology is an important area when the agent is delivered by aerosol. Droplet nuclei remain suspended in the air and are therefore effective for delivery to the lungs; however, the diameter of these droplets must measure $2–5\,\mu m$. If a droplet is too large, it will not remain airborne and will not therefore reach a recipient. If the droplet is too small, it will enter the lungs and then be breathed out. Experiments in the London Underground have shown that non-pathogenic *Bacillus* spores can travel long distances due to the airflow in underground systems. Although the concentration of spores reduced significantly from station to station, the numbers at the fifth station were still sufficient to cause infection if the agent had been pathogenic.

Now that bioterrorism is a real possibility in the modern world, most countries have stepped up their ability to respond to attack. Various agencies within a number of governments are also placing additional resources into effective counter-measures, whether they be surveillance, vaccines or military defence. The modern world continues to change, and the threat of bioterrorism will continue to exist for some time; however, the ability of the western world to avert or respond effectively is changing and will hopefully mean that bioterrorism never becomes a reality.

REFERENCES

Atlas, R.M. (2001). Bioterrorism before and after September 11. *Crit Rev Microbiol* **27**, 355–79.

Benjamin, G.C. (2002). Managing terror. Public health officials learn lessons from bioterrorism attacks. *Physician Exec* **28**, 80–83.

Blendon, R.J., Benson, J.M., DesRoches, C.M., Pollard, W.E., Parvanta, C. and Herrmann, M.J. (2002). The impact of anthrax attacks on the American public. *MedGenMed* **4**, 1.

Clarke, S.C. (2002). Bioterrorism: an overview. *Br J Biomed Sci* **59**, 232–4.

Klietmann, W.F. and Ruoff, K.L. (2001). Bioterrorism: implications for the clinical microbiologist. *Clin Microbiol Rev* **14**, 364–81.

Noah, D.L., Huebner, K.D., Darling, R.G. and Waeckerle, J.F. (2002). The history and threat of biological warfare and terrorism. *Emerg Med Clin North Am* **20**, 255–71.

Owens, S.R. (2002). Waging war on the economy. The possible threat of a bioterrorist attack against agriculture. *EMBO Rep* **3**, 111–13.

Simberkoff, M.S. (2002). Vaccines for adults in an age of terrorism. *J Assoc Acad Minor Phys* **13**, 19–22.

Varkey, P., Poland, G.A., Cockerill, F.R., 3rd, Smith, T.F. and Hagen, P.T. (2002). Confronting bioterrorism: physicians on the front line. *Mayo Clin Proc* **77**, 661–72.

PART II

Bacteriology

14

Plague and other *Yersinia* infections

The genus *Yersinia* is named after Alexandre Yersin, a Swiss doctor who discovered the plague bacillus in June 1894 whilst in Hong Kong during an epidemic of bubonic plague. *Yersinia* are small, Gram-negative bacilli that are non-lactose-fermenting, urease-positive, and motile at 25 °C but not at 37 °C. There are three species of *Yersinia* that are pathogenic to humans:

- *Y. pestis*
- *Y. enterocolitica*
- *Y. pseudotuberculosis*

Y. pestis is responsible for plague and is therefore of interest for historic reasons and because it still causes a significant number of deaths today. *Y. enterocolitica* and *Y. pseudotuberculosis* are causes of gastroenteritis in humans; the latter also causes disease in animals. *Y. pseudotuberculosis* may also be responsible for a number of other conditions in humans and may be isolated from wounds, faeces, sputum and mesenteric lymph nodes.

PLAGUE

Plague is caused by the bacterium *Y. pestis*. Historically, it is one of the most famous diseases known to man due to the epidemics that have occurred, including the Plague of Justinian in 558 AD, the Great Plague of fourteenth-century Europe, the plague of Austria in 1711, the plague of the Balkans between 1770 and 1772, and the recent epidemic in India in 1994 and outbreaks in Africa (Cook, 1995; Drancourt and Raoult, 2002).

Plague is transmitted from animal to animal and from animal to human by fleas (Figure 14.1), although exposure can also occur via infected animal tissue or aerosols (Hinnebusch *et al.*, 2002). Historically, rat fleas (*Xenopsylla cheopis*) were the most common vectors of plague, of which the adult females are the only ones to feed on the host. Epidemics of plague in humans were often due to house rats and occurred more often when disease and death rates increased within a rodent population. Today, however, house rats are rarely implicated in plague transmission. Although rat-borne epidemics of plague no longer occur in western countries (the last epidemic in the USA was in 1924–25), plague still occurs in some developing regions. For example, squirrel fleas are a source of

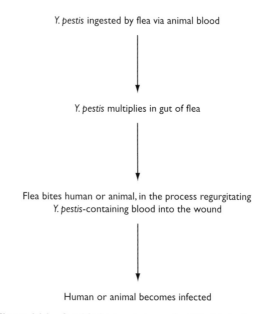

Y. pestis ingested by flea via animal blood

Y. pestis multiplies in gut of flea

Flea bites human or animal, in the process regurgitating Y. pestis-containing blood into the wound

Human or animal becomes infected

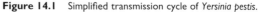

Figure 14.1   Simplified transmission cycle of *Yersinia pestis*.

human plague in North America from the Pacific Coast eastward to Texas and Oklahoma (Huang *et al.*, 2002). Other rodents such as prairie dogs, deer mice and chipmunks occasionally serve as reservoirs of plague. Between outbreaks, it is thought that *Y. pestis* circulates among certain animal populations without causing disease, making such populations long-term reservoirs of infection.

There are thousands of cases of plague worldwide each year (World Health Organization, 1999). Between 1987 and 1996 there was an average of 1920 cases per year. In 1996 and 1997 there were between 3000 and 5000 cases, but in 1999 the number fell to 2600 cases. The majority of plague occurs in Africa, where it is distributed down the eastern side of the continent and in the south, where severe outbreaks have occurred in recent years. There is currently no plague in western Europe or Australia. In Asia and eastern Europe, plague is localized, with few human cases occurring. In North America, as already mentioned, plague is limited to the western side of the continent, from Alberta, Canada down to Mexico. Over a dozen cases of human plague occur each year in North America due to contact with the common flea *Oropsylla montana* from rock squirrels. In South America, plague is limited to two regions, namely Brazil and the Andean mountain region in parts of Bolivia, Peru and Ecuador.

Bubonic plague is an often fatal disease, with up to 75% mortality, characterized by chills, fever, vomiting, diarrhoea, and the formation of buboes. The buboes are formed when *Y. pestis* invades the lymph nodes, causing swelling. Blood vessels break, causing internal bleeding, which dries and turns black under the skin, giving rise to the name Black Death. The incubation period of bubonic plague is two to eight days, and death occurs rapidly after the onset of symptoms, often within two to four days.

Pneumonic plague often develops as a complication of bubonic plague and is characterized by symptoms including lymphadenopathy, cough, chest pains and haemoptysis. The latter is due to *Y. pestis* invading the epithelial lung tissue. Meningitis or gastrointestinal symptoms may also develop.

Death can occur within hours. Person-to-person transmission of pneumonic plague is common during epidemics.

Septicaemic plague is normally spread by direct contact between bodily fluids, although it can also develop from bubonic or pneumonic plague. Occasionally, patients with septicaemic plague develop fever and die rapidly without detectable lymphadenitis characteristic of bubonic plague. Septicaemic plague may account for up to 25% of all plague cases in an epidemic.

The diagnosis of plague involves Gram-staining of bubo aspirates, blood cultures, sputum and cerebrospinal fluid (if meningitis is present). *Y. pestis* can also be stained with the Wayson stain, with which they appear as light-blue bacilli with dark-blue polar bodies. An increased white blood cell count with predominant neutrophils, abnormal liver function tests (LFTs), and disseminated intravascular coagulation (DIC) are also observed.

Early antibiotic therapy is very effective, particularly in bubonic plague. Streptomycin or tetracycline may be used, but if meningitis is present chloramphenicol is the antibiotic of choice. No plague vaccine is currently available. Patients with suspected plague should be isolated to prevent spread of the disease. Such isolation should occur from initial examination through to diagnosis, treatment and clinical outcome.

The prevention of plague is an impossible task due to its existence in wild animals in many parts of the world. Elimination of plague in such populations is pointless. Plague will therefore continue to exist in localized geographic locations even when, in the future, more areas become developed and general living standards improve.

YERSINIA GASTROENTERITIS

Y. enterocolitica and *Y. pseudotuberculosis* are important causes of gastroenteritis worldwide. The incidence of *Yersinia* gastroenteritis has decreased in the UK from around 500 cases each year during the mid-1980s to a few dozen cases in 2000 (source: Health Protection Agency Communicable Disease Surveillance Centre (HPA CDSC)). However, it remains a problem in other countries. Approximately 17 000 cases occur annually in the USA, and there is a greater incidence in northern Europe, Scandinavia and Japan. In the latter, infections have been and continue to be transmitted via water and foods. *Y. enterocolitica* and *Y. pseudotuberculosis* have been isolated from a number of animals, including pigs, birds, cats and dogs; they can also be found in various meats, oysters, fish and raw milk, although only *Y. enterocolitica* has been isolated from the environment. *Y. enterocolitica* is able to grow at 4 °C and therefore refrigerated products can be potential reservoirs of infection. The virulence of *Yersinia* is associated with the presence of a 70-kb virulence plasmid and V and W antigens. Pathogenic strains are resistant to serum complement, are able to invade HeLa (human epithelial) cells, and are cytotoxic. Many strains produce a heat-stable enterotoxin similar to that produced by *Escherichia coli*, but this is probably not an important virulence factor in gastroenteritis.

Yersinia gastroenteritis is most common in those under the age of five years. The organisms can be transmitted zoonotically or from person to person via the faecal-oral route, although the infective dose is unknown. The incubation period may be between one and seven days after ingestion of the organism and is characterized by symptoms such as diarrhoea and vomiting, fever and abdominal pain. The symptoms are due to mucosal ulceration in the terminal ileum, necrotic lesions in Peyer's patches, and enlargement of the mesenteric lymph nodes. Enterocolitis is the presenting feature in two-thirds of reported cases and is associated with the symptoms of infection. Although few complications are associated with infection, unnecessary appendectomy may result from *Yersinia* gastroenteritis due to the fact that one of the main symptoms of infection is abdominal pain in the lower right quadrant, a symptom indicative of appendicitis. Both species have also been associated with reactive arthritis, which starts a few days to one month after the onset of diarrhoea and may involve a number of joints. The condition often lasts for over a month and sometimes for more than four months. It is most common in those individuals with human leukocyte antigen (HLA) type B27 and occurs in 2–3% of cases.

The diagnosis of *Yersinia* gastroenteritis involves the isolation of *Y. enterocolitica* or *Y. pseudotuberculosis* from faeces, blood or vomit, followed by identification using biochemical and serological testing. Infection is usually self-limiting and does not require antibiotic therapy; fluid rehydration is usually sufficient. However, in cases of bacteraemia, antibiotic therapy is required. The antibiotic susceptibilities of *Y. enterocolitica* and *Y. pseudotuberculosis* are similar, but speciation is important due to differences in susceptibility. The former is usually susceptible to gentamicin, chloramphenicol, tetracycline and ciprofloxacin but resistant to ampicillin, whereas the latter is usually susceptible to all these antibiotics. Gentamicin is therefore suggested for treating septicaemia due to *Y. enterocolitica*, whilst ampicillin is suggested for septicaemia due to *Y. pseudotuberculosis*.

Yersinia infections, particularly those caused by *Y. pestis*, are interesting for historic reasons, but they are also potentially devastating. They continue to be a problem worldwide, with plague epidemics still occurring occasionally. Unfortunately, due to their presence in so many animal species, the *Yersinia* will probably never be eradicated and will therefore continue to cause human disease.

REFERENCES

Cook, G.C. (1995). Plague: past and future implications for India. *Public Health* 109, 7–11.

Drancourt, M. and Raoult, D. (2002). Molecular insights into the history of plague. *Microbes Infect* 4, 105–9.

Hinnebusch, B.J., Rudolph, A.E., Cherepanov, P., Dixon, J.E., Schwan, T.G. and Forsberg, A. (2002). Role of *Yersinia* murine toxin in survival of *Yersinia pestis* in the midgut of the flea vector. *Science* 296, 733–5.

Huang, X.Z., Chu, M.C., Engelthaler, D.M. and Lindler, L.E. (2002). Genotyping of a homogeneous group of *Yersinia pestis* strains isolated in the United States. *J Clin Microbiol* **40**, 1164–73.

World Health Organization (1999). Human plague in 1997. *Wkly Epidemiol Rec* **74**, 340–44.

15

Anthrax infection

Anthrax has been known as a cause of disease in animals and humans for hundreds of years. In 1876, Koch proved that *Bacillus anthracis* was the cause of anthrax. *B. anthracis* is a Gram-positive bacillus that is facultatively anaerobic. This means that the bacterium performs fermentation only under anaerobic conditions; other bacteria are obligately anaerobic, i.e. can exist only in oxygen-free environments. It produces a polypeptide capsule in vivo and is also able to enter a spore state. Anthrax has been well studied over the past few hundred years, and the first bacterial vaccines to be produced were against anthrax. These vaccines were produced by a number of workers, including Pasteur, in 1881. Surprisingly, anthrax is not genetically diverse (Keim and Smith, 2002).

There are two virulence factors of *B. anthracis* – its polypeptide capsule (Makino *et al.*, 2002) and its toxin (Ascenzi *et al.*, 2002) – which are encoded for by genes on separate plasmids (Koehler, 2002). If one of these plasmids is not present in a strain of *B. anthracis*, then the bacterium is less virulent. The toxin comprises the oedema factor, the protective antigen, and the lethal factor. The overall effect of the toxin is to depress the cerebral cortex of the central nervous system, resulting in respiratory distress, cardiac collapse, shock, and finally death.

Anthrax is primarily a disease of herbivores, although it has been reported in some carnivores (Table 15.1). Before the advent of the anthrax vaccine, anthrax was a major cause of cattle, sheep and goat loss worldwide. However, the overall importance of anthrax throughout the world has decreased in the past century due to the development of a livestock vaccine in 1937 and the use of

Table 15.1 Animals in which anthrax has been reported

Herbivores	Carnivores
Antelope	Cheetah
Bison	Dingo
Boar	Jackal
Buffalo	Leopard
Cattle	Lion
Deer	Lynx
Elephant	Mink
Elk	Puma
Giraffe	Raccoon
Goat	
Hare	
Hippopotamus	
Impala	
Moose	
Pig	
Rhinoceros	
Sheep	
Waterbuck	
Zebra	

antibiotics. Anthrax is no longer a problem in developed countries for these reasons, but in developing countries endemic for anthrax and where there is no efficient vaccination policy, large losses still occur. In 1985, 168 countries reported anthrax from various herbivore hosts. It is estimated by the

World Health Organization (WHO) that 20 000 to 100 000 cases of anthrax occur in humans each year, although figures may be inaccurate due to difficulties in reporting in developing countries (Hugh-Jones, 1999). A massive outbreak of anthrax occurred in Zimbabwe between 1978 and 1980, with 9711 human cases and 151 deaths. This outbreak was caused by a breakdown in animal and human health programmes and indicates the importance of such schemes.

Animals usually acquire anthrax by ingesting contaminated foodstuffs such as feed, grass or water or by ingesting spores present in soil. Spores of anthrax are able to survive in the environment for prolonged periods of time, sometimes as long as 60 years. Water and soil can become contaminated further by haemorrhagic effusions from an animal dying of anthrax. The usual presentation of anthrax in animals is gastrointestinal disease, although cutaneous anthrax can occur via insect bites. Anthrax is often seen as a hyperacute infection where symptoms may be present only just before death. Such symptoms include a toxaemic appearance and occasional mild seizures, leading to a comatose state and death. Alternatively, a less acute disease course may occur for two or three days.

The diagnosis of anthrax can be made easily in animals who have died from the disease. The blood is dark and haemolysed, and it clots slowly or not at all. The spleen is also large and haemorrhagic. High numbers of anthrax bacilli are present in the blood at the time of death, often in the region of 10^8 bacilli per millilitre. Fixed blood smears may be stained with polychrome methylene blue to visualize the anthrax bacilli. These appear deep blue, with the capsule staining reddish-purple. This appearance is known as the M'Fadyean reaction. Bloodborne bacilli can also be grown on nutrient agar as long as antibiotic therapy has not been given.

In comparison to herbivores, humans are thought to be relatively resistant to anthrax. This evidence is based upon exposure–infection rates in humans and primates. In high-risk occupations, such as in the wool, leather and meat industries, cases of anthrax infection in past decades have been few relative to exposure. The ability of anthrax to cause disease by the respiratory route is low; the parenteral or cutaneous route of inoculation requires fewer bacilli to cause infection although disease is less severe. Human anthrax is almost always acquired by exposure to an infected animal (dead or alive). Person-to-person transmission is very rare; however, laboratory-acquired infection has been reported in the past.

There are three form of anthrax disease in humans: cutaneous, intestinal and pulmonary. Cutaneous anthrax occurs after infection of a cut, lesion or bite in the skin (Ciftci et al., 2002; Oncul et al., 2002; Tutrone et al., 2002; Vijaikumar et al., 2002). Symptoms of the disease occur two to three days after infection and initially consist of a small boil-like papule followed by the development of a ring of vesicles around the original papule. The papule ulcerates to form an eschar (a hard plaque covering an ulcer), which enlarges, turns black in colour, and results in localized oedema. This eschar covers the surrounding vesicles, resulting in a lesion usually measuring about 2 cm in diameter, although it may be 10 cm or more in some cases. If uncomplicated, the anthrax bacilli remain localized. Adenitis is common, but fever is mild or absent. After ten days, the eschar begins to resolve, although total resolution can take two to six weeks. The main complications of cutaneous anthrax are meningitis (Tasyaran et al., 2002), septicaemia and secondary bacterial infection. Meningitis occurs in approximately 5% of cutaneous anthrax cases.

Intestinal anthrax occurs two to five days after the ingestion of anthrax spores from infected meat or milk (Sirisanthana and Brown, 2002). The eschar, as described for cutaneous anthrax, often occurs in the terminal ileum or caecum, although it may occur in other sites of the gastrointestinal tract. Symptoms include nausea, vomiting, anorexia, fever, abdominal pain and bloody diarrhoea.

Pulmonary, or inhalation, anthrax is the most severe form of the disease. Again, the symptoms occur two to five days after infection (Cullamar and Lutwick, 2002). Initial symptoms include mild fever, fatigue and malaise. After the mild initial phase, an acute illness develops, during which the patient may vomit or cough blood, followed by dyspnoea, cyanosis, severe pyrexia and disorientation. This acute illness is followed rapidly by coma and is invariably fatal.

The diagnosis of anthrax in humans is difficult except in cases of cutaneous anthrax. The lesion associated with this form is readily recognizable, and smears of material from the lesion can be stained using polychrome methylene blue. The diagnosis of pulmonary or intestinal anthrax is difficult clinically and can be achieved only when there is evidence of exposure to anthrax.

The control of anthrax in animals relies heavily upon the live-spore vaccine developed by Sterne in 1937. In humans, cell-free vaccines have been available for use since work was done in the 1950s and 1960s; formalin-inactivated and live-spore vaccines are also available, but these are not licensed for use in the UK. Anthrax can be treated with penicillin, tetracycline or chloramphenicol if given early in the disease.

As anthrax is such a devastating disease, it has received interest for use as a biological weapon for some time. If a population could be exposed to spores of *B. anthracis*, then it would be a highly effective weapon. However, to produce the worst form of the disease, the pulmonary form, it is estimated that more than 50 000 spores would need to be inhaled by each individual. If this were achieved, then treatment would be very difficult and the number of casualties would be high. Efforts such as the 1972 Biological Weapons Convention have therefore been made in the last few decades to halt the manufacture of biological weapons. However, as we have seen recently, certain nations continue to pose an international threat through the use of biological weapons (Bartlett *et al.*, 2002).

REFERENCES

Ascenzi, P., Visca, P., Ippolito, G., Spallarossa, A., Bolognesi, M. and Montecucco, C. (2002). Anthrax toxin: a tripartite lethal combination. *FEBS Lett* **531**, 384–8.

Bartlett, J.G., Inglesby, T.V., Jr and Borio, L. (2002). Management of anthrax. *Clin Infect Dis* **35**, 851–8.

Ciftci, E., Ince, E. and Dogru, U. (2002). Traditions, anthrax, and children. *Pediatr Dermatol* **19**, 36–8.

Cullamar, E.K. and Lutwick, L.I. (2002). Inhalational anthrax. *Curr Infect Dis Rep* **4**, 238–43.

Hugh-Jones, M. (1999). 1996–97 Global Anthrax Report. *J Appl Microbiol* **87**, 189–91.

Keim, P. and Smith, K.L. (2002). *Bacillus anthracis* evolution and epidemiology. *Curr Top Microbiol Immunol* **271**, 21–32.

Koehler, T.M. (2002). *Bacillus anthracis* genetics and virulence gene regulation. *Curr Top Microbiol Immunol* **271**, 143–64.

Makino, S., Watarai, M., Cheun, H.I., Shirahata, T. and Uchida, I. (2002). Effect of the lower molecular capsule released from the cell surface of *Bacillus anthracis* on the pathogenesis of anthrax. *J Infect Dis* **186**, 227–33.

Oncul, O., Ozsoy, M.F., Gul, H.C., Kocak, N., Cavuslu, S. and Pahsa, A. (2002). Cutaneous anthrax in Turkey: a review of 32 cases. *Scand J Infect Dis* **34**, 413–16.

Sirisanthana, T. and Brown, A.E. (2002). Anthrax of the gastrointestinal tract. *Emerg Infect Dis* **8**, 649–51.

Tasyaran, M.A., Deniz, O., Ertek, M. and Cetin, K. (2002). Anthrax meningitis: case report and review. *Scand J Infect Dis* **34**, 66–7.

Tutrone, W.D., Scheinfeld, N.S. and Weinberg, J.M. (2002). Cutaneous anthrax: a concise review. *Cutis* **69**, 27–33.

Vijaikumar, M., Thappa, D.M. and Karthikeyan, K. (2002). Cutaneous anthrax: an endemic outbreak in south India. *J Trop Pediatr* **48**, 225–6.

16

Botulism

Botulism is a fairly uncommon disease of humans and animals, but it has a worldwide distribution. The disease was first described in the late eighteenth century, although the causative organism was not isolated until a century later. Botulism is caused by the production of a toxin of *Clostridium botulinum*, an anaerobic, Gram-positive, spore-forming rod. The spores of *C. botulinum* may be found in the environment, such as in the soil and in the sediment of seas and lakes. As with many anaerobic, Gram-positive bacterial spores, those of *C. botulinum* are heat-resistant. Botulism is potentially lethal and is usually due to foodborne intoxication. In infants, the disease may be due to intestinal infection with the organism and often occurs in babies under one year of age (Muensterer, 2000). Infant botulism often occurs at the time of weaning, when the gut's bacterial flora are changing (Brook, 2000). Wound botulism, although very rare, can also occur due to infection of a wound with *C. botulinum*. This is very similar to foodborne botulism, but a fever may also be associated due to the formation of an abscess at the site of the wound.

Botulism occurs with an incidence of around 0.1 per 100 000 people, but this varies considerably according to the country and region. Most cases are due to the ingestion of preformed toxin in foods (Roberts, 2000). There are seven antigenically different types of toxin produced by various strains of *C. botulinum* and they are the most potent natural poisons known to humans (Kessler and Benecke, 1997; Singh, 2000). A fatal human dose has been estimated to be between 0.1 and 1.0 μg. The toxins are named A to G; toxins A to F are involved in human botulism, with toxins A, B and E being the most common (Cherington, 1998).

Type A toxin is associated mostly with vegetables, type B with meat, and type E with fish. The majority of cases are due to home-prepared foods rather than commercially processed foods; therefore, most cases are isolated. Large outbreaks due to the contamination of commercially processed foods are rare but important. The toxins are best produced in anaerobic conditions at 30 °C, are heat-labile, and are destroyed by oxidation. They are also immunogenic and can be transformed as toxoids, which means that they may be used as vaccines. The toxins are neurotoxic, i.e. they affect the nervous system. In the disease, toxin is absorbed through the gastric and upper-intestinal mucosa. It then interferes with neurotransmission at peripheral cholinergic synapses by binding irreversibly to the presynaptic nerve surfaces of neuromuscular junctions. After internalization, this leads to blockage of acetylcholine release.

The incubation period of foodborne botulism is between six hours and 16 days, with a mean time of two to three days. The initial stage of the disease is short and is often characterized by nausea and vomiting followed by bilateral and symmetrical paralytic ocular manifestations. As the disease progresses, the patient is afebrile with normal consciousness but has difficulty in swallowing, difficulty in speaking, and often double vision. Persistent constipation is common, and urinary tract disorders such as dysuria and retention may cause further problems. Respiratory problems due to paralysis are less frequent but may be serious when they occur. Secondary bacterial infections may create problems, and artificial ventilation may be necessary. Morbidity of foodborne botulism is 100%, and mortality is between 10 and 50%.

Most patients recover from botulism without any sequelae, although this takes weeks to months, depending on the intake of toxin. This is due to the time it takes for new nerve terminals to grow.

Infant botulism is characterized by an acute flaccid paralysis that begins with the muscles of the head, face and throat. Paralysis then extends symmetrically to involve the trunk and extremities. The mortality is low – around 2% – if the patient is hospitalized.

The diagnosis of botulism is based on the clinical symptoms. Routine laboratory testing is of little use. The toxin may be detected in serum or suspected foods by use of the mouse sero-neutralization test. This test remains the gold standard in toxin detection. Symptomatic treatment of botulism is essential (Robinson and Nahata, 2003). This may include artificial tears, humidification of the respiratory tract, feeding by gastric tube, and prevention of secondary infection by using antibacterial or antifungal agents. Specific treatment is of dubious value. The use of botulinum toxoid has been suggested, but its value is doubted because of the time it takes for an immunological response to be produced. Immune serum may be given but is reserved for severe cases only and needs to be used early on in the disease.

Type A botulinum toxin is now used to alleviate temporarily the symptoms of many muscle disorders, mostly focal disorders, such as blepharospasm, spasmodic torticollis and hemifacial spasm, It is also used for cosmetic reasons (Mendez-Eastman, 2000; Simpson, 1999). It has been used since the late 1970s and, although the toxin is expensive and requires three to six injections per year, it is of such value that it is now used routinely. The toxin is injected in minute quantities into the required area within a muscle, where it is taken up by nerve terminals. This results in a temporary blocking of neuromuscular transmission that usually lasts between two and four months depending on the time it takes for new axons and acetylcholine receptors to grow.

Botulism will no doubt remain a rare but serious disease. The low number of cases does not warrant use of a national vaccination programme, but the presence of spores in the everyday environment means that eradication is not possible. Early vaccines were developed in the 1940s, but improved vaccines have since been developed (Byrne and Smith, 2000). Outbreaks from commercially processed foods are becoming less and less frequent due to improved production methods. Therefore, only rare, sporadic cases will remain. However, the current global climate, with potential acts of bioterrorism, mean that we must remain aware of the incidence and implications of botulism (Robinson-Dunn, 2002; Varkey *et al.*, 2002).

REFERENCES

Brook, I. (2000). Anaerobic infections in children. *Adv Pediatr* **47**, 395–437.

Byrne, M.P. and Smith, L.A. (2000). Development of vaccines for prevention of botulism. *Biochimie* **82**, 955–66.

Cherington, M. (1998). Clinical spectrum of botulism. *Muscle Nerve* **21**, 701–10.

Kessler, K.R. and Benecke, R. (1997). Botulinum toxin: from poison to remedy. *Neurotoxicology* **18**, 761–70.

Mendez-Eastman, S.K. (2000). BOTOX: a review. *Plast Surg Nurs* **20**, 60–65, quiz 66–7.

Muensterer, O.J. (2000). Infant botulism. *Pediatr Rev* **21**, 427.

Roberts, J.A. (2000). Economic aspects of food-borne outbreaks and their control. *Br Med Bull* **56**, 133–41.

Robinson, R.F. and Nahata, M.C. (2003). Management of botulism. *Ann Pharmacother* **37**, 127–31.

Robinson-Dunn, B. (2002). The microbiology laboratory's role in response to bioterrorism. *Arch Pathol Lab Med* **126**, 291–4.

Simpson, L.L. (1999). Botulinum toxin: potent poison, potent medicine. *Hosp Pract (Off Ed)* **34**, 87–91, quiz 163.

Singh, B.R. (2000). Intimate details of the most poisonous poison. *Nat Struct Biol* **7**, 617–19.

Varkey, P., Poland, G.A., Cockerill, F.R., 3rd, Smith, T.F. and Hagen, P.T. (2002). Confronting bioterrorism: physicians on the front line. *Mayo Clin Proc* **77**, 661–72.

17

Tetanus

Tetanus is caused by the Gram-positive bacterium *Clostridium tetani*. It is a serious disease that causes uncontrollable muscular spasms and results in death in the absence of medical support. The disease was described in the time of Hippocrates, but it was little understood until 1884. The organism is normally found in the soil and as a commensal in human and animal intestines.

Infection can occur after any skin puncture wound, such as a splinter, insect bite, needle injection, or everyday minor skin abrasion (Cook *et al.*, 2001; Farrar *et al.*, 2000). Bacterial spores enter the wound and survive in anaerobic conditions, particularly in areas of dead tissue. The incubation time for symptoms can be between two days and two months but is usually around two weeks. The incubation time is often shorter when the infection site is in the head area. The bacteria multiply in the infection site and produce an endotoxin. This endotoxin, known as tetanospasmin, along with other toxins produced by related clostridia, are among the most poisonous substances known to man. The production of this endotoxin varies between strains, such that some do not produce at all whilst others are highly toxigenic. The toxin is a protein with a molecular weight of 150 000 Da; its function is plasmid-mediated (Ahnert-Hilger and Bigalke, 1995). It is toxic when introduced into tissue but not when ingested (Singh *et al.*, 1995). The toxic effect is thought to occur after the toxin has ascended the motor nerves, resulting in an interaction between the nerve and muscle at the neuromuscular junction (Montecucco and Schiavo, 1995). The toxin induces increased nerve signals to the muscle tissue, resulting in continuous contraction or spasm. All large muscles are affected, and breathing becomes difficult. A common symptom of the disease is lockjaw, which often occurs as an early sign of the disease; tetanus is therefore sometimes known as lockjaw. The bloodstream is not the delivery mechanism for the toxin, as intravenous infection requires more toxin than subcutaneous infection. In humans, tetanus is often descending, meaning that it begins with muscle stiffness in the head and neck region, followed by muscle stiffness in the upper body and then the lower body. The case fatality rate depends on a number of factors, including age, sex, type of wound, and the time and type of treatment given.

The clinical diagnosis of tetanus is often difficult, particularly if the site of infection is not obvious. Obvious wounds may therefore aid in diagnosis. In the laboratory, microscopy of pus or necrotic tissue from the wound site may indicate the presence of Gram-positive bacilli with round, terminal spores (drumstick bacilli). The presence of such bacilli does not, however, confirm infection with *C. tetani*. Culture of pus or tissue is important on standard blood agar incubated anaerobically at 37 °C. Enrichment in cooked-meat medium should also be performed, followed by subculture on blood agar as before.

Tetanus remains a serious disease worldwide, particularly in Africa, Asia and South America, even with the availability of immunization. The infection is not transmissible from case to case, so it is not considered to be an epidemic disease. The disease is most common in non-vaccinated or inadequately vaccinated individuals and, in developing countries, the majority of cases occur in infants and young children (Kurtoglu *et al.*, 1998; Oyelami *et al.*, 1996; Thayaparan and Nicoll, 1998).

However, the overall incidence of the disease worldwide is declining slowly due to improved standards of living, urbanization and immunization. In developed countries, tetanus is now uncommon. In the UK, it is estimated that around 100 cases occurred annually during the 1960s, but this is now down to single figures (Figure 17.1). In the USA, 124 cases of the disease were reported between 1995 and 1997 (Bardenheier *et al.*, 1998), but only 35 cases were reported in 2000 (source: US CDC). An estimated 400 000 deaths occur worldwide annually (Maple and al-Wali, 2001).

The administration of anti-toxin after a wound has occurred, in cases where the risk of tetanus is known to be high, will increase the incubation time of the disease. It does not, however, prevent the disease completely. When tetanus is confirmed, free toxin in the patient should be neutralized by using human tetanus immunoglobulin (HTIG). Antibiotic therapy should be given to control bacterial growth and the production of further toxin. Penicillin and metronidazole are commonly used. The wound should be cleaned thoroughly and all necrotic tissue removed. Supportive treatment including anticonvulsive therapy and artificial respiration should also be provided.

Tetanus can be prevented by immunization, and this plays an important role in prevention in many countries around the world. Children in developed countries now receive vaccination against tetanus as part of their childhood immunization schedule. Boosters should be given every ten years unless skin injury occurs, at which time re-immunization should take place and the ten-year period reset. All individuals can reduce the risk of infection by wearing protective clothing and shoes, particularly in areas or countries where the risk may be greater. For individuals with occupational risk, additional protective clothing may be worn. Passive immunization with gammaglobulin (HTIG) can be given to selected cases when required.

REFERENCES

Ahnert-Hilger, G. and Bigalke, H. (1995). Molecular aspects of tetanus and botulinum neurotoxin poisoning. *Prog Neurobiol* 46, 83–96.

Bardenheier, B., Prevots, D.R., Khetsuriani, N. and Wharton, M. (1998). Tetanus surveillance – United States, 1995–1997. *Mor Mortal Wkly Rep CDC Surveill Summ* 47, 1–13.

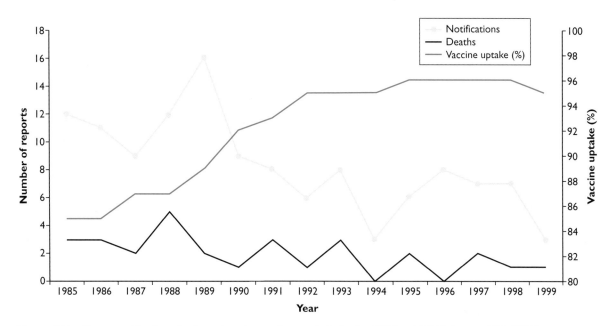

Figure 17.1 Tetanus notifications, deaths, and vaccine uptake rates in England and Wales, 1985–99 (source: HPA CDSC).

Cook, T.M., Protheroe, R.T. and Handel, J.M. (2001). Tetanus: a review of the literature. *Br J Anaesth* **87**, 477–87.

Farrar, J.J., Yen, L.M., Cook, T., *et al.* (2000). Tetanus. *J Neurol Neurosurg Psychiatry* **69**, 292–301.

Kurtoglu, S., Caksen, H., Ozturk, A., Cetin, N. and Poyrazoglu, H. (1998). A review of 207 newborn with tetanus. *J Pak Med Assoc* **48**, 93–8.

Maple, P.A. and al-Wali, W. (2001). The prevention of tetanus in England and Wales. *Commun Dis Public Health* **4**, 106–13.

Montecucco, C. and Schiavo, G. (1995). Structure and function of tetanus and botulinum neurotoxins. *Q Rev Biophys* **28**, 423–72.

Oyelami, O.A., Aladekomo, T.A. and Ononye, F.O. (1996). A 10 year retrospective evaluation of cases of post neonatal tetanus seen in a paediatric unit of a university teaching hospital in south western Nigeria (1985 to 1994). *Cent Afr J Med* **42**, 73–5.

Singh, B.R., Li, B. and Read, D. (1995). Botulinum versus tetanus neurotoxins: why is botulinum neurotoxin but not tetanus neurotoxin a food poison? *Toxicon* **33**, 1541–7.

Thayaparan, B. and Nicoll, A. (1998). Prevention and control of tetanus in childhood. *Curr Opin Pediatr* **10**, 4–8.

18

Other anaerobic infections

Anaerobes receive much less attention than other clinically important microbes. This is probably due to a number of reasons. First, true anaerobes require special growth conditions for them to be isolated from clinical specimens. Second, most anaerobes, except some clostridia, are not associated with any major diseases. Finally, the identification of anaerobes is perhaps not as straightforward as it is for most other bacteria. However, anaerobic bacteria are responsible for a range of infections, and they may be found in or on almost any part of the body, causing abscesses, septicaemia, endocarditis, pericarditis, fistulas, urinary tract infections, ear infections, and general wound and tissue infections (Brook, 2000; Brook, 2002a; Brook, 2002b; Brook, 2002c; Brook, 2002d; Brook, 2002e). A number of bacteria, such as *Streptococcus pyogenes*, are anaerobic but can also tolerate aerobic conditions. This chapter deals only with true anaerobes.

Anaerobes are distributed widely in nature, although their main habitat is the soil. Another main habitat is the intestines of humans and animals. It is also important to note that anaerobes are an important part of the human microflora. For example, *Veillonella* are found in the mouth, particularly on the tongue, whereas *Bacteroides* are found in the alimentary tract in large numbers. Anaerobes are defined by their ability or inability to grow in the presence of oxygen:

- *Obligate anaerobes* are bacteria that are unable to grow in the presence of oxygen.
- *Facultative anaerobes* are bacteria that will grow in the presence or absence of oxygen.

For some anaerobes, this causes great difficulty in laboratory isolation. Many anaerobes are pleomorphic, and therefore their morphologic identification may be difficult. This is particularly so for the Gram-positive anaerobes, which, when stained by the Gram method, are easily decolourized and therefore appear to be Gram-negative.

CLOSTRIDIA

Perhaps the most well-known and the most widely studied of the anaerobic bacteria are the clostridia. There are a number of diseases caused by the genus and over a dozen toxigenic species, but the two most important diseases are tetanus and botulism, caused by *Clostridium tetani* and *C. botulinum*, respectively. Tetanus is an ancient disease dating back to the time of Hippocrates. It presents most commonly as a localized disease at the site of wound infection, resulting in muscle rigidity and spasms (Maple and al-Wali, 2001). Progression to generalized tetanus usually occurs, which affects muscles of the whole body. Neonatal tetanus is caused by infection of the umbilical stump; this disease is always severe and often fatal. The symptoms of tetanus are caused by the tetanus toxin, which blocks inhibitory synapses of the spinal cord motor neurons, allowing uncontrolled stimulation of the muscles (Rossetto *et al.*, 2001). The toxin does not remain localized and instead can spread via the lymphatic system or the nerves, or by diffusion to other muscles.

Botulism is generally a foodborne disease, although it can also be established via wound infection. It is a paralytic disease resulting from the action of the botulinum toxin on the receptors of the peripheral nerve endings, leading to an inability to respond to nerve impulses (Cox and Hinkle, 2002). Botulism and tetanus and are described in more detail in Chapters 16 and 17, respectively.

In addition, there are two other clinically important clostridia: *C. perfringens* and *C. difficile*. The former may be associated with a spectrum of diseases, including gas gangrene, food poisoning, and general wound infections (Stevens and Bryant, 2002). There are five toxin types *of C. perfringens*, named A to E; human disease is associated most commonly with *C. perfringens* type A.

C. difficile may be associated with intestinal infection after broad-spectrum antibiotic use for other conditions (Moyenuddin *et al.*, 2002). The resident microflora of the colon are destroyed, enabling *C. difficile*, if resistant to the antibiotics used, to flourish in the colon. This condition is known as pseudomembranous colitis and is caused by toxins that are released by the bacterium; two toxins are released, an enterotoxin and a cytotoxin.

Although the clostridia cause these important diseases, in wound infections less than 1% of anaerobes isolated from pus are clostridia. As abdominal infections are often caused by anaerobes, it is not surprising that the remaining percentage of anaerobes, mostly Gram-negative bacilli, may be isolated from abdominal pus, although extended incubations in the laboratory are often necessary for their isolation.

ANAEROBIC COCCI

Anaerobic cocci are generally isolated less often than anaerobic Gram-negative bacilli from clinical specimens. Anaerobic cocci tend to be associated with organ abscesses, respiratory infections, and female genital tract infections (Murdoch, 1998). Furthermore, anaerobic cocci are rarely isolated in pure culture, and it is therefore difficult to ascertain whether they are the cause of infection. Before the introduction of antibiotics, anaerobic cocci were a common cause of severe or fatal puerperal infections, and mixed infections were not uncommon. These infections had case fatality rates of about 40%. Historically, it was usual to divide the anaerobic

Gram-positive cocci into two genera, the *Peptostreptococci* and the *Peptococci*. However, it is now known that such casual division is not useful. Instead, anaerobic Gram-positive cocci can be divided into about six genera (Table 18.1). Many of the species within these genera may be found as part of the normal human or animal faecal or intestinal flora. The anaerobic Gram-negative cocci may be divided into three genera: *Acidaminococcus, Megasphaera* and *Veillonella*. Anaerobic cocci account for approximately 30% of anaerobic bacteria isolated from clinical samples, with *Peptostreptococci* being the most commonly isolated from a variety of sites, including the lungs, intestine, urogenital sites, and sebaceous cysts. Isolation rates of Gram-negative cocci are lower because their recovery is more difficult. Of the Gram-negative cocci, *Veillonella* are the most frequently isolated (Wren, 1996).

Table 18.1 Anaerobic bacterial genera[a]

	Gram-negative	Gram-positive
Cocci	Acidaminococcus	Atopobium
	Megasphaera	Coprococcus
	Veillonella	Peptococcus
		Peptostreptococcus
		Ruminococcus
		Sarcina
Bacilli	Bacteroides	Clostridium
	Fusobacterium	Bifidobacterium
	Wolinella	Propionibacterium

[a]This is not a comprehensive list.

LABORATORY ISOLATION AND ANTIBIOTIC THERAPY

Anaerobes may be isolated on standard 5–7% blood agar incubated in anaerobic conditions. There are various methods of creating an anaerobic atmosphere in the laboratory, the most common being the anaerobic jar and anaerobic cabinet. However, isolation rates of Gram-positive and Gram-negative anaerobic cocci may increase if the media is supplemented with Tween 80 and sodium pyruvate, respectively. Incubation should continue for at least 48 hours, as some anaerobes are slow-growing. Although identification capabilities may be limited in many laboratories, identification to genus level is often sufficient for most anaerobic wound infections. For serious infections caused by the clostridia, more detailed studies can include spore location and toxin studies. In addition to anaerobic culture, a number of methods are available for direct detection of the bacteria or toxins they may produce in clinical samples. The most commonly available methods for this purpose are latex agglutination and enzyme-linked immunosorbent assay (ELISA) tests for the detection of *C. difficile*.

Metronidazole remains the main anti-anaerobe therapy, although it may also be used in combination with other antibiotics, such as gentamicin and co-amoxiclav, for some bacteria (Bryskier, 2001). Generally, quinolones are not suitable for treating anaerobic infections, although some quinolones with anti-anaerobic activity are now becoming available (Appelbaum, 1999). If sepsis is present, then treatment with other suitable antibiotics may be warranted, particularly for blind therapy. Most Gram-positive anaerobic cocci are susceptible to penicillin, although such an antibiotic would not be chosen for treating infection with Gram-negative anaerobic bacilli. Therefore, broad-spectrum antibiotics, in line with local antibiotic policy, are more suitable.

REFERENCES

Appelbaum, P.C. (1999). Quinolone activity against anaerobes. *Drugs* 58 (suppl 2), 60–64.

Brook, I. (2000). Anaerobic infections in children. *Adv Pediatr* 47, 395–437.

Brook, I. (2002a). Endocarditis due to anaerobic bacteria. *Cardiology* 98, 1–5.

Brook, I. (2002b). Microbiology and management of polymicrobial female genital tract infections in adolescents. *J Pediatr Adolesc Gynecol* 15, 217–26.

Brook, I. (2002c). Cutaneous and subcutaneous infections in newborns due to anaerobic bacteria. *J Perinat Med* 30, 197–208.

Brook, I. (2002d). Joint and bone infections due to anaerobic bacteria in children. *Pediatr Rehabil* 5, 11–19.

Brook, I. (2002e). Pericarditis due to anaerobic bacteria. *Cardiology* 97, 55–8.

Bryskier, A. (2001). Anti-anaerobic activity of antibacterial agents. *Expert Opin Investig Drugs* 10, 239–67.

Cox, N. and Hinkle, R. (2002). Infant botulism. *Am Fam Physician* 65, 1388–92.

Maple, P.A. and al-Wali, W. (2001). The prevention of tetanus in England and Wales. *Commun Dis Public Health* 4, 106–13.

Moyenuddin, M., Williamson, J.C. and Ohl, C.A. (2002). *Clostridium difficile*-associated diarrhea: current strategies for diagnosis and therapy. *Curr Gastroenterol Rep* 4, 279–86.

Murdoch, D.A. (1998). Gram-positive anaerobic cocci. *Clin Microbiol Rev* 11, 81–120.

Rossetto, O., Seveso, M., Caccin, P., Schiavo, G. and Montecucco, C. (2001). Tetanus and botulinum neurotoxins: turning bad guys into good by research. *Toxicon* 39, 27–41.

Stevens, D.L. and Bryant, A.E. (2002). The role of clostridial toxins in the pathogenesis of gas gangrene. *Clin Infect Dis* 35, S93–100.

Wren, M.W. (1996). Anaerobic cocci of clinical importance. *Br J Biomed Sci* 53, 294–301.

19

Tuberculosis

Of all the known infectious diseases that affect mankind, tuberculosis (TB) is today the leading cause of death in adults, although the disease may affect individuals of any age. A resurgence of TB has taken place in recent years, compounding the epidemic that already existed (Brennan, 1997; Inoue and Matoba, 2001; Murray, 1991). The World Health Organization (WHO) declared TB a global emergency some years ago, and now estimates that one-third of the world's population is infected with TB (Murray, 1991), although not all infected individuals develop the disease. About 3 million people have dual infection with human immunodeficiency virus (HIV) (Sepkowitz et al., 1995). It is estimated that a further 300 million individuals will become infected with TB, 90 million will develop disease, and 30 million will die from the disease in the next ten years. As with many infectious diseases, TB is a particular problem in developing countries, where it is responsible for over 25% of all preventable adult deaths.

A number of factors, such as changes in human social behaviour and an increase in foreign travel, have led to the emergence or re-emergence of some infectious diseases, including TB. When new infections are introduced into a susceptible population, there is a typical initial sharp rise in the number of infected individuals, which reaches a peak before declining gradually, usually over a period of weeks or months. The decline seen with TB, however, occurs over decades or centuries; for example, the longstanding epidemic of TB in the UK (and in many other parts of the world) began in the sixteenth century and reached its peak in the late eighteenth century. The epidemic has since declined in

the UK, although there have been recent concerns associated with a slight increase and antibiotic resistance. In developing countries, however, the epidemic peak has not been reached.

In the UK between 1947 and 1987, notifications of TB declined from 51 725 to 5086 cases per year. From the 1940s, the risk of infection to healthy young individuals became very small due to the availability of effective antibiotic therapy. The bacille Calmette-Guérin (BCG) vaccine, although developed in 1921, was not introduced until the mid-1950s. This vaccine has played an essential role in the reduction of TB in the UK and many other countries, although its true efficacy remains in question. It is thought that the BCG vaccine has its greatest efficacy if given in young individuals; booster vaccinations are not thought to increase the vaccine's protective efficacy. In England and Wales, there were between 385 and 564 cases of TB per year between 1982 and 1998 (source: HPA CDSC). However, over 40% of all cases in England and Wales now occur in London. In the USA, there were over 16 000 reported cases of TB in 2000. Although this is a large number, this represents a 7% decrease from 1999 and a 39% decrease compared with 1992 (source: US CDC).

In recent years in the UK, and in other developed countries, an increase in ethnic populations has occurred. Some of these populations have a higher rate of TB carriage, and therefore a general increase in TB cases has been seen in the UK. Generally in the UK, the majority of TB cases are seen in older individuals who were exposed at any early age before vaccination. However, cases may also be seen in children and pose a diagnostic problem due to the diverse presentations of the disease:

meningitis, pulmonary infection or miliary infection may present. In all cases of TB, an investigation must be carried out and contacts identified to minimize further spread of the disease. There are a number of methods available for the laboratory diagnosis of TB, such as standard TB culture, automated blood culture systems, and molecular methods such as the polymerase chain reaction (PCR) (Drobniewski *et al.*, 2000; Johansen *et al.*, 2002; Miller *et al.*, 2002; Yates *et al.*, 2002). The latter may be quicker but they are available only in specialist reference laboratories, not in routine district general laboratories. Molecular methods can also be used for the detection of antibiotic resistance and epidemiological analyses (Fluit *et al.*, 2001; Murray and Nardell, 2002). Whatever method is used, a rapid diagnosis is required to minimize spread of the disease. Once TB has been diagnosed, antibiotic therapy may be started. However, the treatment of TB is a lengthy process compared with other infectious diseases. Even so, it is regarded as the most cost-effective health intervention due to the long-term savings in monetary, morbidity and mortality terms. Appropriate antibiotic treatment given early on in the disease is highly effective if the course is completed, limits further transmission of the disease, and prevents the development of multi-drug-resistant tuberculosis (MDR-TB) (Musser, 1995). If the antibiotic course is not completed, then the condition of the infected individual is likely to deteriorate rapidly, transmission of TB to other individuals is more likely, and there is a greater risk of the TB strain developing resistance to the prescribed antibiotics.

TB is very much a social disease associated with poverty. For this reason, TB has been in decline in developed countries, whereas it has increased in developing countries where sanitation levels have not improved and populations have continued to rise substantially, leading to increased poverty. TB can be transmitted only by symptomatic individuals; it cannot be transmitted by vectors such as insects. The transmission of TB from an infected individual to an uninfected individual requires only casual contact and may occur when TB bacilli contained within tiny water droplets are expelled from the lungs after coughing or sneezing. These water droplets may remain suspended in the environment for hours and are then inhaled deep into the lungs of the uninfected individual. The water droplets and bacilli contained within each one are small enough to escape the usual ciliary action that removes foreign debris from the air passages. Only up to 10% of individuals infected with TB develop disease, and this is due most often to the patient having a poor immune system.

Recently, the incidence of TB has increased in developed countries where vaccination has previously resulted in a major reduction in the number of TB infections and resultant deaths. In these countries, TB has been thought to no longer pose a significant risk to the health of such nations. However, international travel in the past few decades has allowed the global spread of TB. For example, one-third of all TB cases in the USA are in foreign-born individuals. A major contributory factor to the current resurgence of TB is thought to be the HIV pandemic. It is estimated that one-quarter of all HIV-positive individuals around the world are also infected with TB. This is of particular importance because, in the long term, HIV infection results in an immunocompromised state and leads to acquired immune deficiency syndrome (AIDS). This means that TB infection is more likely to result in disease in those infected with HIV; TB is currently the leading cause of death in HIV-infected individuals.

As with many infectious diseases today, some antibiotic-resistant strains of *Mycobacterium tuberculosis* have emerged. MDR-TB is a widespread problem in immunocompromised and HIV-infected individuals and has received much attention in the USA and Europe. Some strains of *M. tuberculosis* have developed resistance against one or more antibiotics commonly used for treatment of TB, and therefore new antibiotics are needed urgently (Dye *et al.*, 2002; Maartens, 2002). MDR-TB poses a major threat to the global control of TB, particularly if it becomes widespread, as TB would then, once again, be virtually incurable as it was before the 1940s. Such antibiotic resistance is due to chromosomal mutation;

plasmid-mediated resistance is not thought to occur in TB. Those individuals with MDR-TB are less likely to be cured and the cost of treatment is significantly greater.

The current resurgence of TB in developed countries and the continuing increase in developing countries may continue. Over the coming decade, the disease will have to be monitored closely to enable swift and effective measures to be taken. The WHO has set up the Global Tuberculosis Programme to address the problem, and it remains to be seen what can be done in the coming years. In addition, as with many major bacterial diseases, the genome of *M. tuberculosis* has been sequenced. Whole-genome comparisons have been made between different strains of *M. tuberculosis*, and such research could lead to improved therapies, including antibiotics and vaccines (Fleischmann *et al.*, 2002; Khasnobis *et al.*, 2002).

REFERENCES

Brennan, P.J. (1997). Tuberculosis in the context of emerging and reemerging diseases. *FEMS Immunol Med Microbiol* **18**, 263–9.

Drobniewski, F.A., Watterson, S.A., Wilson, S.M. and Harris, G.S. (2000). A clinical, microbiological and economic analysis of a national service for the rapid molecular diagnosis of tuberculosis and rifampicin resistance in *Mycobacterium tuberculosis*. *J Med Microbiol* **49**, 271–8.

Dye, C., Williams, B.G., Espinal, M.A. and Raviglione, M.C. (2002). Erasing the world's slow stain: strategies to beat multidrug-resistant tuberculosis. *Science* **295**, 2042–6.

Fleischmann, R.D., Alland, D., Eisen, J.A., *et al.* (2002). Whole-genome comparison of *Mycobacterium tuberculosis* clinical and laboratory strains. *J Bacteriol* **184**, 5479–90.

Fluit, A.C., Visser, M.R. and Schmitz, F.-J. (2001). Molecular detection of antimicrobial resistance. *Clin Microbiol Rev* **14**, 836–71.

Inoue, K. and Matoba, S. (2001). Counterattack of re-emerging tuberculosis after 38 years. *Int J Tuberc Lung Dis* **5**, 873–5.

Johansen, I.S., Thomsen, V.O., Johansen, A., Andersen, P. and Lundgren, B. (2002). Evaluation of a new commercial assay for diagnosis of pulmonary and nonpulmonary tuberculosis. *Eur J Clin Microbiol Infect Dis* **21**, 455–60.

Khasnobis, S., Escuyer, V.E. and Chatterjee, D. (2002). Emerging therapeutic targets in tuberculosis: post-genomic era. *Expert Opin Ther Targets* **6**, 21–40.

Maartens, G. (2002). Advances in adult pulmonary tuberculosis. *Curr Opin Pulm Med* **8**, 173–7.

Miller, J.M., Jenny, A.L. and Payeur, J.B. (2002). Polymerase chain reaction detection of *Mycobacterium tuberculosis* complex and *Mycobacterium avium* organisms in formalin-fixed tissues from culture-negative ruminants. *Vet Microbiol* **87**, 15–23.

Murray, J.F. (1991). An emerging global programme against tuberculosis: agenda for research, including the impact of HIV infection. *Bull Int Union Tuberc Lung Dis* **66**, 207–9.

Murray, M. and Nardell, E. (2002). Molecular epidemiology of tuberculosis: achievements and challenges to current knowledge. *Bull World Health Organ* **80**, 477–82.

Musser, J. (1995). Antimicrobial agent resistance in mycobacteria: molecular genetic insights. *Clin Microbiol Rev* **8**, 496–514.

Sepkowitz, K., Raffalli, J., Riley, L., Kiehn, T. and Armstrong, D. (1995). Tuberculosis in the AIDS era. *Clin Microbiol Rev* **8**, 180–99.

Yates, M.D., Drobniewski, F.A. and Wilson, S.M. (2002). Evaluation of a rapid PCR-based epidemiological typing method for routine studies of *Mycobacterium tuberculosis*. *J Clin Microbiol* **40**, 712–14.

20

Leprosy

Leprosy is a disease that has afflicted humans for thousands of years (Lechat, 1999). Records from 600 BC suggest that leprosy originated in India; there is also palaeopathological evidence of leprosy in Egyptian mummies from 200 BC. Other evidence indicates that leprosy was recognized in the ancient civilizations of China, Egypt and India. Since these times, leprosy has been a terrible and feared disease that originally had a global distribution. Even up to the nineteenth century leprosy was endemic as far as the Arctic Circle and throughout Europe. Today, leprosy remains a public health problem (Stearns, 2002) and is distributed throughout tropical and subtropical regions, such as equatorial Africa, India, north-eastern South America, and the Northern Territory of Australia (World Health Organization, 2002).

Leprosy, like so many other infectious diseases, is most common in people of lower socioeconomic classes, who do not have access to good hygienic conditions, and who often live in crowded conditions. Billions of people live in countries where leprosy is endemic. According to the World Health Organization (WHO), there are now fewer than 600 000 registered cases of leprosy, and more than 11 million people have been cured of the disease since 1982 (Hastings *et al.*, 1988). In endemic areas, leprosy affects one in 10 000 of the population, and new cases total half a million each year. Furthermore, between 1 and 2 million individuals have had leprosy in the past, leaving them visibly and irreversibly disabled. Humans are the main reservoir for leprosy, although armadillos in the southern USA have been found with disease caused by organisms indistinguishable from *Mycobacterium leprae*; however, armadillos do not rep-

resent a major reservoir for human infection. Between humans, leprosy bacilli can be transmitted via the skin and nasal mucosa. The latter is the most important route of transmission because between 10 000 and 10 million bacteria may occur on the nasal mucosa. There is also the possibility that leprosy may be transmitted via insect vectors, although this has not yet been proven.

Leprosy is a chronic disease caused by the bacterium *M. leprae*. The bacterium was discovered in 1873 by Hansen (Sasaki *et al.*, 2001) and was the first bacterium to be identified as a cause of disease in humans. As a member of the mycobacteria, it is an acid-fast rod-shaped bacillus. There is great diversity in the clinical symptoms associated with leprosy. However, two main forms have been described, known as tuberculoid leprosy and lepromatous leprosy (Hastings *et al.*, 1988). The former occurs in individuals who possess high resistance to the disease, perhaps due to previous exposure, and affects the nerves and overlying skin. It is a benign, chronic, and sometimes self-healing disease. Lepromatous leprosy is seen in individuals with low resistance and results in a severe, systemic and progressive disease. It affects the nerves, skin, lymph nodes, eyes, mouth and larynx. Further classification of leprosy is given to borderline forms, known as BB (central borderline), BT (between BB and tuberculoid), and BL (between BB and lepromatous).

The incubation period for both forms of leprosy is unknown, although it has been estimated to be as short as two weeks (Hastings *et al.*, 1988). The incubation period has also been reported to be as long as 30 years in war veterans who were exposed whilst serving in endemic areas but who subsequently lived in non-endemic countries. Leprosy affects all ages and both sexes, although the male/female ratio of disease is 2 : 1. Infection does not always result in clinical disease. Actual disease is determined by a number of host factors, including genetic predisposition, route of initial infection, occurrence of re-infection, prior infection with other mycobacteria, and co-infection with human immunodeficiency virus (HIV) (Fitness *et al.*, 2002). In areas endemic for leprosy, factors such as re-infection, prior infection and co-infection with HIV are not uncommon; more than one factor can occur at any one time, so the chances of developing disease are increased. Mortality in leprosy is difficult to quantify and is often not considered to be important because death usually takes a long time. However, the mortality rate in some areas has been found to be four times greater than that for the general population. Death from leprosy often occurs due to indirect causes, such as secondary infection.

The diagnosis of leprosy is based mostly on the clinical signs and symptoms of the disease, which are easily recognizable (Hastings *et al.*, 1988). The presence of a skin lesion consistent with leprosy and with sensory loss is the main clinical sign. These skin lesions can be single or multiple and are usually less pigmented than the surrounding normal skin. The lesion may exist as a macule, papule or nodule. Thickened nerves are also a sign of leprosy. Alternatively, a skin smear may be performed and stained using the Ziehl–Neelsen technique to confirm leprosy. *M. leprae* cannot be cultured in vitro. However, the organism may be grown in a few animal models, such as the mouse footpad and the nine-banded armadillo, and these models have been used for research purposes. The nine-banded armadillo is particularly useful because widespread dissemination occurs due to the animal's primitive immunological system and low body temperature. As described above, subclinical infection with leprosy can occur. Although these cases may be diagnosed using antibody techniques, they represent an important reservoir of infection.

Treatment for leprosy was introduced in the 1940s with the drug dapsone, but resistance to dapsone became widespread. Today, the regimen of treatment for leprosy depends on the disease form, but multidrug therapy (MDT) is given for both classes (Hastings and Franzblau, 1988). For tuberculoid leprosy, a combination of rifampicin and dapsone should be given; for lepromatous leprosy, a combination of rifampicin, clofazimine and dapsone is used. Rifampicin is the most effective drug, but single-drug treatment should not be given, so as to avoid the development of drug resistance. It is recommended that MDT be given for at least two years. The WHO implemented a global action plan against leprosy in 1992. The MDT regimen is highly effective in curing diseased individuals and in reducing the prevalence of leprosy. Monitoring methods are now standardized, and the WHO, in collaboration with national programmes, has promoted initiatives such as Leprosy Elimination Monitoring. Such initiatives contributed to reducing the number of countries showing leprosy prevalence rates above one per 10 000 population from 122 in 1985 to 55 in 1997. Such control programmes need to be continued so that the incidence of leprosy can be reduced further still on a global scale. Although the WHO aimed to eliminate leprosy by 2000, this did not happen (Marlowe and Lockwood, 2001). Therefore, further work is required and other methods of control may be needed. The genome sequence of *M. leprae* has now been completed, and this will increase the understanding of the bacterium. This should provide novel therapies to combat leprosy (Grosset and Cole, 2001). Until then, leprosy will remain the feared disease that has been with mankind for so many years.

REFERENCES

Fitness, J., Tosh, K. and Hill, A.V. (2002). Genetics of susceptibility to leprosy. *Genes Immun* **3**, 441–53.

Grosset, J.H. and Cole, S.T. (2001). Genomics and the chemotherapy of leprosy. *Lepr Rev* **72**, 429–40.

Hastings, R.C. and Franzblau, S.G. (1988). Chemotherapy of leprosy. *Annu Rev Pharmacol Toxicol* **28**, 231–45.

Hastings, R.C., Gillis, T.P., Krahenbuhl, J.L. and Franzblau, S.G. (1988). Leprosy. *Clin Microbiol Rev* **1**, 330–48.

Lechat, M.F. (1999). The paleoepidemiology of leprosy: an overview. *Int J Lepr Other Mycobact Dis* **67**, 460–70.

Marlowe, S.N. and Lockwood, D.N. (2001). Update on leprosy. *Hosp Med* **62**, 471–6.

Sasaki, S., Takeshita, F., Okuda, K. and Ishii, N. (2001). *Mycobacterium leprae* and leprosy: a compendium. *Microbiol Immunol* **45**, 729–36.

Stearns, A.T. (2002). Leprosy: a problem solved by 2000? *Lepr Rev* **73**, 215–24.

World Health Organization (2002). Leprosy. Global situation. *Wkly Epidemiol Rec* **77**, 1–8.

21

Travellers' diarrhoea

More than 300 million people travel across international boundaries every year, and approximately 35 million of these travel from an industrialized country to the developing world (Lima, 2001). Diarrhoea is the most common illness found in travellers, occurring in 30–50%, depending on a number of factors, e.g. travellers' diarrhoea is common in children (Stauffer *et al.*, 2002). The illness results in inconvenience for both holidaymakers and business travellers (Anon, 2002). Travellers' diarrhoea is defined as the occurrence of three or more unformed stools each day during or after the period of travel, or any number of such stools if accompanied by fever, abdominal cramps or vomiting. Dysentery in travellers is more serious and is characterized by bloody diarrhoea, fever and abdominal cramps. Some changes in bowel habit, often resulting in the symptoms of travellers' diarrhoea, are related to a change in diet or stress and anxiety associated with travelling. However, a causative enteropathogen can be isolated in 50–80% of those cases defined as travellers' diarrhoea.

There are a number of causes of travellers' diarrhoea (Table 21.1). The most common is enterotoxigenic *Escherichia coli* (ETEC), which accounts for around 40% of cases (Bouckenooghe *et al.*, 2002). ETEC is isolated most commonly from people who have travelled to Africa, Central America or the Indian subcontinent (Adachi *et al.*, 2002; Bouckenooghe *et al.*, 2002; Jiang *et al.*, 2002). Other pathogenic *E. coli*, such as enterohaemorrhagic *Escherichia coli* (EHEC) and enteroinvasive *Escherichia coli* (EIEC), may also be isolated, and, along with *Shigella* spp., account for another 20% of travellers' diarrhoea (Clarke,

Table 21.1 Common causes of travellers' diarrhoea

Enterotoxigenic *Escherichia coli*
Enterohaemorrhagic *E. coli*
Enteroinvasive *E. coli*
Campylobacter
Salmonella
Cholera
Cryptosporidium
Cyclospora

2001; Levine, 1987). *Campylobacter* spp. and *Salmonella* spp. are responsible for around 15% of cases, depending mainly on the country of travel (Coker *et al.*, 2002). Although cholera is an important cause of diarrhoea and mortality in the Indian subcontinent and Central and South America, it seldom affects travellers. An estimated 15–20% of cases of travellers' diarrhoea are caused by other bacteria such as *Aeromonas* spp. and *Yersinia* spp. and by viruses, protozoa and helminths. As with any other infection, an enteropathogen cannot always be isolated from cases of travellers' diarrhoea; these account for the remaining 5–10% and may be due to faecal clearance of the organism before resolution of accompanying symptoms, effects of antimicrobial therapy, culture/isolation problems, or the presence of an unknown pathogen. For example, in the past decade, at least three 'new' human enteropathogens have been identified: *Campylobacter* spp., *Cryptosporidium* spp. and *Cyclospora* spp. Although species of these organisms were already known to infect and cause disease in other animals, it was not until recently (particularly recently for *Cyclospora* spp.) that they were identified as human pathogens.

For a traveller to develop the symptoms of travellers' diarrhoea, exposure to a pathogenic micro-organism must occur (Anon, 2002; Clarke, 2001; Hart *et al.*, 1993). The most common sources of travellers' diarrhoea are food and water, although person-to-person transmission may also occur (Backer, 2002). Swimming pools and seawater have also been responsible for some cases. Furthermore, there are numerous risk factors that depend on the destination and mode of travel. For example, travel from one developed country to another carries a low risk of illness, whereas travel from a developed country to a developing area such as Asia and Africa carries a high risk. This is because exposure is linked strongly to personal hygiene and general levels of sanitation. There are also some host factors, such as age, gastric function and diet attitudes, that contribute to the risk of developing travellers' diarrhoea. Most cases of travellers' diarrhoea present as acute, watery diarrhoea. They are often self-limiting and of short duration. Accompanying symptoms may include anorexia, nausea, vomiting, abdominal pain or cramps, faecal urgency and bloating. Fever is an uncommon occurrence and is usually low-grade when it does occur. A small percentage of cases may be more severe, both symptomatically and in duration. With some enteropathogens, symptoms may be recurrent over a period of months.

As with all infections, prevention is better than cure; therefore, pre-travel education is important and minimizes the risk of travellers' diarrhoea. Such education includes simple hygiene matters, mostly linked to cooking and drinking. Prophylaxis is generally not recommended, although many clinical trials have shown that it is effective. There is concern that prophylaxis could lead to increased drug resistance. Resistance to commonly used antibacterial agents has already occurred in some countries. The potential side effects from such drugs also often outweigh the potential benefits if used on a massive scale. Other approaches to the prevention of travellers' diarrhoea include lactobacillus

therapy and vaccination. Certain lactobacilli may be used to protect against infection with other micro-organisms by inhibiting their growth. However, the protection is only short-term. Many vaccines are under development that provide long-term protection against the more common causes of travellers' diarrhoea, and these may soon be available. Antibacterial treatment after the onset of symptoms is recommended for reducing the duration and severity of the illness, although its role is controversial due to the potential side affects, the cost of such drugs, and the development of antibiotic resistance. For example, a single dose of ciprofloxacin is effective if given within 24 hours of the onset of symptoms but otherwise is ineffective. It must also be remembered that antibacterial therapy is effective only against bacterial enteropathogens. Antidiarrhoeal drugs may be used to reduce the frequency of stools. Replacement of fluid and electrolytes is important, especially in infants and young children.

Laboratory diagnosis of travellers' diarrhoea is often unnecessary because most cases are self-limiting, symptomatic treatment alone is often sufficient, and the symptoms often resolve before the patient returns home. However, for those individuals who developed the illness late in their travels or who have a prolonged illness, laboratory investigations may be necessary. These investigations tend to focus on the more serious pathogens or those that may be of public health significance. Routine laboratory investigations include *Salmonella* spp., *Shigella* spp. and *Campylobacter* spp. Parasite investigations are performed routinely in some laboratories or will be included if requested. Culture for the various types of *E. coli* is not performed routinely because it is fairly specialized due to the requirement of serotyping. Similarly, virus investigations are not performed routinely.

Until good oral vaccines are available routinely, it would appear that the occurrence of travellers' diarrhoea will continue. As discussed, the best measure for preventing illness is good hygiene; antibacterial agents are useful when an individual is symptomatic. It will be interesting to note whether more enteropathogens are discovered over the next decade and whether the current epidemiology changes.

REFERENCES

Adachi, J.A., Ericsson, C.D., Jiang, Z.D., DuPont, M.W., Pallegar, S.R. and DuPont, H.L. (2002). Natural history of enteroaggregative and enterotoxigenic *Escherichia coli* infection among US travelers to Guadalajara, Mexico. *J Infect Dis* **185**, 1681–3.

Anon (2002). What to do about traveller's diarrhoea. *Drug Ther Bull* **40**, 36–8.

Backer, H. (2002). Water disinfection for international and wilderness travelers. *Clin Infect Dis* **34**, 355–64.

Bouckenooghe, A.R., Jiang, Z.D., De La Cabada, F.J., Ericsson, C.D. and DuPont, H.L. (2002). Enterotoxigenic *Escherichia coli* as cause of diarrhea among Mexican adults and US travelers in Mexico. *J Travel Med* **9**, 137–40.

Clarke, S.C. (2001). Diarrhoeagenic *Escherichia coli* – an emerging problem? *Diagn Microbiol Infect Dis* **41**, 93–8.

Coker, A.O., Isokpehi, R.D., Thomas, B.N., Amisu, K.O. and Obi, C.L. (2002). Human campylobacteriosis in developing countries. *Emerg Infect Dis* **8**, 237–44.

Hart, C.A., Batt, R.M. and Saunders, J.R. (1993). Diarrhoea caused by *Escherichia coli*. *Ann Trop Paediatr* **13**, 121–31.

Jiang, Z.D., Lowe, B., Verenkar, M.P., *et al.* (2002). Prevalence of enteric pathogens among international travelers with diarrhea acquired in Kenya (Mombasa), India (Goa), or Jamaica (Montego Bay). *J Infect Dis* **185**, 497–502.

Levine, M.M. (1987). *Escherichia coli* that cause diarrhea: enterotoxigenic, enteropathogenic, enteroinvasive, enterohemorrhagic, and enteroadherent. *J Infect Dis* **155**, 377–89.

Lima, A.A. (2001). Tropical diarrhoea: new developments in traveller's diarrhoea. *Curr Opin Infect Dis* **14**, 547–52.

Stauffer, W.M., Konop, R.J. and Kamat, D. (2002). Traveling with infants and young children. Part III: travelers' diarrhea. *J Travel Med* **9**, 141–50.

22

Salmonella

Diarrhoeal disease causes a high level of global morbidity and mortality, particularly in populations of low socioeconomic development. In developed countries, some of the pathogens associated with these diseases are manageable through antimicrobial therapy or supportive measures. However, in developing countries these resources are limited and it is therefore in these countries that the majority of the morbidity and mortality occur. As standards of living increase, there is a reduction in the level of mortality, mainly due to a decrease in the incidence of faecal-oral transmission.

Salmonella is a Gram-negative bacterium of the enterobacteria group that is capable of inducing diarrhoea in infected individuals. There are two major species: *S. enterica* and *S. bongori*. Each species is subdivided into subspecies and serovars (Guard-Petter, 2001). There are over 2500 serovars according to the scheme of Kauffman–White, a serological method for identifying strains of *Salmonella*. Salmonellae are distributed worldwide and can infect a diverse range of animals, including insects, reptiles, birds and mammals, as well as humans. They can persist in the natural environment and in food and water meant for human consumption. In humans, salmonellae can cause acute gastrointestinal disease, which is acquired most commonly by food poisoning. Most cases are caused by various serovars of the subspecies *S. enterica*. A few serovars of *S. enterica*, most notably *S. enterica* serovar Typhi, cause more serious invasive infection; this disease state is quite different. In the UK, salmonellae are the second most common bacterial agents of food poisoning. In 1981, there were over 10 000 cases of human salmonellosis; this increased throughout the 1980s and 1990s, with a peak of over 30 000 cases, although the incidence has since fallen to around 15 000 cases per year (source: HPA CDSC). Most of these infections are associated with some degree of morbidity, but mortality is rare. In the USA, 32 021 isolates of *Salmonella* were reported during 2000 (source: US CDC).

In the majority of cases, salmonellae must be swallowed to cause infection. They enter the stomach and must be able to overcome the host's physiological and immune mechanisms to initiate infection and cause disease. The small intestine normally has a sparse microbial flora due to a number of mechanisms, such as the pH of the gastric acid, the motility of the small bowel, and the production of secretory antibodies. However, if the salmonellae are in sufficient numbers, or if any of the immune or physiological mechanisms have been neutralized to some extent, then they may cause disease in the small intestine. Infection is therefore more common in patients who are hypochlorhydric or who are being treated with antacids. The first stage in the invasion of the intestinal wall depends on the ability of the bacteria to adhere to the epithelial cells. Salmonellae are able to initiate infection partly due to their ability to adhere to the intestinal epithelium. It has been shown that the bacteria possess fimbriae, which are probably mediators in adherence. These may be type 1 or type 3 fimbriae. If both fimbrial types are present, then the bacteria are able to adhere more readily to the gastroepithelium. They are then able to penetrate these cells and migrate through them to be extruded into the lamina propria. Infection is confined to the intestinal mucosa in gastroenteritis; those bacteria that reach extraintestinal sites are phagocytosed. It is only during infection with the more invasive salmonellae, such as *S. typhi*, that invasion of extraintestinal sites occurs, because the bacteria are resistant to phagocytosis.

Due to the invasion of the epithelium and consequent local cellular damage by salmonellae, an acute inflammatory response occurs in the ileum and caecum, sometimes with ulceration. This leads to diarrhoea, abdominal pain, vomiting and low-grade fever. Diarrhoea is usually the main feature of infection and varies greatly in its severity. Three events are responsible for the diarrhoea: the invasion of the intestinal mucosa, the production of a local inflammatory response, and the secretion of fluid and electrolytes following activation of mucosal adenylate cyclase. The amount of fluid exsorption, and therefore diarrhoea, does not always appear to be related to the degree of inflammatory response. The mechanisms involved in fluid exsorption during infection with salmonellae are not clear. Significant advances have been made recently in the understanding of the virulence mechanisms of salmonellae and other enteropathogens, such as those that allow invasion of the gastroepithelium and the survival and multiplication of salmonellae within macrophages (Brumell et al., 2002; Collazo and Galan, 1997; Finlay, 1995; Goosney et al., 1999; Kimbrough and Miller, 2002; Zaharik et al., 2002). There is evidence to suggest that some serotypes of *Salmonella* may produce an enterotoxin that resembles cholera toxin. If salmonellae remain outside the epithelium and do not invade, then it appears that fluid secretion or exsorption is not induced and clinical symptoms are mild.

In most cases, the clinical course of the disease is characterized by gastroenteritis alone. However, enteric fever and bacteraemia do occur rarely. The occurrence of enteric fever and bacteraemia apply especially to immunocompromised patients, to infants, and to the elderly. The initial gastroenteritis is usually more severe in these patients. In a few cases, invasion of the wall of the colon may take place. This results in severe dysenteric symptoms, with blood and mucus in the stools. *Salmonella* gastroenteritis is usually self-limiting and does not require antibiotic treatment. If, however, the symptoms are severe, such as in the very young or the eld-

erly, then appropriate antibiotics such as ciprofloxacin may be given. However, the benefits of antibiotic chemotherapy must be weighed against the potential pitfalls such as side effects and the development of antibiotic resistance (Bager and Helmuth, 2001). In cases of typhoid, then antibiotic treatment and other support are usually required due to the severity of the infection. Although a typhoid vaccine is available, improved vaccines could be developed against salmonellae. Continuing research into the virulence mechanisms of salmonellae as well as the completion of the *S. typhi* genome sequence may lead to improved therapies, including vaccines (Garmory et al., 2002; Wain et al., 2002).

Salmonellae are therefore significant foodborne pathogens that cause considerable morbidity in the form of gastrointestinal disease. Public health measures are important to prevent and control the spread of such disease.

REFERENCES

Bager, F. and Helmuth, R. (2001). Epidemiology of resistance to quinolones in *Salmonella*. *Vet Res* **32**, 285–90.

Brumell, J.H., Perrin, A.J., Goosney, D.L. and Finlay, B.B. (2002). Microbial pathogenesis: new niches for salmonella. *Curr Biol* **12**, R15–17.

Collazo, C.M. and Galan, J.E. (1997). The invasion-associated type-III protein secretion system in *Salmonella* – a review. *Gene* **192**, 51–9.

Finlay, B.B. (1995). Interactions between *Salmonella typhimurium*, enteropathogenic *Escherichia coli* (EPEC), and host epithelial cells. *Adv Dent Res* **9**, 31–6.

Garmory, H.S., Brown, K.A. and Titball, R.W. (2002). Salmonella vaccines for use in humans: present and future perspectives. *FEMS Microbiol Rev* **26**, 339–53.

Goosney, D.L., Knoechel, D.G. and Finlay, B.B. (1999). Enteropathogenic *E. coli*, *Salmonella*, and *Shigella*: masters of host cell cytoskeletal exploitation. *Emerg Infect Dis* **5**, 216–23.

Guard-Petter, J. (2001). The chicken, the egg and *Salmonella enteritidis*. *Environ Microbiol* **3**, 421–30.

Kimbrough, T.G. and Miller, S.I. (2002). Assembly of the type III secretion needle complex of *Salmonella typhimurium*. *Microbes Infect* **4**, 75–82.

Wain, J., House, D., Parkhill, J., Parry, C. and Dougan, G. (2002). Unlocking the genome of the human typhoid bacillus. *Lancet Infect Dis* **2**, 163–70.

Zaharik, M.L., Gruenheid, S., Perrin, A.J. and Finlay, B.B. (2002). Delivery of dangerous goods: type III secretion in enteric pathogens. *Int J Med Microbiol* **291**, 593–603.

23

Diarrhoeagenic *Escherichia coli*

Escherichia coli was first described by the German paediatrician Theodore Escherich in 1885. *E. coli* is a Gram-negative rod-shaped bacterium of the family Enterobacteriaceae and is a gut commensal that is normally excreted in faeces. For many years it was thought that *E. coli* were not pathogenic, but it has been found that *E. coli* may cause a number of diseases in humans, such as diarrhoeal disease, urinary tract infection, meningitis and various wound infections.

E. coli are a cause of diarrhoeal illness around the world, although in developed countries they rarely cause gastroenteritis, except for travellers' diarrhoea and haemorrhagic colitis, the latter of which may be epidemic or sporadic (Clarke, 2001; Hart *et al.*, 1993). Initially, all diarrhoeagenic strains of *E. coli* were termed enteropathogenic *E. coli* (EPEC), but as more has been learnt about the pathogenic mechanisms of these bacteria they have been grouped accordingly. There are now seven classes of diarrhoeagenic *E. coli*, with only the classical serotypes still being termed EPEC. The term 'EPEC' should be reserved for those *E. coli* that do not belong to any of the other diarrhoeagenic *E. coli* classes, do not produce any enterotoxin, but do cause the characteristic virulence lesions in the gut. The seven classes of diarrhoeagenic *E. coli* are:

- enteropathogenic *E. coli* (EPEC);
- enterohaemorrhagic *E. coli* (EHEC);
- enteroinvasive *E. coli* (EIEC);
- enterotoxigenic *E. coli* (ETEC);
- enteroaggregative *E. coli* (EAggEC);
- diffuse-adherent *E. coli* (DAEC);

- cytolethal distending toxin-producing *E. coli* (CDT-EC).

EPEC and ETEC are the most important of these in terms of total diarrhoeal episodes on a global scale. EPEC are a major cause of infantile diarrhoea. Although more has become known about EPEC's virulence mechanisms in recent years, they are still little understood. EHEC has become an important pathogen due to food-associated outbreaks in the USA and the UK. EIEC are the cause of bacillary dysentery; they produce diarrhoeal illness by invasion of the intestine, resulting in a bloody, mucoid diarrhoea. ETEC are a major cause of *E. coli*-associated diarrhoea worldwide and the main aetiology of travellers' diarrhoea. Diarrhoea is caused by the bacteria producing a heat-stable (ST) and a heat-labile (LT) enterotoxin. EAggEC are a more recent addition to the diarrhoeagenic classes of *E. coli*; they are so-called due to their adherence pattern to cultured epithelial cells (Elliot and Nataro, 1995). EAggEC are associated with acute or persistent diarrhoea, particularly in children, which is brought about by the production of an ST enterotoxin that has homology to the ST enterotoxin of ETEC. DAEC have been described recently as a cause of diarrhoea and are so called because of their adherence pattern to cultured epithelial cells (Benz and Schmidt, 1990). Their aetiological role in diarrhoea is a controversial issue because some studies have shown an association of DAEC with diarrhoea, whilst others have not. CDT-EC are the latest diarrhoeagenic *E. coli* to be described (Bouzari and Varghese, 1990). These *E. coli* have been reported to cause the distension and eventual disintegration of certain cell lines. However, the association of CDT-EC with diarrhoea is not clear.

ENTEROHAEMORRHAGIC *ESCHERICHIA COLI*

EHEC are also commonly known as Vero cyto-toxin-producing *E. coli* (VTEC). Not all EHEC produce Vero cytotoxin, and therefore the term 'VTEC' should be reserved solely for those *E. coli* that do produce it. EHEC belong to a number of O serogroups, but those of serogroup 0157 are the most important in human disease. The organism produces a toxin that has cytotoxic activity on Vero cells and is therefore known as Vero cyto-toxin (VT) (Clarke, 2001; Hart *et al.*, 1993). Interest in Vero cytotoxins began in the late 1970s, when it was found that some strains of EPEC produced them; these strains of bacteria were soon reclassified as EHEC. There are two major types of VT, known as VT1 and VT2. VT1 is related closely to the Shiga toxin produced by *Shigella dysenteriae*; VT2 is antigenically distinct from VT1 and Shiga toxin. VT2 is the toxin most commonly isolated from cases of EHEC infection. EHEC also possesses a number of other mechanisms, such as adhesins, which are involved in virulence (Frankel *et al.*, 1998). EHEC was first identified as a human pathogen in 1982 after two outbreaks occurred in the USA. Since then, outbreaks have been reported from various parts of the world, including North America, western Europe, Australia, Asia and South Africa. The first outbreak of haemolytic uraemic syndrome (HUS) associated with EHEC in England was identified by the Public Health Laboratory Service (PHLS) in 1983. The most common phage types (PT) of EHEC isolated in the UK are PT1, PT2, PT4, PT8 and PT49, and there are between 800 and 1000 cases each year (source: HPA CDSC).

Transmission of EHEC may occur by the ingestion of contaminated food (Table 23.1), such as meats, unpasteurized milk and water, by person-to-person contact, or by zoonotic transmission. Cattle appear to be the main reservoir of EHEC, and the

Table 23.1 Foods that have been associated with EHEC outbreaks

Minced beef
Dry-cured salami
Water
Meat pies
Raw vegetables
Cheese
Milk
Unpasteurized apple juice
Yoghurt

organism has been isolated from apparently healthy animals. Faecal carriage of EHEC in a dairy herd has been reported recently as 9%. Infected cattle may therefore introduce infection and contaminate carcasses of healthy animals. Mincing of beef may also transfer EHEC from the meat surface to the interior, and therefore infection can occur when meat is cooked improperly or when raw or undercooked meat contaminates other foods. Meat from a single infected animal may contaminate a large amount of mince. Human infection with EHEC is associated with a range of symptoms, from non-bloody diarrhoea, fever and vomiting through to haemorrhagic colitis and HUS. HUS is characterized by acute renal failure, haemolytic anaemia and thrombocytopenia. Between 2% and 7% of infected individuals usually develop HUS; it is more common in young children. The infectious dose has been estimated to be fewer than 100 organisms. The incubation period is usually one to six days, but it can be up to 14 days. The infection is usually self-limiting, often resolving within eight days. There is no specific treatment for EHEC infection; therapy is symptomatic, and antibiotic treatment, as in many gastrointestinal infections, may not be beneficial. Excretion has been reported up to 62 days after the onset of symptoms, although it is usually approximately two weeks. Diagnosis of EHEC infection is mainly by laboratory detection of the organism in faeces. Alternatively, DNA probes may be used to detect VT genes in faeces, or antibodies can be detected by conventional assays.

Since the early 1990s, there has been a general global increase in the number of EHEC infections, and recent large outbreaks have led to an increased interest in the pathogen. The increase in EHEC infections may be due to a number of factors, such as improved reporting and a general increase in fast-food consumption. Seasonal variation is seen in EHEC isolations, with the organism being isolated most frequently from sporadic cases and outbreaks in the third quarter of the year. Such variation is seen in England and Wales, the USA and other countries.

The first of the recent large outbreaks occurred amongst schoolchildren in the city of Sakai, Japan, in July and August of 1996. The total number of children affected was over 6300, from 62 schools; 92 patients developed HUS, and there were two reported deaths. School lunch was the suspected cause of the outbreak. Over 3000 further cases from outside the city of Sakai occurred in Japan, with 11 deaths by the end of August. In the UK, the annual incidence of EHEC infection varies between less than 1 and 1.0 cases per 100 000 population. Outbreaks, however, can change this figure significantly. For example, the large outbreak of EHEC infection in Scotland in 1996 resulted in over 400 individuals having symptoms of EHEC infection, of which 256 cases were confirmed (Liddell, 1997). The outbreak was attributed to the consumption of cooked meats supplied by a butcher. Recent outbreaks of EHEC infection around the world and the general increase in cases that has occurred in recent years strongly suggest that the organism is an emerging pathogen that is likely to cause further problems in the future.

ENTEROPATHOGENIC *ESCHERICHIA COLI*

The diarrhoeal disease caused by EPEC has been noted for many centuries. The disease was known initially as infantile diarrhoea. Until the early part of the twentieth century, this was a major problem worldwide, with high morbidity and mortality (Clarke, 2001; Clarke *et al.*, 2002). However, the number of deaths due to EPEC infection in babies in developed countries has fallen considerably since the beginning of the twentieth century. This resulted initially in a decline in interest in determining the aetiology of infantile diarrhoea, but during the 1930s a number of severe outbreaks of nosocomial neonatal enteritis occurred in New York, each with a high mortality, which restored interest in the aetiology of infantile diarrhoea.

John Bray reported the isolation of diarrhoeagenic *E. coli* from cases of infantile summer diarrhoea in 1945. The term 'enteropathogenic *Escherichia coli*' was introduced in 1955 to describe strains of *E. coli* that were implicated epidemiologically with infantile diarrhoea (Bray, 1945; Bray and Bevan, 1948; Neter *et al.*, 1955). EPEC are not a homogeneous group of enteropathogens because serotype does not always correlate with pathogenicity. As the early methods of identifying EPEC relied on serotyping alone, there was always some reluctance in accepting the organisms as pathogens. However, the pathogenic ability of EPEC was confirmed in 1978, when it was shown that strains of EPEC that did not produce enterotoxins, were not invasive, and were negative in infant rabbit assays for gross fluid accumulation still caused diarrhoea in adult volunteers.

As little as three or four decades ago, EPEC was still a significant cause of infantile diarrhoea in developed countries. EPEC infection in developed countries is now rare and is no longer regarded as a problem. However, it remains a problem in developing countries, and it is now estimated that there are over 100 million diarrhoeal episodes attributable to EPEC each year in such countries (Clarke *et al.*, 2002). Diarrhoeal disease due to EPEC is age-related, usually occurring in infants less than six months of age. The reason for the age specificity of EPEC infection is not well understood; factors such as mucosal immunity and differences in gut structure between infants and adults (i.e. possession of receptors) could play a part.

EPEC infection results in an acute or persistent watery, non-bloody or mucoid diarrhoea, often accompanied by fever and vomiting. The disease ranges from a subclinical infection to a fulminating diarrhoea, presumably depending on host factors. After colonization of the intestine with EPEC, bacteria can be isolated for about four to seven days before the onset of symptoms and then throughout infection. In most cases, the organisms are also cleared; however in some cases, carriage may occur for some weeks. Most infants with diarrhoea caused by EPEC recover uneventfully if water and electrolyte disturbances are corrected promptly. However, antimicrobial therapy may also be of benefit in those with a life-threatening condition.

EPEC are defined mostly in terms of their negative characteristics. In 1983, Edelman and Levine defined EPEC as 'diarrhoeagenic *E. coli* belonging to serogroups epidemiologically incriminated as pathogens but whose pathogenic mechanisms have not been proven to be related either to LT enterotoxins or ST enterotoxins or to *Shigella*-like invasiveness. EPEC adhere in a seemingly pathognomic way to the intestinal epithelium.' Three main mechanisms of virulence have been determined, which are thought to be involved in colonization, adherence, and host-cell cytoskeleton rearrangement. Colonization is thought to be mediated by a plasmid, termed the EPEC adherence factor (EAF) plasmid. The EAF plasmid possesses genes that encode the bundle-forming pili (Bfp) of EPEC, which create bundles that intertwine with other bacteria to create a three-dimensional network. The Bfp may be partially or wholly responsible for the recruitment of bacteria in the surrounding environment of the host cell, allowing EPEC to attach to epithelial cells in vitro with a localized adherence pattern; such attachment is also thought to occur in vivo. After localized adherence, intimate adherence to the epithelium occurs, which is mediated by a number of proteins associated with a large chromosomal locus, termed the locus of enterocyte effacement (LEE). The LEE encodes many of the genes known to be involved with attaching and effacing (AE), including the *eae* (*E. coli* attaching and effacing) genes. The protein product of one of

the genes, *eae*A, is known as intimin. The *eae* genes are associated with EPEC's ability to adhere intimately to the epithelial surface and to produce a characteristic ultrastructural lesion. Host-cell cytoskeleton rearrangement occurs after attachment and intimate adherence. This is mediated by host-cell protein phosphorylation, resulting in localized destruction of the intestinal brush-border microvilli and distortion of the apical enterocyte membrane. This results in cytoskeletal rearrangement and the formation of an actin-rich cup-like indentation (pedestal) at the site of bacterial contact, termed the attaching and effacing (AE) lesion. The formation of AE lesions results in a reduction in the absorptive capacity of the intestinal mucosa, which leads inevitably to a reduction in electrolyte balance and subsequent diarrhoea. The elucidation of some of the virulence mechanisms of EPEC has led to a greater understanding of not only EPEC but also other bacteria. Other enteric bacteria, previously thought to be non-pathogenic, possess genes that code for virulence factors in EPEC.

Diagnosis and identification of EPEC may be attained by routine biochemical and serotyping methods. However, these tests are not 100% sensitive or specific, and other methods are therefore required. A test that may be employed to identify EPEC from either intestinal biopsies or cultured cell lines is the fluorescent actin-staining (FAS) test. The test utilizes the fact that phalloidin (a fungal toxin) binds to filamentous actin, which accumulates at the sites of EPEC AE lesions. Fluorescein-conjugated phalloidin is used so that the results of the test may be visualized by standard ultraviolet microscopy.

ENTEROTOXIGENIC *ESCHERICHIA COLI*

ETEC were first identified as a cause of diarrhoea in 1970. They are now considered a major cause of *E. coli*-associated diarrhoea worldwide (Clarke, 2001). The symptoms of ETEC infection are due to the production of one or both of two enterotoxins by the bacterium: a heat-stable (ST) enterotoxin and a heat-labile (LT) enterotoxin. The genes encoding these enterotoxins are located on transferable plasmids. Like EPEC, ETEC are associated with poor hygiene and sanitation and are therefore of most importance in developing countries. In such countries, the number of diarrhoeal episodes due to ETEC is on a level with those caused by EPEC. Many individuals visiting developing countries suffer from ETEC infection during their stay or upon their return. Most of these cases probably occur due to the ingestion of water or food contaminated with ETEC. Outbreaks can occur in hotels after person-to-person spread. The illness is known as 'travellers' diarrhoea' and is usually an acute illness with symptoms consisting of loose stools, nausea, vomiting and abdominal cramps. In developing countries, the most severe form of acute infection is a cholera-like illness, which occurs in areas where *Vibrio cholerae* are already endemic. This may occur in all age groups, and it is difficult to distinguish clinically from true cholera. ETEC is not usually a problem in developed countries, although it has been linked with outbreaks, some of which have been large, with approximately 2000 individuals being infected. ETEC has been associated with a few outbreaks of infantile enteritis in hospitals and also with larger outbreaks due to contaminated water or food.

EPEC and ETEC are the most important of the diarrhoeagenic *E. coli* in terms of total diarrhoeal episodes on a global scale. For example, in one study in Bangladesh, ETEC and EPEC were the only pathogenic *E. coli* associated with diarrhoea in children under five years of age. Therefore, research must continue to elucidate the virulence mechanisms of these two organisms, whilst sanitation and hygiene provisions must improve in developing countries where they cause the most morbidity and mortality.

OTHER PATHOGENIC
ESCHERICHIA COLI

Molecular techniques have allowed the identification of adhesins and toxins produced by other diarrhoeagenic *E. coli* in the other classes of

diarrhoeagenic *E. coli* – EIEC, EAggEC, DAEC and CDT-EC. EIEC are an important cause of diarrhoeal disease. They are responsible for a bacillary dysentery-like illness and, not surprisingly, therefore share some of the virulence properties associated with *Shigella dysenteriae*. EIEC are a significant cause of morbidity and mortality in young children in developed countries, although, like most enteropathogens, they are more important in developing countries where sanitation and hygiene levels are of a poor standard. EIEC are able to invade the intestinal epithelium; this is dependent upon the possession of a 120–140-MDa plasmid that encodes all the genes necessary for such virulence. Infection with EIEC results in a diarrhoeal illness characterized by bloody, mucoid diarrhoea.

EAggEC are a more recent addition to the diarrhoeagenic classes of *E. coli*. They are so-called due to their adherence pattern to cultured epithelial cells (Chan *et al.*, 1994; Germani *et al.*, 1996). Such an adherence pattern provides the gold standard for the definition of EAggEC and is seen as bacteria adhering in a stacked brick-line formation on the cell surface. EAggEC are a significant cause of diarrhoea in developing countries and are associated epidemiologically with an acute or persistent diarrhoea. This illness, which often lasts for more than 14 days, is of particular significance in children. However, a high rate of asymptomatic carriage occurs with EAggEC infection, and therefore the presence of other pathogens should be excluded. EAggEC do not induce attaching/effacing lesions characteristic of EPEC, and do not produce cholera-like or Shiga-like toxins. Little is known of their pathogenicity, except that they produce a toxin known as the enteroaggregative heat-stable enterotoxin (EAST1). This enterotoxin, although partly homologous and functionally similar to, is distinct from the ST enterotoxin. EAST1 is thought to be responsible for the symptoms of infection. The production of a heat-labile (LT) toxin has also been reported from EAggEC, which is related antigenically to *E. coli* haemolysin.

Early studies on DAEC could not find an association between the organism and diarrhoeal illness; however, more recent studies have found such an association. DAEC are so-called because of their adherence pattern to cultured epithelial cells (Germani *et al.*, 1996; Jallat *et al.*, 1994). Like EAggEC, their adherence to these cells provides a gold standard for their definition. People infected with DAEC may experience mucoid watery stools and suffer from fever and vomiting. The mean duration of illness is about eight days. DAEC has been reported as a cause of diarrhoeal illness in both developed and developing countries. Their pathogenic mechanisms are poorly understood, although it is thought that DAEC may produce one or more toxins, one of which is a haemolysin. However, their aetiological role in diarrhoea remains controversial.

CDT-EC are the most recently described class of diarrhoeagenic *E. coli*. These *E. coli* have been reported in a number of studies in developing countries. They cause the distension and eventual disintegration of certain cell lines (Albert *et al.*, 1996; Ghilardi *et al.*, 2001). In one report, CDT-EC additionally possessed the virulence factors of EPEC or EAggEC. However, the association of CDT-EC with diarrhoea is not clear, because in one report from Bangladesh there was no statistically significant association of carriage with diarrhoea. Therefore, results of further studies are required to confirm or disprove the diarrhoeagenic potential of CDT-EC and to determine whether they really are another separate class.

As research continues into the diarrhoeagenic *E. coli*, more virulence determinants associated with these organisms will be discovered. It remains to be seen whether more classes of diarrhoeagenic *E. coli* will be named, although this is now probably unlikely. The true impact of the more recently named classes on global diarrhoea remains to be elucidated. Meanwhile, strategies are required to control all classes of diarrhoeagenic *E. coli* so that the burden on the health of individuals, particularly in developing countries, can be reduced.

REFERENCES

Albert, M.J., Faruque, S.M., Faruque, A.S., *et al.* (1996). Controlled study of cytolethal distending toxin-producing *Escherichia coli* infections in Bangladeshi children. *J Clin Microbiol* **34**, 717–19.

Benz, I. and Schmidt, M.A. (1990). Diffuse adherence of enteropathogenic *Escherichia coli* strains. *Res Microbiol* **141**, 785–6.

Bouzari, S. and Varghese, A. (1990). Cytolethal distending toxin (CLDT) production by enteropathogenic *Escherichia coli* (EPEC). *FEMS Microbiol Lett* **59**, 193–8.

Bray, J. (1945). Isolation of antigenically homogenous strains of *Bact. coli* neapolitanum from summer diarrhoea of infants. *J Pathol* **57**, 239–47.

Bray, J. and Bevan, T.E.D. (1948). Slide agglutination of *Bacterium coli* var. neopolitanum in summer diarrhoea. *J Pathol Bacteriol* **60**, 395–401.

Chan, K.N., Phillips, A.D., Knutton, S., Smith, H.R. and Walker-Smith, J.A. (1994). Enteroaggregative *Escherichia coli*: another cause of acute and chronic diarrhoea in England? *J Pediatr Gastroenterol Nutr* **18**, 87–91.

Clarke, S.C. (2001). Diarrhoeagenic *Escherichia coli* – an emerging problem? *Diagn Microbiol Infect Dis* **41**, 93–8.

Clarke, S.C., Haigh, R.D., Freestone, P.P. and Williams, P.H. (2002). Enteropathogenic *Escherichia coli* infection: history and clinical aspects. *Br J Biomed Sci* **59**, 123–7.

Edelman, R. and Levine, M.M. (1983). Summary of a workshop of enteropathogenic *Escherichia coli*. *J Infect Dis* **147**, 1108–18.

Elliot, S.J. and Nataro, J.P. (1995). Enteroaggregative and diffusely adherent *Escherichia coli*. *Rev Med Microbiol* **6**, 196–206.

Frankel, G., Phillips, A.D., Rosenshine, I., Dougan, G., Kaper, J.B. and Knutton, S. (1998). Enteropathogenic and enterohaemorrhagic *Escherichia coli*: more subversive elements. *Mol Microbiol* **30**, 911–21.

Germani, Y., Begaud, E., Duval, P. and Le Bouguenec, C. (1996). Prevalence of enteropathogenic, enteroaggregative, and diffusely adherent *Escherichia coli* among isolates from children with diarrhea in new Caledonia. *J Infect Dis* **174**, 1124–6.

Ghilardi, A.C., Gomes, T.A. and Trabulsi, L.R. (2001). Production of cytolethal distending toxin and other virulence characteristics of *Escherichia coli* strains of serogroup O86. *Mem Inst Oswaldo Cruz* **96**, 703–8.

Hart, C.A., Batt, R.M. and Saunders, J.R. (1993). Diarrhoea caused by *Escherichia coli*. *Ann Trop Paediatr* **13**, 121–31.

Jallat, C., Darfeuille-Michaud, A., Rich, C. and Joly, B. (1994). Survey of clinical isolates of diarrhoeogenic *Escherichia coli*: diffusely adhering *E. coli* strains with multiple adhesive factors. *Res Microbiol* **145**, 621–32.

Liddell, K.G. (1997). *Escherichia coli* O157: outbreak in central Scotland. *Lancet* **349**, 502–3.

Neter, E., Westphal, O., Luderitz, R., Gino, M. and Gorzynski, E. A. (1955). Demonstration of antibodies against enteropathogenic *Escherichia coli* in sera of children of various ages. *Paediatrics* **16**, 801–7.

24

Campylobacter enteritis

A German paediatrician, Theodore Escherich, reported what is now known as *Campylobacter* enteritis in 1886, around the same time that he described *Escherichia coli*. He described the presence of spiral bacteria in the faeces of children, although these bacteria could not be cultured on solid media. It was not until 1913 that *Campylobacter* were first isolated from domestic animals. For the next half-century they were thought to be solely of veterinary importance (Skirrow, 1981). In 1963, the genus was defined, but it was another decade before a detailed system of classification was proposed. Species of *Campylobacter* were implicated as human gastrointestinal pathogens in 1973, and they are now the most commonly reported bacterial cause of enteritis in developing and developed countries (Coker *et al.*, 2002; Skirrow, 1991).

The genus name *Campylobacter* is derived from the Greek word for curved rod; it was proposed to describe microaerophilic bacteria that were different from *Vibrios*. Species of *Campylobacter* are Gram-negative, 5–8 μm long and 0.2–0.5 μm wide, and curved, spiral or S-shaped. They possess a single polar flagellum or a flagellum at either end, making the bacteria highly motile, with a characteristic rapid corkscrew movement. Relative to other Gram-negative bacteria, their nucleotide G+C content is low, ranging from 28% to 38%. The general characteristics of the *Campylobacter* are not defined across the genus but are widely variable throughout the species, regardless of whether they are pathogenic or non-pathogenic (On, 1996). Their differences in biochemical reactions are limited due to their general inability to ferment common carbohydrates. However, all species of *Campylobacter* are oxi-

dase-positive and reduce nitrates. Most species are microaerophilic, but their growth temperatures are wide-ranging: some species are able to grow at 15 °C while others grow at 42 °C. Even individual species have a wide tolerance of temperature, e.g. *C. fetus* subsp. *fetus* is able to grow at 25 °C but can also be cultured at 37 °C or sometimes higher.

Species of *Campylobacter* found to be pathogenic in humans were first discovered in 1973 and later confirmed in 1977 (Skirrow, 1977). Since then, a huge interest in the genus has developed in both research and diagnostic terms. From 1977, many diagnostic laboratories started to culture *Campylobacter*, and reporting national surveillance centres were set up. Since then, laboratories have improved in isolating *Campylobacter*. Over the past few decades, the number of isolates reported to surveillance centres in Europe and the USA has increased significantly, probably due to a number of factors including better diagnosis, increased reporting, and an increased number of actual cases. In the UK, for example, almost 25 000 cases of *Campylobacter* infection were reported in 1986, increasing to over 55 000 in 2001 (source: HPA CDSC). *Campylobacter* enteritis is seasonal, with the peak of reports being in late May or early June; this is in contrast to *Salmonella* infection, which peaks in July. It is not known why these peaks occur and why they are different between the two organisms.

Campylobacter are both environmental and zoonotic, having been isolated from water, wild birds, and domestic animals such as poultry, cattle, pigs, sheep, dogs and cats. Milk, water and poultry are thought to be the main reservoirs of *Campylobacter* (Corry and Atabay, 2001).

However, the majority of *Campylobacter* are not serotyped, and it is therefore difficult to determine the number of outbreaks and also the reservoir of infection. Unlike *Salmonella*, *Campylobacter* cannot multiply on food at ambient temperatures and must be inside a living host to multiply (Park, 2002). Unlike many other gastrointestinal diseases, once human infection with *Campylobacter* has occurred, person-to-person transmission is uncommon.

The species pathogenic to humans are thermophilic and prefer to grow at 42–43 °C. A selective agar medium was developed by Skirrow (1977) that provided laboratories with the ability to isolate *Campylobacter* from clinical samples. This medium, or improvements of it, is still used today. Most cases of *Campylobacter* enteritis in humans are due to *C. jejuni* and *C. coli*, although other species, including *C. lari* and *C. upsaliensis*, have also been isolated from humans with enteritis. However, some species require special isolation procedures and growth temperatures, so such species may be more common causes of enteritis than is currently proposed. *Campylobacter* appear to be phenotypically diverse (Wareing *et al.*, 2002), although at present only a small percentage are identified genotypically. However, a multi-locus sequence typing (MLST) scheme has been described, which may be useful for typing and epidemiological studies (Dingle *et al.*, 2002; Dingle *et al.*, 2001). This is in contrast to *Salmonella*, for which most isolates are serotyped.

Symptoms of *Campylobacter* enteritis occur between two and ten days after exposure to the bacteria. Illness usually lasts for over a week, but prolonged illness is infrequent (Andrews, 1998). Symptoms include profuse, watery diarrhoea, nausea, abdominal pain and cramps, which may be accompanied by fever. Symptoms recur in about 25% of individuals and persist in up to 5% for as long as three months after initial infection. Even so, *Campylobacter* enteritis, like other gastrointestinal infections, is usually self-limiting and does not require antibiotic treatment. Such treatment is indicated only in serious infections, in which case erythromycin is the antibiotic of choice; ciprofloxacin may be a suitable alternative for adults. However, resistance to both these antibiotics is emerging. *Campylobacter* enteritis can also lead to bacteraemia, although the number of cases per year is small compared with that caused by *Salmonella*. One of the most serious sequelae of infection with *Campylobacter* is Guillain–Barré syndrome (GBS) (Nachamkin, 2002). Most cases of GBS occur one to three weeks after a gastrointestinal or urinary tract infection, although the aetiology of the syndrome is not known. There is strong serological evidence implicating *Campylobacter* as a significant cause of GBS.

Campylobacter enteritis cannot be diagnosed solely on clinical grounds because many of the symptoms are common to other gastrointestinal infections. Laboratory diagnosis is required, which is usually achieved by culture on a derivative of the medium designed by Skirrow, or a modern alternative. Such culture media contain charcoal and often lysed horse blood, with the addition of between one and four antibiotics to prevent the growth of other faecal bacteria. Identification from such media is fairly straightforward; it can be limited to colony morphology, Gram stain and oxidase positivity, or it can be more detailed, using further biochemical testing. Serodiagnosis can be performed using a number of methods, including enzyme-linked immunosorbent assay (ELISA), tube agglutination and complement fixation, although the former is the most sensitive. However, a host immune response cannot be detected until five to ten days after initial infection; also, raised antibody titres can exist in healthy individuals who have had previous exposure to *Campylobacter*. Serodiagnosis is therefore useful only for epidemiological purposes or where faecal samples are unavailable for culture. More recently, DNA probes have been used that can detect a number of species in faecal samples within hours. The *Campylobacter* genome has also been sequenced, which is leading to improved diagnostic and typing methods as well as improved understanding of the virulence aspects of the bacterium (Bereswill and Kist, 2002; Wren *et al.*, 2001). This should also lead to improved therapies.

Like so many other gastrointestinal diseases, *Campylobacter* infection can be avoided by simple measures. As the main reservoirs of infection are milk, water and poultry, and the organisms are rarely transmitted from person to person, then proper milk and water treatment and adequate storage and cooking of foodstuffs should be sufficient to avoid infection. However, public education relating to these measures is difficult and expensive, although such measures would, in the long term, prove to be cost-effective.

REFERENCES

Andrews, G.P. (1998). The enteric *Campylobacter*: they are everywhere. *Clin Lab Sci* **11**, 305–8.

Bereswill, S. and Kist, M. (2002). Molecular microbiology and pathogenesis of *Helicobacter* and *Campylobacter* updated: a meeting report of the 11th conference on *Campylobacter*, *Helicobacter* and related organisms. *Mol Microbiol* **45**, 255–62.

Coker, A.O., Isokpehi, R.D., Thomas, B.N., Amisu, K.O. and Obi, C.L. (2002). Human campylobacteriosis in developing countries. *Emerg Infect Dis* **8**, 237–44.

Corry, J.E. and Atabay, H.I. (2001). Poultry as a source of *Campylobacter* and related organisms. *Symp Ser Soc Appl Microbiol* (suppl 30), 96–114S.

Dingle, K.E., Colles, F.M., Wareing, D., *et al.* (2001). Multilocus sequence typing system for *Campylobacter jejuni*. *J Clin Microbiol* **39**, 14–23.

Dingle, K.E., Colles, F.M., Ure, R., *et al.* (2002). Molecular characterization of *Campylobacter jejuni* clones: a basis for epidemiologic investigation. *Emerg Infect Dis* **8**, 949–55.

Nachamkin, I. (2002). Chronic effects of *Campylobacter* infection. *Microbes Infect* **4**, 399–403.

On, S. (1996). Identification methods for campylobacters, helicobacters, and related organisms. *Clin Microbiol Rev* **9**, 405–22.

Park, S.F. (2002). The physiology of *Campylobacter* species and its relevance to their role as foodborne pathogens. *Int J Food Microbiol* **74**, 177–88.

Skirrow, M.B. (1977). *Campylobacter* enteritis: a 'new' disease. *Br Med J* **2**, 9–11.

Skirrow, M.B. (1981). *Campylobacter* enteritis in dogs and cats: a 'new' zoonosis. *Vet Res Commun* **5**, 13–19.

Skirrow, M.B. (1991). Epidemiology of *Campylobacter* enteritis. *Int J Food Microbiol* **12**, 9–16.

Wareing, D.R., Bolton, F.J., Fox, A.J., Wright, P.A. and Greenway, D.L. (2002). Phenotypic diversity of *Campylobacter* isolates from sporadic cases of human enteritis in the UK. *J Appl Microbiol* **92**, 502–9.

Wren, B.W., Linton, D., Dorrell, N. and Karlyshev, A.V. (2001). Post genome analysis of *Campylobacter jejuni*. *Symp Ser Soc Appl Microbiol* (suppl 30), 36–44S.

25

Shigellosis

Diarrhoeal disease is an important cause of morbidity and mortality around the world and is the second most common disease in children after respiratory disease. Other bacterial diarrhoeal diseases have been described in previous chapters, including salmonella and diarrhoeagenic *Escherichia coli*. Another common diarrhoeal disease is described in this chapter, namely *Shigella* infection, or shigellosis.

Shigellosis is caused by *Shigella*, a bacterium related closely to *E. coli* and salmonellae (Lan and Reeves, 2002). They are therefore members of the Enterobacteriaceae. There are four *Shigella* species or subgroups, namely *S. dysenteriae* (subgroup 1), *S. flexneri* (subgroup 2), *S. boydii* (subgroup 3) and *S. sonnei* (subgroup 4). Subgroups 1 to 4 may also be termed A to D. These species, except for *S. sonnei*, are divided into serotypes based on their lipopolysaccharide (O antigen); there are 12 serotypes of *S. dysenteriae*, six of *S. flexneri* and 18 of *S. boydii*. *S. dysenteriae* is the main cause of bacillary dysentery, although enteroinvasive *E. coli* causes essentially the same disease and is very similar in its characteristics and virulence mechanisms. *S. dysenteriae* serotype 1 is otherwise known as Shiga's bacillus, and *S. dysenteriae* serotype 2 is also known as Schmitz's bacillus. All *Shigellae* can be identified readily in the laboratory using standard biochemical tests, although they are similar in many respects to *E. coli* (Edwards, 1999). Due to the variability of carbohydrate metabolism between species and strains, serological methods for speciation are best. Further identification may be performed by bacteriophage or colicin typing as well as toxin production analysis.

Shigellosis can be transmitted by infection with as few as ten bacteria. The incubation period after infection is between 16 and 72 hours, with the symptomatic infection lasting up to two weeks if left untreated. Infection generally results in diarrhoea, abdominal cramps, fever, nausea and vomiting, although this varies according to the species involved; stools may be bloody or mucoid (Edwards, 1999; Masoumi *et al.*, 1995). *Shigella* is most common in children aged between two and three years and is surprisingly uncommon in those under six months of age. Severe shigellosis may be seen in children, resulting in convulsions, stiff neck, headache, lethargy and confusion (symptoms that are not dissimilar to those of other infections, such as meningitis). The diarrhoea associated with shigellosis often causes dehydration and complications such as kidney failure. Not all individuals are symptomatic upon infection with *Shigella*, and some have only mild symptoms. As with many infections, it is the young and the elderly who often have the most severe symptoms.

In general, *Shigella* affect the epithelium and mesenteric lymph glands of the large bowel. The effects of *Shigella* infection, ranging from acute inflammation to severe ulceration, result from the bacteria adhering to cells, followed by their subsequent invasion causing host cell death. *Shigellae* possess a number of virulence mechanisms that, among other things, enable them to move from one cell to another thereby causing spread of infection within the epithelium without exposure to external host pressures (Adam, 2001; Bourdet-Sicard *et al.*, 2000; Ingersoll *et al.*, 2002; Nhieu and Sansonetti, 1999; Niebuhr and Sansonetti, 2000). *S. dysenteriae*, also known as Shiga's bacillus, is the traditional cause of bacillary dysentery; it releases a toxin known as Shiga toxin, also termed Vero-cytotoxin (VT) and Shiga-like toxin (SLT). This is a heat-labile toxin that consists of two subunits known as A and B. Subunit B is responsible for binding of the toxin to host cells, and subunit A is responsible for the toxic activity, namely the inhibition of protein synthesis. The other *Shigella* species, as well as *S. dysenteriae*, possess genes contained on virulence plasmids or on the chromosome that are responsible for the expression of factors that enable *Shigella* to survive within the host gastrointestinal tract, to invade host cells, and to survive within them.

It is estimated that over 160 million episodes of shigellosis occur each year, with the majority being in developing countries (Kotloff *et al.*, 1999). Almost three-quarters of all episodes of shigellosis occur in children under five years of age. *S. flexneri* is most common in developing countries, whilst *S. sonnei* is most common in developed countries. More than one million deaths can be attributed to shigellosis each year (Philpott *et al.*, 2000). Most cases, and particularly deaths, occur in developing countries due to poor hygiene and inadequate water supplies, although shigellosis is also common in developed countries (Edwards, 1999). In temperate climates the disease is most common during the summer months, whereas in tropical regions it occurs during the rainy season. In crowded areas, such as those seen throughout many parts of developing countries, *S. dysenteriae* type 1 is most common, resulting in large outbreaks of dysentery. In *Shigella*-endemic areas, *S. flexneri* accounts for approximately 50% of culture-positive infections.

During 2000, almost 13 000 cases of shigellosis were reported in the USA (Source: US CDC). As in other developed countries, *S. sonnei* is the most common species in the UK, accounting for over 90% of reported isolates. The infection was particularly common before and during the First World War, at which point dysentery was made notifiable. The incidence of shigellosis has varied from less than 1000 notifications after the war, to 44 000 in the mid 1950s, falling to consistently fewer than 5000 notifications since 1995 (Figure 25.1).

Shigella can be spread via food and water. Many foods have been associated with *Shigella*, including salads, raw vegetables, milk products and poultry. In addition, water or food may be contaminated with human waste or via poor handling. Importantly, *Shigella* infection may be passed from person to person; this is one of the factors that distinguishes it from other gastrointestinal infections, because as few as ten individual *Shigellae* are required for infection. Outbreaks in nurseries and schools are therefore frequent due to the relative ease of person-to-person transmission.

As only a few bacteria are required to spread disease, the main preventive measure for shigellosis is good hygiene. Hand-washing is highly effective at stopping spread of infection, as is stopping the sharing of toys in child settings when diarrhoeal disease is suspected. Antibiotic therapy with tetracycline, ampicillin or co-trimoxazole can shorten

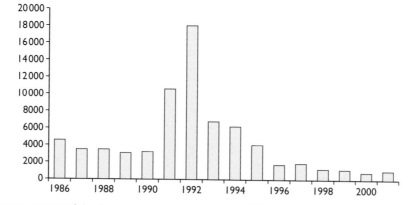

Figure 25.1 Laboratory reports of shigellosis (faecal isolates) in England and Wales 1986–2001 (source: HPA CDSC).

the duration of illness and also prevent its spread to others, although treatment of infected individuals is concerned primarily with preventing dehydration. There is no vaccine available for any *Shigella* species; both live oral and subunit parental vaccines are being developed, but it will be years before either vaccine, if proven effective, will be approved for use. In the meantime, molecular methods are improving our understanding of *Shigellae* in terms of their virulence and epidemiology (Dorman *et al.*, 2001; Taylor and Echeverria, 1993).

REFERENCES

Adam, T. (2001). Exploitation of host factors for efficient infection by *Shigella*. *Int J Med Microbiol* **291**, 287–98.

Bourdet-Sicard, R., Egile, C., Sansonetti, P.J. and Tran Van Nhieu, G. (2000). Diversion of cytoskeletal processes by *Shigella* during invasion of epithelial cells. *Microbes Infect* **2**, 813–19.

Dorman, C.J., McKenna, S. and Beloin, C. (2001). Regulation of virulence gene expression in *Shigella flexneri*, a facultative intracellular pathogen. *Int J Med Microbiol* **291**, 89–96.

Edwards, B.H. (1999). *Salmonella* and *Shigella* species. *Clin Lab Med* **19**, 469–87.

Ingersoll, M., Groisman, E.A. and Zychlinsky, A. (2002). Pathogenicity islands of *Shigella*. *Curr Top Microbiol Immunol* **264**, 49–65.

Kotloff, K.L., Winickoff, J.P., Ivanoff, B., *et al.* (1999). Global burden of *Shigella* infections: implications for vaccine development and implementation of control strategies. *Bull World Health Organ* **77**, 651–66.

Lan, R. and Reeves, P.R. (2002). *Escherichia coli* in disguise: molecular origins of *Shigella*. *Microbes Infect* **4**, 1125–32.

Masoumi, J.P., Anwar, M.S. and Bokhari, S.R. (1995). Clinical features of infantile diarrhea associated with single or multiple enteric pathogens. *J Pak Med Assoc* **45**, 266–9.

Nhieu, G.T. and Sansonetti, P.J. (1999). Mechanism of *Shigella* entry into epithelial cells. *Curr Opin Microbiol* **2**, 51–5.

Niebuhr, K. and Sansonetti, P.J. (2000). Invasion of epithelial cells by bacterial pathogens the paradigm of *Shigella*. *Subcell Biochem* **33**, 251–87.

Philpott, D.J., Edgeworth, J.D. and Sansonetti, P.J. (2000). The pathogenesis of *Shigella flexneri* infection: lessons from in vitro and in vivo studies. *Philos Trans R Soc Lond B Biol Sci* **355**, 575–86.

Taylor, D.N. and Echeverria, P. (1993). Diarrhoeal disease: current concepts and future challenges. Molecular biological approaches to the epidemiology of diarrhoeal diseases in developing countries. *Trans R Soc Trop Med Hyg* **87** (suppl 3), 3–5.

26

Cholera

Vibrio cholerae is a Gram-negative rod-shaped bacterium. It is the causative agent of cholera, a gastrointestinal disease that results in a secretory, non-inflammatory diarrhoeal illness (Shears, 2001). Profuse watery diarrhoea is stimulated due to the production of an enterotoxin by the cholera bacilli. The disease is transmitted mainly via food and water, although person-to-person transmission can occur (Estrada-Garcia and Mintz, 1996). Cholera is distributed globally and has been reported in the Indian subcontinent, South-East Asia, the Middle East, South America, South Africa and parts of Europe. There have been eight pandemics of cholera in the past 200 years, the seventh and eighth of which still continue. These two pandemics are due to different serogroups of *V. cholerae*, namely 01 and 0139 (Reeves and Lan, 1998): the pandemic caused by the former serogroup started in Indonesia in 1961 and has spread to Africa and South America; that caused by the 0139 serogroup began in 1991 in southern Asia.

V. cholerae must be swallowed (usually by the ingestion of contaminated food or water) to gain entry to the stomach. The bacteria are sensitive to the pH of gastric acid, and therefore a large infective dose (10^{11} organisms) is often required before infection can be initiated. However, if the pH of the gastric acid is neutralized to any extent, then the infective dose is much lower. Once in the small intestine, the bacilli are able to adhere to the microvilli of the intestinal epithelium. Upon adherence, the bacteria colonize and multiply. Attachment and colonization probably takes between 12 and 24 hours following ingestion. Motility is also of considerable importance in the virulence of *V. cholerae*, allowing the bacteria to penetrate the mucosal layer of the small intestine. However, the symptoms of the disease still occur without cell invasion.

V. cholerae is able to produce one of the most profound physiological responses known to occur in any human infection: the induction of gross fluid exsorption from the small intestine without causing any significant cellular damage and without invasion of the gastroepithelium. The loss of fluid is so great that it can cause collapse or death within a few hours. These dramatic effects are due to the production of an enterotoxin by the infecting bacteria. Once multiplication begins, the bacteria produce the enterotoxin that mediates the disease process. To bring about the loss of fluid, the enterotoxin must be able to interact with the epithelial cells. Specific binding substances, namely membrane-bound gangliosides, have been identified as mediators of this interaction. The production of the enterotoxin begins between one and three days after ingestion of the bacteria.

A toxin is a component or a product of a bacterium that, when extracted and purified, can reproduce the disease associated with that toxin. Many enzymes and chemicals produced by bacteria are solely determinants of virulence and do not produce any of the symptoms of disease. The term 'enterotoxin' is used for a group of exotoxins, of which cholera toxin is the major example; these are proteins found outside the cell and whose site of action may be some distance from the site of infection. They have specific effects at low concentrations and usually have an enzymatic function. Cholera toxin is produced as a determinant of virulence, but it also produces all the symptoms of the disease (de Haan and Hirst, 2000; Reidl and Klose, 2002). It acts locally, primarily in the interference of cellular function, and is not disseminated around the body. The toxin consists of one A subunit and five B subunits. The A subunit contains the enzyme adenosine diphosphate (ADP) ribosyl transferase and is composed of two parts, A_1 and A_2; the B subunit is involved in receptor binding. The A subunit is the active protein that enters the cell. The toxin causes an increase in the intracellular levels of cyclic adenosine monophosphate (AMP). This results in an inhibition of the uptake of sodium and chloride ions by cells lining the microvilli and stimulates hypersecretion of chloride and bicarbonate ions. The uptake of water is blocked, and the secretion of electrolytes causes the exsorption of water across the epithelium. Hypersecretion of sodium, potassium, chloride and bicarbonate ions, with accompanying water, leads to the production of large volumes of isotonic diarrhoea.

Other enterotoxins, namely heat-stable toxins, may also be produced by V. cholerae, but these do not produce such severe symptoms as those associated with cholera toxin. Strains of V. cholerae have been isolated that do not produce any of the conventional enterotoxins known to be associated with intestinal secretion, including cholera toxin and heat-stable toxins. However, the strains still induce severe acute watery diarrhoea and dehydration, thereby suggesting that there are other toxins involved in the pathogenesis of diarrhoea by some or all strains of V. cholerae.

The clinical course of the disease may be characterized by vomiting, poor skin turgor, sunken eyes, intense peripheral vasoconstriction, and deep breathing. It is only a matter of time before shock and death follow. It is the severity of the saline depletion that is the primary determinant of mortality, which, in untreated patients, may approach 70%. Active management of patients is therefore crucial to their survival and is based primarily on urgent rehydration (Shears, 2001). Management may also include the use of antibiotics, although the incidence of antimicrobial resistance is increasing (Lolekha, 1986).

In treated patients, mortality decreases to about 1%. The massive fluid and electrolyte loss results in decreased cardiac output and blood pressure, leading to hypovolaemic shock. The passing of urine may cease altogether, with acute renal failure and uraemia. Secondary effects have also included third-trimester abortions. Asymptomatic infection with V. cholerae is common (about 75%), and carrier states occur frequently in recovered cases of cholera. This provides a reservoir of infection for further transmission of the disease through the faecal–oral route.

The genome of V. cholerae has been sequenced. This, along with other molecular and epidemiological data, is providing information useful for the development of new therapies (McNicholl et al., 2000). It is now known, for example, that a pathogenicity island is present in epidemic and pandemic strains of cholera but not environmental strains (Karaolis et al., 1998). However, it has also been found that some environmental strains of cholera carry virulence genes previously thought to occur only in 01 and 0139 serogroups (Deriu et al., 2002; Faruque and Nair, 2002). In addition, the association of cholera with plankton is now well acknowledged and could warn of future large epidemics through the use of satellite imaging (Colwell, 1996; Lipp et al., 2002). Although genomics is leading to the development of new vaccines (Ryan and Calderwood, 2000), current vaccines do not provide good immunological protection and do not protect against both major serogroups (Chaturvedi, 1997).

Although parenteral vaccination is available against cholera, protection lasts only three to six months and is effective in only 50% of those vaccinated. Oral vaccines are being developed against serogroups 01 and 0139. Fluid replacement therapy is adequate and is currently the mainstay to alleviate many of the symptoms associated with cholera. Better vaccination preparations are being sought, which would provide long-lasting immunity and cost-effectiveness to prevent such high levels of mortality.

REFERENCES

Chaturvedi, S. (1997). Oral vaccines for cholera control. *Natl Med J India* **10**, 17–18.

Colwell, R.R. (1996). Global climate and infectious disease: the cholera paradigm. *Science* **274**, 2025–31.

De Haan, L. and Hirst, T.R. (2000). Cholera toxin and related enterotoxins: a cell biological and immunological perspective. *J Nat Toxins* **9**, 281–97.

Deriu, A., Sechi, L.A., Molicotti, P., Spanu, M.L. and Zanetti, S. (2002). Virulence genes in halophilic *Vibrio* spp. isolated in common mussels. *New Microbiol* **25**, 93–6.

Estrada-Garcia, T. and Mintz, E.D. (1996). Cholera: foodborne transmission and its prevention. *Eur J Epidemiol* **12**, 461–9.

Faruque, S.M. and Nair, G.B. (2002). Molecular ecology of toxigenic *Vibrio cholerae*. *Microbiol Immunol* **46**, 59–66.

Karaolis, D.K., Johnson, J.A., Bailey, C.C., Boedeker, E.C., Kaper, J.B. and Reeves, P.R. (1998). A *Vibrio cholerae* pathogenicity island associated with epidemic and pandemic strains. *Proc Natl Acad Sci USA* **95**, 3134–9.

Lipp, E.K., Huq, A. and Colwell, R.R. (2002). Effects of global climate on infectious disease: the cholera model. *Clin Microbiol Rev* **15**, 757–70.

Lolekha, S. (1986). Consequences of treatment of gastrointestinal infections. *Scand J Infect Dis Suppl* **49**, 154–9.

McNicholl, J.M., Downer, M.V., Udhayakumar, V., Alper, C.A. and Swerdlow, D.L. (2000). Host–pathogen interactions in emerging and re-emerging infectious diseases: a genomic perspective of tuberculosis, malaria, human immunodeficiency virus infection, hepatitis B, and cholera. *Annu Rev Public Health* **21**, 15–46.

Reeves, P.R. and Lan, R. (1998). Cholera in the 1990s. *Br Med Bull* **54**, 611–23.

Reidl, J. and Klose, K.E. (2002). *Vibrio cholerae* and cholera: out of the water and into the host. *FEMS Microbiol Rev* **26**, 125–39.

Ryan, E.T. and Calderwood, S.B. (2000). Cholera vaccines. *Clin Infect Dis* **31**, 561–5.

Shears, P. (2001). Recent developments in cholera. *Curr Opin Infect Dis* **14**, 553–8.

27

Helicobacter pylori

Although bacteria have been found in many different environments, some of them extreme, the human stomach was previously considered an inhospitable environment for bacteria due to its acidic pH. However, in 1983, Barry Marshall and J. Robin Warren at the Royal Perth Hospital in Australia showed that bacteria do inhabit the stomach, after culturing a spiral-shaped bacterium from the human gastric mucosa. Furthermore, they showed an association between the presence of this bacterium and gastric inflammation (Marshall and Warren, 1984). These Gram-negative, curved, flagellated, micro-aerophilic bacteria were initially classified as a species of the genus *Campylobacter*, but after further studies it was decided that there were sufficient differences between this 'new' organism and other members of the genus to warrant the designation of a new genus, *Helicobacter* (Marshall, 2002; Marshall, 1993). The bacterium was named *Helicobacter pylori*. Since then, over a dozen other species of *Helicobacter* have been isolated from the gastrointestinal tract of a number of animals (Corry and Atabay, 2001):

- *H. pylori*
- *H. cinaedi*
- *H. canis*
- *H. pulorum*
- *H. fennelliae*
- *H. trogontum*
- *H. hepaticus*
- *H. muridarum*
- *H. bilis*
- *H. mustelae*

- *H. cholecystus*
- *H. bizzozeronii*
- *H. felis*
- *H. acinonychis*
- *H. nemestrinae*
- *H. rodentium*

H. pylori infection is probably the second most common bacterial infection known to man, after the bacteria that cause tooth decay. Interestingly, *H. pylori* have also been found in low numbers in dental plaque (Kilmartin, 2002). Perhaps more surprisingly, *H. pylori* has a restricted host specificity as determined by binding specificity. It has been shown that *H. pylori* will bind only to human gastric epithelium and that of some primates. The acquisition of *H. pylori* is thought to be by person-to-person contact. The bacterium has been isolated from faeces and dental plaque, so either faecal-oral or oral-oral transmission may be possible. Initial infection results in an acute gastritis, which resembles gastritis of many other aetiologies. This results in an influx of acute inflammatory cells and the degeneration of gastric epithelial cells, leading to a cease in the production of acid. It may take weeks for acid production to restart and, of course, during this time the stomach is open to infection by other organisms that are normally intolerant of the acidic environment. This initial infection is self-limiting and usually lasts only a few weeks. However, acute inflammatory cells remain in the gastric epithelium in reduced numbers and there is an influx of chronic inflammatory cells. This leads to chronic superficial gastritis, which is the primary disease associated with *H. pylori* infection, although clinical symptoms are not seen in the majority of individuals with the disease at this stage. The *H. pylori* bacterium is carried in the individual's stomach for many years without any apparent symptoms and probably persists for life once acquired. It is estimated that 40% of individuals in developed countries are infected with *H. pylori* by adulthood, whilst in developing countries an astounding 80% are infected. There are currently thought to be over 20 million individuals infected with *H. pylori* in the UK. There is now plenty of evidence that *H. pylori* is the cause of a number of chronic gastric diseases. Individuals with chronic superficial gastritis have been shown to have a predisposition for developing peptic ulcer disease, gastric lymphoma and chronic atrophic gastritis; the latter may lead to gastric adenocarcinoma. The most controversial issue regarding *Helicobacter* infection is its association with non-steroidal anti-inflammatory drugs (NSAIDs) (Chan and Leung, 2002; Laine, 2002), as these are the two main causes of peptic ulcers.

H. pylori possesses a number of virulence determinants that are probably necessary for gastric colonization and subsequent infection (Marshall, 2002). Such virulence determinants include flagella, adhesins, and the production of enzymes such as catalase and urease. These determinants have specific functions; for example, the flagella enable the bacteria to remain in the gastric epithelium and not get cleansed out with dead epithelia, whilst urease acts as a buffer in the bacterium's microenvironment. A toxin, namely vacuolating cytotoxin, has also been described from *H. pylori*. Approximately 50% of *H. pylori* strains produce this toxin, which induces the formation of acidic vacuoles in the cytoplasm of host gastric cells. This process may be involved in the cause of gastric mucosal ulceration.

There are a number of tests available for the diagnosis of *H. pylori* infection. A presentation of dyspepsia does not necessarily warrant testing for *Helicobacter* (Meurer and Bower, 2002; Wu and Sung, 2002), but before treatment testing is generally recommended. Tests have an estimated accuracy of 95%, but each test is suited to a particular clinical problem. Direct methods include the demonstration of *H. pylori* by histological staining or culture of gastric biopsy samples. Such samples are obtained by endoscopy, an invasive procedure, which, if unnecessary, should be avoided. Indirect methods include the urea breath test, enzyme-linked immunosorbent assay (ELISA), and the urease test, which is an invasive procedure. The urea breath test utilizes the ability of *H. pylori* to hydrolyse urea. Labelled urea is given to the patient and labelled carbon dioxide is exhaled if the patient is infected. The ELISA test is used to detect serum antibodies against *H. pylori*. Other serological tests have been developed but have been found to be less sensitive than ELISA. Molecular techniques are also available, including DNA hybridization and the polymerase chain reaction (PCR) (Kisa *et al.*, 2002).

H. pylori is susceptible to a number of antibiotics in vitro. In theory, the treatment of *H. pylori* infection could be a problem because of the environment in which they inhabit. Before the discovery of *H. pylori*, the treatment of duodenal ulcers relied upon symptomatic therapies, often with acid-suppressing drugs. Since the discovery of *H. pylori*, the use of antibiotics has been the obvious choice. Due to the acidic conditions, if antibiotics are given as treatment, then most of them become wholly or partially inactive and only low doses normally reach the bacteria, resulting in a reduction of therapeutic success and the possibility of the bacteria developing resistance. However, suitable antibiotic regimens have now been in use for a number of years (Godshall, 2002; Meurer and Bower, 2002). Triple therapy is generally recommended and is better than dual therapy (Ohlin *et al.*, 2002). In the UK, triple therapy involves the administration of a proton pump inhibitor, clarithromycin, and either metronidazole or amoxicillin. Unlike therapy with acid-suppressing drugs, antibiotic treatment results in an approximate 87% success of eradication of *H. pylori*. Relapse of duodenal ulcers after antibiotic treatment is also greatly reduced, with estimated relapse rates of 0–3%. However, the triple therapy antibiotic regime does give rise to a number of side effects, including malaise, sore mouth, diarrhoea and nausea. Therefore, a single drug that is totally effective against *H. pylori* in the acidic environment is sought.

A massive amount of research has been carried out on *H. pylori* since its first description. At one time, *Helicobacter* research was increasing year on year at a tremendous rate, but it has since levelled out as more has been discovered. However, a lot remains to be learned about its true epidemiology, virulence properties, and links with gastric cancer. There is now strong evidence that *Helicobacter* infection can lead to cancer (Lax and Thomas, 2002; Miwa *et al.*, 2002; Peek and Blaser, 2002). This is most often after chronic infection, although the rate of cancer is still low. However, it is more likely that genomic sequence data will result in a greater understanding of *Helicobacter* and lead to therapies for infection and complications such as cancer (Bereswill and Kist, 2002).

REFERENCES

Bereswill, S. and Kist, M. (2002). Molecular microbiology and pathogenesis of *Helicobacter* and *Campylobacter* updated: a meeting report of the 11th conference on *Campylobacter*, *Helicobacter* and related organisms. *Mol Microbiol* **45**, 255–62.

Chan, F.K. and Leung, W.K. (2002). Peptic-ulcer disease. *Lancet* **360**, 933–41.

Corry, J.E. and Atabay, H.I. (2001). Poultry as a source of *Campylobacter* and related organisms. *Symp Ser Soc Appl Microbiol*, 96–114S.

Godshall, C.J. (2002). Treatment of *Helicobacter pylori* infection in patients with peptic ulcer disease. *Am J Surg* **183**, 2–3.

Kilmartin, C.M. (2002). Dental implications of *Helicobacter pylori*. *J Can Dent Assoc* **68**, 489–93.

Kisa, O., Albay, A., Mas, M.R., Celasun, B. and Doganci, L. (2002). The evaluation of diagnostic methods for the detection of *Helicobacter pylori* in gastric biopsy specimens. *Diagn Microbiol Infect Dis* **43**, 251–5.

Laine, L. (2002). Review article: the effect of *Helicobacter pylori* infection on nonsteroidal anti-inflammatory drug-induced upper gastrointestinal tract injury. *Aliment Pharmacol Ther* **16** (suppl 1), 34–9.

Lax, A.J. and Thomas, W. (2002). How bacteria could cause cancer: one step at a time. *Trends Microbiol* **10**, 293–9.

Marshall, B.J. (1993). *Helicobacter pylori*: a primer for 1994. *Gastroenterologist* **1**, 241–7.

Marshall, B. (2002). *Helicobacter pylori*: 20 years on. *Clin Med* **2**, 147–52.

Marshall, B.J. and Warren, J.R. (1984). Unidentified curved bacilli in the stomach of patients with gastritis and peptic ulceration. *Lancet* **1**, 1311–15.

Meurer, L.N. and Bower, D.J. (2002). Management of *Helicobacter pylori* infection. *Am Fam Physician* **65**, 1327–36.

Miwa, H., Go, M.F. and Sato, N. (2002). H. pylori and gastric cancer: the Asian enigma. *Am J Gastroenterol* **97**, 1106–12.

Ohlin, B., Cederberg, A., Kjellin, T., *et al.* (2002). Dual versus triple therapy in eradication of *Helicobacter pylori*. *Hepatogastroenterology* **49**, 172–5.

Peek, R.M., Jr and Blaser, M.J. (2002). *Helicobacter pylori* and gastrointestinal tract adenocarcinomas. *Nat Rev Cancer* **2**, 28–37.

Wu, J.C. and Sung, J.J. (2002). Ulcer and gastritis. *Endoscopy* **34**, 104–10.

28

Listeriosis

Listeria are Gram-positive, flagellated bacteria that are cocco-bacillary or rod-shaped in nature. Over the past decade or so, they have received much interest as an uncommon but important cause of human infection. Hayem was probably the first to describe a case of human listeriosis in 1881; this was followed by a description in 1918 by Cotoni of a case of meningitis that was later confirmed to be caused by *Listeria monocytogenes*. However, little work was done until 1926, when Murray and colleagues described *Listeria* as a cause of mononuclear leukocytosis in rabbits and guinea pigs. They isolated a Gram-positive bacterium that they called *Bacterium monocytogenes*, renamed *Listeria* in 1940. There are at least eight species, the type species being *L. monocytogenes* (Table 28.1). *L. monocytogenes* is the major pathogen of the genus in both humans and animals, although infection may occur with other species of the genus. *Listeria* are ubiquitous organisms with a worldwide distribution. The bacteria have been isolated from almost all environments and a wide range of animals, including mammals, birds, fish and invertebrates.

As mentioned, *Listeria* infection can occur in both humans and animals (Low and Donachie, 1997). However, in many animals, carriage of the bacteria has not been associated with disease. *Listeria* can cause mastitis in cows, and large numbers of the bacteria may be passed in milk. In sheep and cattle, listeriosis commonly presents as encephalitis, septicaemia, abortion, diarrhoea or purulent conjunctivitis. Encephalitis is most common; it lasts up to 14 days and is fatal. The infection often presents as meningoencephalitis in swine, as monocytosis and liver necrosis in rabbits, and as heart disease in chickens.

In humans, carriage of *Listeria* can occur in the gastrointestinal and genital tract at varying rates, most commonly around 5–10%. Infection can lead to abortion, can affect the central nervous system, and can cause septicaemia. It is an uncommon infection, however, and accounts for only around 2% of all cases of bacterial meningitis in the UK. Although Burn in 1936 first suggested that *Listeria* infection in cattle may be transmitted to humans through the ingestion of milk, it is only in recent years that *Listeria* has gained attention as a cause of foodborne illness (Nieman and Lorber, 1980). Soft cheeses and other milk products that contain contaminated milk may be sources of infection, particularly because *Listeria* are able to multiply at refrigeration temperatures (Farber and Peterkin, 1991). Other food products, such as chicken, seafood and salad products, may also be the source of infections, as the bacteria have been isolated from these foods (Ben Embarek, 1994). Neonatal

Table 28.1 Species of *Listeria*

L. denitrificans
L. grayi
L. innocua
L. ivanovii
L. monocytogenes
L. murrayi
L. seeligeri
L. welshimeri

listeriosis results in a number of clinical manifestations, depending on the age of the fetus at the time of infection. During early pregnancy, infection may result in abortion or stillbirth. The mother may be infected without any signs of infection. Also, infection in the mother does not necessarily lead to infection of the fetus. In adults, infection may occur at any age, but it appears more frequently in the elderly and in people with a predisposition to infection, such as those on immunosuppressive therapy and alcoholics. Infection of the central nervous system results in meningitis, meningoencephalitis or encephalitis (Armstrong and Fung, 1993; Bartt, 2000). A raised temperature, stiff neck, seizures and fluctuating consciousness are often apparent. The onset may be so sudden that the patient dies in hours. Other complications of listeriosis have also been reported (Adeonigbagbe *et al.*, 2000; Bourgeois *et al.*, 1993; Braun *et al.*, 1993). It is estimated that around 2000 individuals become seriously ill with listeriosis in the USA each year; this figure does not include those with minor illness, which may account for thousands more. Of those with serious with serious illness, around a quarter die.

The diagnosis of listeriosis can be difficult in humans because the clinical signs are not characteristic. Laboratory confirmation is therefore necessary using standard methods for diagnosing other causes of meningitis or septicaemia. *Listeriae* are able to grow on most standard non-selective bacteriological media, particularly in the presence of blood or serum (Brackett and Beuchat, 1989; Curtis and Lee, 1995). After overnight incubation, *Listeria* colonies measure between 1 and 2 mm in diameter and are generally round and translucent. All species have a characteristic sour milk smell, and all except *L. denitrificans* have a blue colour when colonies are observed under transmitted light. Some species, including *L. monocytogenes*, demonstrate beta-haemolysis when grown on blood agar, and can be differentiated further by a number of tests, including nitrate reduction, carbohydrate hydrolysis, and the Christie–Atkins–Munch–Peterson (CAMP) test. In neonatal infections, appropriate tissue or blood samples are used for diagnosis, depending on the clinical outcome. Treatment for listeriosis is with standard antibiotics, usually in combination, such as ampicillin and gentamicin (Crum, 2002). The mortality rate remains high, even after treatment, in immunocompromised individuals. Although listeriosis has not yet emerged as a major health problem in developed countries, surveillance of the infection should be continued as food habits continue to change.

REFERENCES

Adeonigbagbe, O., Khademi, A., Karowe, M., Gualtieri, N. and Robilotti, J. (2000). *Listeria monocytogenes* peritonitis: an unusual presentation and review of the literature. *J Clin Gastroenterol* 30, 436–7.

Armstrong, R.W. and Fung, P.C. (1993). Brainstem encephalitis (rhombencephalitis) due to *Listeria monocytogenes*: case report and review. *Clin Infect Dis* 16, 689–702.

Bartt, R. (2000). Listeria and atypical presentations of *Listeria* in the central nervous system. *Semin Neurol* 20, 361–73.

Ben Embarek, P.K. (1994). Presence, detection and growth of *Listeria monocytogenes* in seafoods: a review. *Int J Food Microbiol* 23, 17–34.

Bourgeois, N., Jacobs, F., Tavares, M.L., *et al.* (1993). *Listeria monocytogenes* hepatitis in a liver transplant recipient: a case report and review of the literature. *J Hepatol* 18, 284–9.

Brackett, R.E. and Beuchat, L.R. (1989). Methods and media for the isolation and cultivation of *Listeria monocytogenes* from various foods. *Int J Food Microbiol* 8, 219–23.

Braun, T.I., Travis, D., Dee, R.R. and Nieman, R.E. (1993). Liver abscess due to *Listeria monocytogenes*: case report and review. *Clin Infect Dis* 17, 267–9.

Crum, N.F. (2002). Update on *Listeria monocytogenes* infection. *Curr Gastroenterol Rep* 4, 287–96.

Curtis, G.D. and Lee, W.H. (1995). Culture media and methods for the isolation of *Listeria monocytogenes*. *Int J Food Microbiol* 26, 1–13.

Farber, J.M. and Peterkin, P.I. (1991). *Listeria monocytogenes*, a food-borne pathogen. *Microbiol Rev* 55, 476–511.

Low, J.C. and Donachie, W. (1997). A review of *Listeria monocytogenes* and listeriosis. *Vet J* 153, 9–29.

Nieman, R.E. and Lorber, B. (1980). Listeriosis in adults: a changing pattern. Report of eight cases and review of the literature, 1968–1978. *Rev Infect Dis* 2, 207.

29

Syphilis

Sexually transmitted diseases (STDs) occur worldwide, affecting people in both developing and developed countries. Such diseases have important repercussions on reproductive health and have been shown to increase the risk of infection with human immunodeficiency virus (HIV). The estimated annual incidence of curable STDs (not including AIDS and other viral STDs) is 333 million cases worldwide (Gerbase *et al.*, 1998). At present, the four most common STDs are those that can be cured easily: syphilis, chlamydia, trichomoniasis and gonorrhoea (Gerbase *et al.*, 1998).

The high incidence of STDs worldwide is a serious public health concern. The increasing mobility of populations, urbanization, poverty, demographic changes, and changes in sexual behaviour

are some of the factors that have placed an ever increasing proportion of the population at risk for STD infection. The prevention and control of STDs is one of the main priorities of the World Health Organization (WHO). Strategies to fulfil these priorities include the promotion of responsible sexual behaviour, general access to condoms at affordable prices, and prompt and appropriate management of STDs.

Syphilis is an important STD caused by the spirochaete *Treponema pallidum*. It is thought to affect more than 2.5 million people (Antal *et al.*, 2002). Despite a general decline over the past few decades, there are still hundreds of cases of syphilis in the UK each year (Figure 29.1). In the USA, there are approximately 6000 cases of primary and

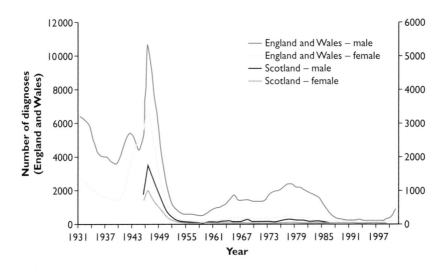

Figure 29.1 Diagnosis of syphilis (primary, secondary and latent in the first two years of infection) seen in genitourinary medicine clinics in England, Scotland and Wales 1931–2001* (source: HPA CDSC).

#Equivalent Scottish data are not available before 1945 and for 2000–2001.

*As Northern Ireland data for the time period 1931–2000 are incomplete, they have been excluded from this figure.

secondary syphilis reported each year (source: US CDC). Most cases are contracted during sexual intercourse, as congenital syphilis is now extremely rare (Walker and Walker, 2002). The disease can be divided into four main stages: primary, secondary, latent and late syphilis (Adler, 1984). On host penetration, the spirochaete multiply at the site of entry; it is usually about three weeks before clinical symptoms become apparent. Primary syphilis results in the formation of a single lesion that contains a large number of spirochaetes. Local lymph nodes also become enlarged. Secondary syphilis occurs if the infection is left untreated and involves invasion of the bloodstream and the development of widespread papular rashes; patients may also complain of malaise, fever, headache and sore throat. These symptoms may last for as long as four or five years. After secondary syphilis, there is a period of quiescence known as latent syphilis, during which the patient is clinically well. Up to 10 or 20 years later, complications of late syphilis may develop in two stages. Tertiary syphilis is characterized by the formation of chronic granulomata, which may affect the skin, bones, joints or mucous membranes of the upper respiratory tract. More serious complications, such as aortic aneurysms or meningovascular syphilis (Holmes *et al.*, 1984), may develop in quaternary syphilis due to the involvement of the cardiovascular system and central nervous system, the latter of which may lead to psychiatric problems (Hutto, 2001).

Serological testing is the most common method of demonstrating infection with *T. pallidum* (Larsen *et al.*, 1995). Cultivation in artificial culture media, chick embryo or tissue culture is not possible, and microscopy can be misleading if the results are negative. There are a number of serological methods – some more specific than others – which detect antibodies produced in response to syphilis infection. There are two main categories of serological test methods. The first type detects antibodies produced against cardiolipid, a non-specific treponemal antigen. The classical Wasserman complement fixation test was the most commonly used method, but this has since been replaced by modern flocculation tests such as the Venereal Disease Reference Laboratory (VDRL) test and rapid plasma reagin (RPR) test. Due to their simplicity and accuracy, these tests are used as screening or first-line tests for both routine and mass screening programmes. The tests become positive 10–14 days after the appearance of symptoms, the titre rising gradually.

The second type of serological test detects antibodies produced against antigens specific for pathogenic treponemes. The two most commonly used tests are the *T. pallidum* haemagglutination assay (TPHA) and the fluorescent treponemal antibody absorbed (FTA-ABS) test. The TPHA is very sensitive and is very simple to perform; however, it is often negative in untreated primary syphilis. The FTA-ABS test is both highly specific and highly sensitive at all stages of syphilis infection and is therefore an accepted reference test. An older test within this category is the *T. pallidum* immobilization (TPI) test; this has now been superseded by the TPHA and the FTA-ABS test because it was time-consuming, expensive and technically demanding.

The role of the ELISA in the serological diagnosis of syphilis is currently limited. Only a few companies are able to offer tests that detect anti-syphilis immunoglobulin G (IgG) and anti-syphilis immunoglobulin M (IgM). It must be noted that with the RPR test, certain physiological factors may give false-positive results, known as 'biological false-positives'; these may be caused by recent immunization, pregnancy or chronic infection. A lack of test specificity may also result in false-positives. The pattern of results obtained with the VDRL/RPR, TPHA and FTA-ABS tests can indicate the stage of infection, but clinical and epidemiological details should also be taken into consideration. Quantitative results of the VDRL/RPR and TPHA tests may be of further assistance in determining the stage of infection.

The use of serological tests can therefore provide a laboratory diagnosis of syphilis. If several types of test are used, and the results are interpreted collectively, then the stage of syphilis may also be determined. Serological tests also allow the rapid screening of patients, such as those attending antenatal clinics. Were serological testing not available, then laboratory diagnosis would be far more difficult and less reliable through the use of microscopy. Improved serological assays and new molecular tests such as the polymerase chain reaction (PCR) will help to improve the diagnosis of syphilis (Larsen *et al.*, 1995; Morse, 2001; Wicher *et al.*, 1999).

In order to control syphilis, different methods of disease management have taken place (Green *et al.*, 2001; Pao *et al.*, 2002). However, a more integrated approach may improve control measures. During such time, the availability of the genome sequence of *T. pallidum* should lead to an improved understanding of this spirochaete. New therapies and vaccine may be developed, which will help to reduce the number of cases of syphilis worldwide (Barbosa-Cesnik *et al.*, 1997; Norris *et al.*, 2001) and possibly lead to its eradication (Rompalo, 2001).

REFERENCES

Adler, M.W. (1984). ABC of sexually transmitted diseases. Syphilis: clinical features. *Br Med J (Clin Res Ed)* 288, 468–71.

Antal, G.M., Lukehart, S.A. and Meheus, A.Z. (2002). The endemic treponematoses. *Microbes Infect* 4, 83–94.

Barbosa-Cesnik, C.T., Gerbase, A. and Heymann, D. (1997). STD vaccines – an overview. *Genitourin Med* 73, 336–42.

Gerbase, A.C., Rowley, J.T., Heymann, D.H., Berkley, S.F. and Piot, P. (1998). Global prevalence and incidence estimates of selected curable STDs. *Sex Transm Infect* 74 (suppl 1), S12–16.

Green, T., Talbot, M.D. and Morton, R.S. (2001). The control of syphilis, a contemporary problem: a historical perspective. *Sex Transm Infect* 77, 214–17.

Holmes, M.D., Brant-Zawadzki, M.M. and Simon, R.P. (1984). Clinical features of meningovascular syphilis. *Neurology* 34, 553–6.

Hutto, B. (2001). Syphilis in clinical psychiatry: a review. *Psychosomatics* 42, 453–60.

Larsen, S.A., Steiner, B.M. and Rudolph, A.H. (1995). Laboratory diagnosis and interpretation of tests for syphilis. *Clin Microbiol Rev* 8, 1–21.

Morse, S.A. (2001). New tests for bacterial sexually transmitted diseases. *Curr Opin Infect Dis* 14, 45–51.

Norris, S.J., Cox, D.L. and Weinstock, G.M. (2001). Biology of *Treponema pallidum*: correlation of functional activities with genome sequence data. *J Mol Microbiol Biotechnol* 3, 37–62.

Pao, D., Goh, B.T. and Bingham, J.S. (2002). Management issues in syphilis. *Drugs* 62, 1447–61.

Rompalo, A.M. (2001). Can syphilis be eradicated from the world? *Curr Opin Infect Dis* 14, 41–4.

Walker, D.G. and Walker, G.J. (2002). Forgotten but not gone: the continuing scourge of congenital syphilis. *Lancet Infect Dis* 2, 432–6.

Wicher, K., Horowitz, H.W. and Wicher, V. (1999). Laboratory methods of diagnosis of syphilis for the beginning of the third millennium. *Microbes Infect* 1, 1035–49.

30

Chlamydia

Chlamydiae are obligate intracellular organisms. They are best classified as bacteria, although in some respects they resemble large viruses. The genus *Chlamydia* contains four species: *C. pneumoniae*, *C. trachomatis*, *C. abortus* and *C. pecorum* (Poppert *et al.*, 2001). The former three species are now recognized as being of pathogenic importance to humans. Human infection of the respiratory tract due to *Chlamydia* was first described in 1879.

C. pneumoniae causes mild community-acquired respiratory disease and accounts for the majority of human chlamydial infections (Campbell and Kuo, 2002; Hindiyeh and Carroll, 2000). However, around 70% of cases are mild or asymptomatic (Hahn *et al.*, 2002). The incidence of infection with *C. pneumoniae* is greatest during adolescence and early adulthood. The symptoms associated with infection are similar to those of mycoplasma respiratory infection, namely fever, malaise and headache, but may also include pharyngitis, sinusitis, otitis media and acute wheezing. *C. pneumoniae* has also been implicated in some cases of endocarditis. Reinfection can occur after the development of antibodies; 20–70% of adults have serological evidence of previous exposure to *C. pneumoniae*. The organism is thought to be transmitted from person to person, with no intermediate host or animal reservoir.

C. trachomatis is responsible for a number of different diseases (Coonrod, 2002). Of the 11 serotypes, serotypes A–C are responsible for trachoma (Tabbara, 2001). This disease is the leading cause of preventable blindness in developing countries and occurs throughout the tropics and subtropics. The prevalence of trachoma is approximately 500 million cases, with an estimated 5 million cases of visual impairment and blindness. The rate of blindness in developing countries is five to 10 times greater than in developed countries. Trachoma occurs due to acute *C. trachomatis* infection at an early age (about two years), with the rate of acute infection falling by the mid-teens. Spread of infection is from eye to eye. Trachoma is characterized by the appearance of pale-coloured nodules on the eyelid conjunctiva. Reinfection with *C. trachomatis* occurs and leads to chronic infection. Opacification of the cornea then takes place, and in later stages of the disease scarring occurs. After time, due to shrinkage of the cornea and extensive scarring, blindness may occur. In the Nile Delta, 90% of individuals over the age of 25 years have conjunctival scarring, and almost a fifth over 50 years of age are blind.

C. trachomatis is also the most common bacterial sexually transmitted disease (STD) in the developed world, particularly in women (Coonrod, 2002; Mardh and Novikova, 2001). In the UK and other countries, the incidence has increased in recent years (Figure 30.1). In the USA, there were 702 093 cases of genital chlamydial infection in 2000 (source: US CDC). Serotypes D–K are sexually transmitted and cause a variety of diseases. In men, infection causes up to 50% of all cases of acute non-gonococcal urethritis and 30% of acute epididymitis cases. Many cases are asymptomatic, and infected men therefore act as a large reservoir for potential chlamydial transmission. Up to 70–80% of cases in women are asymptomatic, but infection causes up to half of all cases of cervicitis and up to 60% of pelvic inflammatory disease cases in developed countries. The most common site of

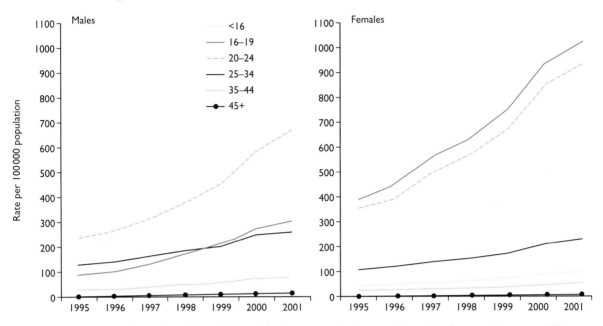

Figure 30.1 Diagnoses of uncomplicated genital chlamydial infection in genitourinary medicine clinics by sex and age group, UK, 1995–2001* (source HPA CDSC).

*Data are unavailable for Scotland for 2000–2001.

infection in females is the endocervix. In symptomatic cases, features often include a vaginal discharge and dysuria. If infection ascends from the lower genitourinary tract to the endometrium and fallopian tubes, then lower abdominal pain and menstrual abnormalities may occur. Some infections may persist for months; in such cases, there is a risk of ectopic pregnancy and infertility (Watson et al., 2002). Transmission of C. trachomatis to neonates during birth may lead to conjunctivitis or pneumonia. Neonatal conjunctivitis due to C. trachomatis usually appears 3–13 days after birth. It may resolve after a few months, but it must be treated to avoid the potential of conjunctival scarring. Pneumonia due to C. trachomatis is one of the most common causes of pneumonia in the newborn. It occurs 4–12 weeks after birth; symptoms include dyspnoea and coughing. Again, the infection may resolve, but if left untreated decreased pulmonary function may be seen later in childhood.

Lymphogranuloma venereum (LGV) is another disease caused by infection with certain serotypes of C. trachomatis and spread via sexual contact (Mabey and Peeling, 2002). It differs from trachoma and other urogenital diseases due to C. trachomatis in that the LGV serotypes infect lymphatic tissue rather than epithelial cells. The disease is rare in developed countries and is most prevalent in the tropics and subtropics. LGV occurs in three stages: the first stage involves the formation of a lesion, most commonly in the genital region. The secondary stage begins once the lesion has healed, and results in swelling of the inguinal lymph nodes. Accompanying symptoms may include fever and joint pains, and complications may include conjunctival infection, meningitis and pneumonitis. The third stage develops if the disease is left untreated, resulting in ulceration or proctitis. Elephantiasis of the vulva or scrotum may also occur.

C. abortus (formerly C. psittaci) causes respiratory disease and is acquired by contact with psittacine birds such as parrots (Poppert et al., 2001); other bird species and even farm animals have also been implicated in C. abortus infection (Nietfeld, 2001). The incubation period ranges from four to 29 days, but is usually between seven and 10 days. Symptoms include headache, chills, fever and a non-productive cough. Some patients present with central nervous system features. There may also be extrapulmonary features, such as abdominal pain, vomiting, myalgia and hepatitis. Complications involving the heart have included endocarditis, myocarditis and pericarditis.

Laboratory diagnosis of all chlamydial infections is similar, depending on the site of infection (Hindiyeh and Carroll, 2000; Watson *et al.*, 2002). All three species that are pathogenic to humans may be isolated in tissue culture. Antigen detection techniques can also be employed, such as direct immunofluorescence and enzyme immunoassay (EIA). The most frequently used method in the UK is serological diagnosis by the complement fixation test (CFT). Acute and convalescent sera are tested for the presence of immunoglobulin M (IgM) or immunoglobulin G (IgG). However, the CFT is only genus-specific and therefore only of real use for infection screening. Other tests, such as the polymerase chain reaction (PCR), PCR-EIA, micro-immunofluorescence, and the whole-cell inclusion immunofluorescence test (WHIF), may also be used for diagnosis. The ligase chain reaction (LCR) has also been described recently for the diagnosis of genitourinary infection with *C. trachomatis* (Watson *et al.*, 2002).

Chlamydial infections may persist for months or years if left untreated, and subsequently lead to complications. Infection is able to continue within the host by transfer of the *Chlamydiae* to other cells during cell division. Therefore, therapy is essential to prevent complications. Treatment of chlamydial infection is often with tetracycline, doxycycline or erythromycin. However, *C. pneumoniae* may not respond as quickly as *C. abortus* to these drugs. In the case of *C. trachomatis* infection of the genital tract, both sexual partners should be treated. Molecular genomics and genome sequencing are now providing improved methods for the diagnosis of chlamydial infections (Stephens and Lammel, 2001); hopefully, therapies and vaccines will also be developed in the future (Igietseme *et al.*, 2002).

REFERENCES

Campbell, L.A. and Kuo, C.C. (2002). *Chlamydia pneumoniae* pathogenesis. *J Med Microbiol* **51**, 623–5.

Coonrod, D.V. (2002). Chlamydial infections. *Curr Womens Health Rep* **2**, 266–75.

Hahn, D.L., Azenabor, A.A., Beatty, W.L. and Byrne, G.I. (2002). *Chlamydia pneumoniae* as a respiratory pathogen. *Front Biosci* **7**, e66–76.

Hindiyeh, M. and Carroll, K.C. (2000). Laboratory diagnosis of atypical pneumonia. *Semin Respir Infect* **15**, 101–13.

Igietseme, J.U., Black, C.M. and Caldwell, H.D. (2002). Chlamydia vaccines: strategies and status. *BioDrugs* **16**, 19–35.

Mabey, D. and Peeling, R.W. (2002). *Lymphogranuloma venereum*. *Sex Transm Infect* **78**, 90–92.

Mardh, P.A. and Novikova, N. (2001). *Chlamydia trachomatis* infections – a major concern for reproductive health. Where do we stand regarding epidemiology, pathogenesis, diagnosis and therapy? *Eur J Contracept Reprod Health Care* **6**, 115–26.

Nietfeld, J.C. (2001). Chlamydial infections in small ruminants. *Vet Clin North Am Food Anim Pract* **17**, 301–14.

Poppert, S., Marre, R. and Essig, A. (2001). Biology and clinical significance of chlamydiae. *Contrib Microbiol* **8**, 51–71.

Stephens, R.S. and Lammel, C.J. (2001). Chlamydia outer membrane protein discovery using genomics. *Curr Opin Microbiol* **4**, 16–20.

Tabbara, K.F. (2001). Trachoma: a review. *J Chemother* **13** (suppl 1), 18–22.

Watson, E.J., Templeton, A., Russell, I., *et al.* (2002). The accuracy and efficacy of screening tests for *Chlamydia trachomatis*: a systematic review. *J Med Microbiol* **51**, 1021–31.

31

Gonorrhoea

The disease gonorrhoea has a long history, dating back to biblical times or before, with the first documented scientific observation being made by Hippocrates (460–355 BC). The term 'gonorrhoea' was first used by Galen (AD 120–200). The bacterium was discovered much later, in 1879, by Neisser, after whom the genus was named. It was later grown and its pathogenicity proven through human inoculation experiments by Bumm in 1885. Gonorrhoea is caused by the bacterium *Neisseria gonorrhoeae* (also known as the 'gonococcus'), a fragile, Gram-negative, intracellular diplococcus that requires carbon dioxide and a complex nutrient surrounding for survival. Its only host is humans, outside which it does not survive. The disease is transmitted from person to person, almost exclusively through sexual intercourse, although it can also be acquired orally or anally by sexual contact or self-inoculation. It is among the most common and widely recognized sexually transmitted diseases (STDs) throughout the world, with an estimated annual incidence of 62 million cases (Gerbase *et al.*, 1998). A dramatic increase in gonorrhoea has occurred since 1955, due to major social changes, such as increased promiscuous activity and travel, thereby leading to a change in attitudes towards sexual relationships. Extramarital, homosexual and casual relationships are now more common, and gonorrhoea is therefore considered a social disease as well as a bacterial disease. At its peak, over 10^6 new infections were being reported each year in the USA, and around 60 000 in the UK. However, the current worldwide epidemic shows signs of control due to rapid detection and treatment of infection and prompt tracing of contacts; for example, 358 995 cases of gonorrhoea were reported in the USA during 2000 (source: US CDC).

Gonorrhoea affects primarily the columnar epithelial cells of the urethral or endocervical mucosa. Extragenitourinary sites, including the rectum, oropharynx and eyes, may also be involved. Gonorrhoea may be transmitted from mother to baby during birth, resulting in a severe eye infection known as ophthalmia neonatorum. This is caused by an intense inflammatory response, which can result in blindness.

After infection, the incubation period is usually two to five days, although this can vary from one to 14 days. In females, up to 50–75% of infections may be asymptomatic. The cervix is the most common site of initial infection, which, due to the production of an inflammatory response, often results in the production of a purulent discharge. Involvement of the urethra causes dysuria and increased urinary frequency. Cervical gonorrhoea may sometimes occur due to gonococcal bacteria ascending into the uterus and fallopian tubes, resulting in salpingitis or pelvic inflammatory disease (PID). In male patients, infection occurs in the urethra and is characterized by a copious and purulent discharge, which may be accompanied by dysuria. Infection can extend to the posterior urethra, causing severe pain on urination, with urgency and frequency. Spread to the upper genital tract can lead to epididymitis and possibly sterility. In both males and females, proctitis may be asymptomatic or may result in anal discharge, pruritus, tenesmus and rectal bleeding. Infection of the pharynx may lead to erythema and a purulent exudate. Conjunctivitis, a result of rubbing the eyes with contaminated fingers, usually results in a purulent discharge. Complications in female patients include disseminated gonorrhoea, bartholinitis and pelvic infection; in men, they include urethral stricture, prostatitis and disseminated gonococcaemia. The spread of gonorrhoea from the genital region can sometimes lead to a characteristic illness consisting of arthritis, skin lesions and sometimes fatal endocarditis.

A few diseases result in the same symptoms as, but are not caused by, gonorrhoea. Such diseases are known collectively as non-gonococcal urethritis and may be caused by *Chlamydia trachomatis* and mycoplasmas. Distinguishing between gonorrhoea and non-gonococcal urethritis is important due to the use of different antibiotic treatment.

The discharge associated with gonorrhoea is the hallmark of the disease, from which a laboratory diagnosis using microscopy can often be made. A Gram stain of such discharge will reveal Gram-negative diplococci inside polymorphonuclear leukocytes. However, although this method detects approximately 95% of male infections, it detects only 50–60% of female infections. A number of other methods can also be employed to diagnose gonorrhoea, such as fluorescent antibody tests and culture (Young, 1978a; Young, 1978b). *N. gonorrhoeae* is not a commensal in any numbers and should therefore never be reported as such. However, other Gram-negative cocci may be present in clinical samples and may cause difficulties in the diagnosis of gonorrhoea. A national standard for typing gonococci has not been reached, and the advancement of molecular methods has confused matters. However, outer-membrane genes such as *opa* and *por*B can be used for typing purposes (Kohl *et al.*, 1990; Moyes & Young, 1991; O'Rourke *et al.*, 1995; Unemo *et al.*, 2002; Van Looveren *et al.*, 1999).

Gonorrhoea is a treatable disease, although this has not always been the case. Before the advent of antibiotics, there was no treatment for gonorrhoea. This changed dramatically after the introduction of the sulphonamides in the 1930s. However, resistant strains developed rapidly and the sulphonamides became largely ineffective. Luckily, the penicillins soon became available, and gonorrhoea has been treatable ever since. Even today, the drugs used for treatment are cheap and readily available, and therefore patients with symptoms can be cured easily. The problem that exists, however, is that many infected individuals do not have significant symptoms. Approximately one-third of infected women and 10% of infected men are asymptomatic. Therefore, disease can be spread readily via sexual activities. Asymptomatic carriers are not aware of having gonorrhoea unless a sexual contact has symptomatic infection, and disease can spread unwittingly, especially through promiscuous activity. It is for this reason that so much effort has been diverted towards the development of a vaccine. However, the production of a vaccine has been challenging due to the strategies possessed by *N. gonorrhoeae* in avoiding the host immune response. *N. gonorrhoeae*, like *N. meningitidis*, is able to vary its surface antigenic structure in order to avoid the host immune response. An effective vaccine is therefore some time away, although the need for one is becoming more urgent due to the emergence of antibiotic-resistant strains. Although most strains are susceptible to beta-lactam antibiotics and tetracyclines, the incidence of resistant strains has been increasing in recent years (Ison *et al.*, 2001; Ison, 1996; Tapsall, 2002). Some strains are resistant to both classes of antibiotics, although they remain susceptible to other antibiotics; however, these other antibiotics are more expensive. Two types of beta-lactam resistance have been found in strains of *N. gonorrhoeae*. The first is mediated chromosomally by a gene encoding a penicillin-binding protein that no longer binds penicillin. The second is plasmid-mediated by a gene encoding a beta-lactamase. Tetracycline resistance is plasmid-mediated by a gene encoding ribosome protection (tetracycline affects protein synthesis).

Gonorrhoea is a disease that is preventable by education and treatable with antibiotic therapy. The disease remains a global problem and will do so until education measures are strictly enforced or an effective vaccine is made available. The gonococcal genome has been sequenced, and this may lead to improved therapies or development of a vaccine (Moxon and Rappuoli, 2002). Although the current worldwide epidemic appears to be receding, we should not be complacent over the need to continue enforcing control measures.

REFERENCES

Gerbase, A.C., Rowley, J.T., Heymann, D.H., Berkley, S.F. and Piot, P. (1998). Global prevalence and incidence estimates of selected curable STDs. *Sex Transm Infect* 74 (suppl 1), S12–16.

Ison, C., Martin, I., Ivens, D., Philip, S. and Greene, L. (2001). Ciprofloxacin resistance in gonococci. *Lancet* 357, 803.

Ison, C.A. (1996). Antimicrobial agents and gonorrhoea: therapeutic choice, resistance and susceptibility testing. *Genitourin Med* 72, 253–7.

Kohl, P.K., Ison, C.A., Danielsson, D., Knapp, J.S. and Petzoldt, D. (1990). Current status of serotyping of *Neisseria gonorrhoeae*. *Eur J Epidemiol* 6, 91–5.

Moxon, R. and Rappuoli, R. (2002). Bacterial pathogen genomics and vaccines. *Br Med Bull* 62, 45–58.

Moyes, A. and Young, H. (1991). Epidemiological typing of *Neisseria gonorrhoeae*: a comparative analysis of three monoclonal antibody serotyping panels. *Eur J Epidemiol* 7, 311–19.

O'Rourke, M., Ison, C.A., Renton, A.M. and Spratt, B.G. (1995). Opa-typing: a high-resolution tool for studying the epidemiology of gonorrhoea. *Mol Microbiol* 17, 865–75.

Tapsall, J. (2002). Current concepts in the management of gonorrhoea. *Expert Opin Pharmacother* 3, 147–57.

Unemo, M., Olcen, P., Berglund, T., Albert, J. and Fredlund, H. (2002). Molecular epidemiology of *Neisseria gonorrhoeae*: sequence analysis of the porB gene confirms presence of two circulating strains. *J Clin Microbiol* 40, 3741–9.

Van Looveren, M., Ison, C.A., Ieven, M., *et al.* (1999). Evaluation of the discriminatory power of typing methods for *Neisseria gonorrhoeae*. *J Clin Microbiol* 37, 2183–8.

Young, H. (1978a). Cultural diagnosis of gonorrhoea with modified New York City (MNYC) medium. *Br J Vener Dis* 54, 36–40.

Young, H. (1978b). Identification and penicillinase testing of *Neisseria gonorrhoeae* from primary isolation cultures on modified New York City medium. *J Clin Microbiol* 7, 247–50.

32

Whooping cough

Whooping cough (pertussis) is an infectious childhood disease of the respiratory tract caused by a small Gram-negative bacillus, *Bordetella pertussis* (Girard, 2002; Heininger, 2001a). At the beginning of the twentieth century, whooping cough was a fatal disease in the UK, killing approximately 10 000 children each year. In developed countries, both morbidity and mortality have declined in recent years, and in the UK there are now hundreds rather than thousands of cases (Figure 32.1). In the USA, there were 7867 cases of whooping cough in 2000 (source: US CDC). In developing countries, however, whooping cough remains a common disease. Whooping cough may occur at any time of the year, but in the UK it is more common in late winter and spring. Peaks of prevalence occur at three- to four-year intervals.

The incubation period of whooping cough is difficult to determine because there is no characteristic rash or symptom associated with the disease (Birkebaek, 2001; Postels-Multani *et al.*, 1995). It has been estimated to be between seven and 10 days, although some cases have reported incubation periods as short as three days and others as long as 21 days. At its height, the symptoms of whooping cough can be diagnosed at sight, but in the early stages the symptoms are similar to those of a common cold. The disease usually begins with a mild fever, which lasts a few days before symptoms of a common cold develop. This is called the catarrhal stage. The symptoms persist for 7–10 days, after which the spasmodic stage develops. When a spasm occurs, the child may cough 20 or 30 times; as the glottis relaxes, air sweeps past into

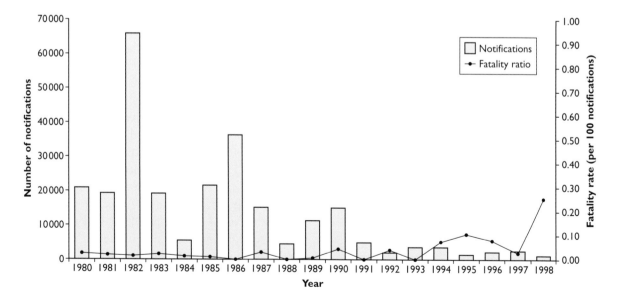

Figure 32.1 Notifications and deaths of whooping cough in England and Wales, 1980–98 (source: HPA CDSC).

the almost empty lungs with a characteristic 'whoop'. During coughing, the child's face becomes congested and red, the eyes bulge from their sockets, and the veins of the neck and scalp swell. Spasms might be repeated almost immediately. In young infants, the glottis might close completely at the end of the spasm, resulting in apnoea, cyanosis and sometimes convulsions. Death from asphyxiation does not occur often. The frequency of the spasms varies from patient to patient and may range from three to four in a day to the same number in an hour. The spasmodic stage of the disease may last from one to four weeks, although slight coughing may persist for a few months.

Many complications are associated with whooping cough. The most common respiratory complication is lung collapse. This is rarely diagnosed on clinical grounds, and only radiological examination of the lungs reveals its presence. The effects of pressure from the spasmodic coughing may result in the appearance, or increase in size, of umbilical or inguinal herniae. Convulsions are also more frequent and persistent in whooping cough than in any other infectious disease. Sometimes the child may pass into coma, which may range from hours to weeks; the outlook in these cases is serious, and at least half of such children die. Paralysis, mental retardation and epilepsy are frequent sequelae for those who survive the coma. However, many children recover to be both physically and mentally normal. Bronchopneumonia is a serious complication and may be caused by *B. pertussis* itself or by other respiratory pathogens such as *Streptococcus pneumoniae* or *Haemophilus influenzae*.

Age is probably the most significant deciding factor in assessing prognosis in whooping cough. It is estimated that as many as 75% of deaths from whooping cough occur in infants under one year of age, and almost all deaths are in children under the age of three years. Infants under one year of age, and especially those less than three months old, suffer severely from the disease. They are at their most vulnerable at this age, and the disease interferes with their growth and development. Neurological disorders are most common in the first year of life,

and persistent lung collapse is less frequent. The total mortality in the developed world is probably under 1%, but in developing countries mortality it is much greater.

Diagnosis is achieved mainly on clinical grounds because the symptoms of the spasmodic cough are so characteristic of whooping cough (Hindiyeh and Carroll, 2000). Early diagnosis is difficult clinically but can be achieved bacteriologically. Bacterial culture confirmation is difficult in the spasmodic stage because *B. pertussis* may not be present in the upper respiratory tract after the catarrhal stage. Pernasal swabs are preferred for bacterial culture and nasopharyngeal secretions for immunofluorescence, although postnasal secretions, postnasal swabs and cough plate methods may also be used. The polymerase chain reaction (PCR) may also be used (Qin *et al.*, 2002; von Konig *et al.*, 2002).

B. pertussis produces a number of toxic products (Antoine *et al.*, 2000), although they also possess a number of virulence mechanisms common to other pathogens (Bock and Gross, 2001; Coote, 2001; Cotter and DiRita, 2000; Konig *et al.*, 2002; Locht *et al.*, 2001). One particular isolated toxin, pertussis toxin, has several biological effects and may be central to pathogenesis. This toxin is able to induce lymphocytosis and increase sensitivity to histamine and anaphylaxis. It is also possible that *B. pertussis* secretes a soluble adenylate cyclase, which leads to depression of the antibacterial functions of neutrophils. However, the role of these toxins in the pathogenesis of whooping cough is still not understood fully.

The single most effective protective agent against whooping cough is the pertussis vaccine (Girard, 2002). This does not prevent disease in all vaccinated individuals, but it lessens the severity of the illness and the frequency of complications in people who get the disease. A decline in vaccine uptake occurred in the mid-1970s and resulted in two large epidemics of whooping cough, but recovery in the uptake of the vaccine between 1978 and 1992 resulted in a major reduction in the incidence of the disease and in the proportion of cases occurring in preschool children. New vaccines are being developed using information from molecular research, particularly that gained from the genome sequence (Heininger, 2001a; Heininger, 2001b).

REFERENCES

Antoine, R., Raze, D. and Locht, C. (2000). Genomics of *Bordetella pertussis* toxins. *Int J Med Microbiol* **290**, 301–5.

Birkebaek, N.H. (2001). *Bordetella pertussis* in the aetiology of chronic cough in adults. Diagnostic methods and clinic. *Dan Med Bull* **48**, 77–80.

Bock, A. and Gross, R. (2001). The BvgAS two-component system of *Bordetella* spp.: a versatile modulator of virulence gene expression. *Int J Med Microbiol* **291**, 119–30.

Coote, J.G. (2001). Environmental sensing mechanisms in *Bordetella*. *Adv Microb Physiol* **44**, 141–81.

Cotter, P.A. and DiRita, V.J. (2000). Bacterial virulence gene regulation: an evolutionary perspective. *Annu Rev Microbiol* **54**, 519–65.

Girard, D.Z. (2002). Which strategy for pertussis vaccination today? *Paediatr Drugs* **4**, 299–313.

Heininger, U. (2001a). Pertussis: an old disease that is still with us. *Curr Opin Infect Dis* **14**, 329–35.

Heininger, U. (2001b). Recent progress in clinical and basic pertussis research. *Eur J Pediatr* **160**, 203–13.

Hindiyeh, M. and Carroll, K.C. (2000). Laboratory diagnosis of atypical pneumonia. *Semin Respir Infect* **15**, 101–13.

Konig, J., Bock, A., Perraud, A.L., Fuchs, T.M., Beier, D. and Gross, R. (2002). Regulatory factors of *Bordetella pertussis* affecting virulence gene expression. *J Mol Microbiol Biotechnol* **4**, 197–203.

Locht, C., Antoine, R. and Jacob-Dubuisson, F. (2001). *Bordetella pertussis*, molecular pathogenesis under multiple aspects. *Curr Opin Microbiol* **4**, 82–9.

Postels-Multani, S., Schmitt, H.J., Wirsing von Konig, C.H., Bock, H.L. and Bogaerts, H. (1995). Symptoms and complications of pertussis in adults. *Infection* **23**, 139–42.

Qin, X., Turgeon, D.K., Ingersoll, B.P., *et al.* (2002). *Bordetella pertussis* PCR: simultaneous targeting of signature sequences. *Diagn Microbiol Infect Dis* **43**, 269–75.

Von Konig, C.H., Halperin, S., Riffelmann, M. and Guiso, N. (2002). Pertussis of adults and infants. *Lancet Infect Dis* **2**, 744–50.

33

Acute bacterial meningitis

Meningitis is the term used to describe inflammation of the membranes surrounding the brain and spinal cord (Booy and Kroll, 1994; Segreti and Harris, 1996). The disease may be caused by bacteria, viruses, fungi and protozoa; however, most cases are of bacterial or viral origin, therefore only these will be described here. Acute bacterial meningitis is an important worldwide cause of morbidity and mortality, with a mortality of 30–50%. Epidemics of meningitis have not occurred in developed countries since the Second World War, but epidemics lasting several years still occur in developing countries. The most common bacterial causes of meningitis are *Streptococcus pneumoniae*, *Haemophilus influenzae*, *Neisseria meningitidis*, group B streptococci and *Escherichia coli* (Ferguson *et al.*, 2002; Meli *et al.*, 2002; Rosenstein and Perkins, 2000; Segreti and Harris, 1996). The incidence of meningitis caused by these bacteria varies with age. Group B streptococcal and *E. coli* meningitis are most common in neonates and babies less than three months of age. *H. influenzae* meningitis occurs between the ages of three months and five years, although the Hib vaccine, introduced in a number of countries in the early 1990s, has led to a dramatic decrease in disease. Meningitis caused by *N. meningitidis* and *S. pneumoniae* may occur at any age, although the former is most common in children and young adults. Other less common causes of meningitis include *Staphylococcus aureus* and *Listeria monocytogenes*, although many other bacteria may also cause meningitis.

Bacterial meningitis results from the invasion of bacteria into the cerebrospinal fluid (CSF) when the pathogenic virulence factors overcome the host defence mechanisms. This involves colonization of the host mucosal epithelium, which means that the bacteria must be able to attach and invade the epithelium effectively by evading secretory immunoglobulin A (IgA) and avoiding the ciliary mechanisms of the mucosa. In some bacteria, this process is aided partly by the possession of fimbriae. Once colonization is attained, the bacteria must be capable of invasion and survival in the intravascular space. The main host defence here is the alternative complement pathway, and the bacteria must therefore possess a polysaccharide capsule to survive. The next stage involves crossing the blood–brain barrier and surviving in the CSF. The CSF contains sufficient nutrients for the bacteria to multiply if they are able to withstand the influx of host immune defence mechanisms.

Clinical meningitis arises from the host response to the presence of bacteria in the CSF. The classic symptoms of acute bacterial meningitis are headache, photophobia and neck stiffness. Other typical symptoms include lethargy, anorexia, vomiting and convulsions. The latter are particularly common in young children. Listlessness and diarrhoea are the symptoms often seen in neonates. Haemorrhagic rash may be present and is characteristic of meningococcal meningitis, although it may also occur in meningitis caused by other bacteria. Overall, the symptoms of meningitis depend on the age of the patient and the duration of the illness. Septic shock may also occur due to the presence of Gram-negative bacteria, such as *N. meningitidis*, in the blood. This results in hypotension and is due to the release of endotoxins, which stimulate the host production of proteins such as tumour necrosis factor (TNF). Surviving patients may suffer from hearing or neurological damage.

Rapid chemotherapy is essential to reduce both morbidity and mortality (Cuevas and Hart, 1993; Foster and Nadel, 2002). Currently, penicillin is the recommended treatment if the patient is first seen by a general practitioner. Upon admittance to hospital, and on reflection of microbiology results, therapy may be changed to a more suitable drug. Bactericidal rather than bacteriostatic therapy is preferable. The rapid lysis of bacterial cells present in the CSF may lead to exacerbation of the inflammation due to the release of inflammatory bacterial fragments.

Laboratory investigation is essential for the confirmation of meningitis and for determining its aetiology (Diggle et al., 2001). However, the interpretation of laboratory results may be complicated if chemotherapy is administered early on in the disease. Microscopy and cell counts are performed on the CSF. A centrifuged deposit should be stained by Gram's method for the presence of bacteria. Atypical bacterial morphology is common, especially if chemotherapy has been started before obtaining the CSF. If abnormal numbers of leukocytes are present in the cell count (usually >5/mm^3), then a differential stain should be performed from a centrifuged deposit or a cytospin preparation to determine the ratio of polymorphonuclear leukocytes to mononuclear leukocytes. A predominant number of polymorphonuclear leukocytes often indicates acute bacterial meningitis, and the CSF usually contains 1000–10 000/mm^3 of these. Erythrocytes may also be present, especially if there was trauma when obtaining the CSF. In such cases, the ratio of leukocytes to erythrocytes must be determined.

Laboratory tests performed for the investigation of meningitis include:

- CSF microscopy;
- Gram stain of CSF;
- CSF biochemistry;
- CSF culture;
- polymerase chain reaction (PCR) on CSF.

Biochemical analysis of the CSF is also performed. The glucose and protein concentrations are determined: the former is reduced and the latter is raised in acute bacterial meningitis. However, the CSF glucose concentration should be interpreted only in relation to the blood glucose. If acute bacterial meningitis is indicated by biochemical and microbiological results, but no bacteria are seen in stained microscopy, then antigen detection may be of value. This may be done using commercially available latex agglutination tests. CSF culture is performed regardless of the presence or absence of bacteria or leukocytes. Bacteria are frequently not seen in microscopy; more rarely, leukocytes may be absent but organisms may be present in quite high numbers. Culture is important for the identification of the causative bacteria and for antimicrobial susceptibility testing.

Individuals who are at increased risk of acquiring bacterial meningitis may receive chemoprophylaxis (Peltola, 1999). Such patients include close contacts of an index case. Rifampicin is usually the drug of choice. Vaccines are also available for people who are at long-term risk, such as those who are asplenic and people working in close communities where epidemics are common. Vaccines have been developed against S. pneumoniae, N. meningitidis and H. influenzae (Buttery and Moxon, 2000; Peltola, 1999). However, vaccines should not be used to replace chemoprophylaxis in those exposed to an index case.

The morbidity and mortality of this disease will inevitably remain at their current levels unless we are able to recognize meningitis earlier, initiate chemotherapy at an early stage, and recognize and treat the consequences associated with the accompanying septicaemia. Improved diagnostic methods are enhancing the surveillance of meningitis, which is leading to a better understanding of the epidemiology of meningitis. However, the use of genome sequences will be the mainstay of improved therapies and vaccines in the future (Rappuoli, 2001).

REFERENCES

Booy, R. and Kroll, S. (1994). Bacterial meningitis in children. Curr Opin Pediatr 6, 29–35.

Buttery, J.P. and Moxon, E.R. (2000). Designing meningitis vaccines. *J R Coll Physicians Lond* **34**, 163–8.

Cuevas, L.E. and Hart, C.A. (1993). Chemoprophylaxis of bacterial meningitis. *J Antimicrob Chemother* **31** (suppl B), 79–91.

Diggle, M.A., Edwards, G.F. and Clarke, S.C. (2001). Developments in the diagnosis of meningococcal disease and the characterization of *Neisseria meningitidis*. *Rev Med Microbiol* **12**, 211–17.

Ferguson, L.E., Hormann, M.D., Parks, D.K. and Yetman, R.J. (2002). *Neisseria meningitidis*: presentation, treatment, and prevention. *J Pediatr Health Care* **16**, 119–24.

Foster, C. and Nadel, S. (2002). New therapies and vaccines for bacterial meningitis. *Expert Opin Investig Drugs* **11**, 1051–60.

Meli, D.N., Christen, S., Leib, S.L. and Tauber, M.G. (2002). Current concepts in the pathogenesis of meningitis caused by *Streptococcus pneumoniae*. *Curr Opin Infect Dis* **15**, 253–7.

Peltola, H. (1999). Prophylaxis of bacterial meningitis. *Infect Dis Clin North Am* **13**, 685–710.

Rappuoli, R. (2001). Conjugates and reverse vaccinology to eliminate bacterial meningitis. *Vaccine* **19**, 2319–22.

Rosenstein, N.E. and Perkins, B.A. (2000). Update on *Haemophilus influenzae* serotype b and meningococcal vaccines. *Pediatr Clin North Am* **47**, 337–52.

Segreti, J. and Harris, A.A. (1996). Acute bacterial meningitis. *Infect Dis Clin North Am* **10**, 797–809.

34

Meningococcal disease

Meningitis was first described by Socrates, although the cause of the condition remained unknown until the late nineteenth century. With the rapid progression of laboratory methods and the development of bacteriology from an art into a science in the last 25 years of the nineteenth century, microbiologists made repeated attempts to isolate an organism from patients who had died of meningitis. A number of reports in the medical literature described various microscopic findings, but for several years none of them attempted to culture the meningococcus. Some workers did not find the organisms in cerebrospinal fluid (CSF), while others described organisms similar to pneumococci. In the 1870s, Marchiafava and Celli identified and described micrococci within the cytoplasm of leukocytes, but cultures were negative.

The breakthrough came in 1887, when Anton Weichselbaum, working in Vienna, isolated a coccoid bacterium from meningeal exudate. Since he had isolated pneumococci from other cases of meningitis, he was cautious in his interpretation of these findings. However, he later called this organism *Diplococcus intracellularis meningitidis*, which later became known as *Neisseria meningitidis*. Jaeger later investigated a small epidemic of meningitis in the military, and reported an intracellular bacterium that resembled the coccoid bacterium described by Weichselbaum. Cultures yielded a Gram-positive chain of cocci similar to streptococci. There were supporters of both men, and confusion remained for some time, but eventually a series of further reports were published confirming Weichselbaum's findings and confirming the association between the meningococcus and meningitis. After Weichselbaum's report, the diagnosis of meningitis was improved by the introduction of lumbar puncture by Quincke. Soon after, meningococci were isolated for the first time from the CSF of patients who were ill with meningitis.

Isolation of the causative organism and the introduction of lumbar puncture as a routine clinical procedure led the way for intraspinal immunotherapy in the early years of the twentieth century. At about the same time, it was predicted that patients with meningococcal meningitis could also carry the organism in the oropharynx.

German microbiologists showed that rabbits and horses immunized with meningococci developed agglutinating antibodies. This led to the first human trials of antiserum for the treatment of meningococcal meningitis. Flexner and Jobling, of the Rockefeller Institute in New York, were working in parallel with the German team, and by 1908 they were able to report a series of 400 cases from Europe and the USA who had been treated with the meningococcal antiserum; the overall mortality had been reduced to 25%. However, there were complications with this immunotherapy, such as fever, skin eruptions, arthritis and digestive disturbances. Intraspinal immunotherapy remained in use until the 1930s, but it was superseded by the introduction of the sulphonamide antibiotics. Shortly after the antiserum trials, Rupert Waterhouse, a physician working in Bath, reported a case of suprarenal apoplexy on post-mortem examination of a fatal case of fulminant meningococcal septicaemia. This was followed by a report of similar cases by Friderichsen in Copenhagen in 1918, and the syndrome was termed Waterhouse–Friderichsen syndrome.

It is now known that there are 13 serogroups of *N. meningitidis* (Diggle *et al.*, 2001). These are subdivided further on the basis of analysis of outer-membrane proteins PorB and PorA, which provide a serotype and serosubtype, respectively. The serogroups most commonly isolated worldwide are A, B and C, although serogroups Y and W135 can also be associated with certain symptoms or outbreaks.

Due to the improved understanding of the meningococcus in the first half of the twentieth century, its epidemiology was beginning to be understood. Much has been learned from its high incidence in army recruits due to it spreading in people living in cramped conditions. There were thousands of notified cases of meningococcal disease during the First World War. When cases of cerebrospinal fever began to occur in British and colonial army recruits in the winter of 1914–15, the Medical Research Council's Special Advisory Committee suggested that the causative organism was a new strain of meningococcus introduced into the UK by Canadian troops. Britain and Canada were not the only nations to experience outbreaks of meningitis: there were also cases in Australian and New Zealand troops, increased disease rates in Germany in 1915, and numerous outbreaks in US recruit training camps in 1917. In Britain, the winter of 1914 was unusually wet, and cases of meningitis began to occur frequently, with outbreaks in Portsmouth and Winchester and, in particular, among troops stationed on Salisbury Plain. The environment for these troops was overcrowded and was ideal for the spread of meningococci; the patients were later treated by inhalation of 1% zinc sulphate solution.

In 1915, Gordon and Murray, microbiologists in the Royal Army Medical Corps, published a system of meningococcal classification based on antisera raised in rabbits. Their scheme, which divided meningococci into four groups (I, II, III and IV), was adopted widely in English-speaking countries. Other systems were devised elsewhere. At the end of the First World War, interest in meningococcal disease subsided. At that time, most infections were due to serogroup A, but serogroup B strains began to be isolated more frequently. In 1919, long before the era of antibiotics and intensive care, Herrick

described meningococcal disease with the words: 'no other infection so quickly slays'. More than 80 years later, this still holds true. Because healthy young children are primarily the victims of this disease, its incidence continues to increase.

The first group of specific antimicrobial agents, the sulphonamides, were discovered in the 1930s. The prevention of meningococcal infection in mice by using sulphonamides was reported in 1936. As in the First World War, meningitis at this time was common in recruit camps, particularly affecting new recruits, and was less common in troops who had completed their basic training. During the Second World War, the meningococcal epidemic was primarily a civilian one, in both the USA and the UK. Sulphonamides provided the mainstay of specific treatment during the war years. The superiority of sulphonamide treatment alone was demonstrated in 1939. The introduction of sulphonamides not only had a dramatic effect on reducing mortality in meningococcal meningitis; they were also used for the first time during the war to clear nasopharyngeal carriage of meningococci. Later in the Second World War, penicillin became available. Most strains of meningococci remain sensitive to penicillin even today (Cartwright et al., 1992; Tapsall et al., 2001).

In the post-war years, because of the introduction of a polysaccharide vaccine for US military recruits, meningococcal disease became less of a problem for the military. The pace of work on the meningococcus has not slowed since 1945. During the past decade, however, the incidence of the disease has increased in many parts of Europe; much of this increase was due to the emergence of serogroup C strains after the decline in group B disease in the early 1990s (Figure 34.1). Many of the serogroup C strains that occur in Europe belong to the ET-37 strain complex, which is often associated with clusters or outbreaks (Vogel et al., 2000; Wang et al., 1993). Due to the introduction of the meningococcal serogroup C conjugate (MenC) vaccine in the UK and some other European countries, the incidence of serogroup C disease has decreased in those age groups who have received immunization (Figure 34.2) (Finn and Lakshman, 2002;

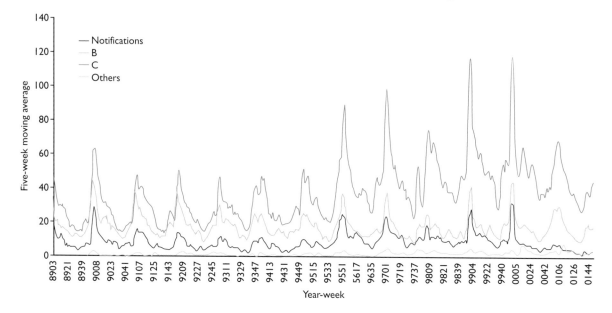

Figure 34.1 Meningococcal disease in England and Wales, 1989–2001; five-week moving average (source: HPA CDSC).

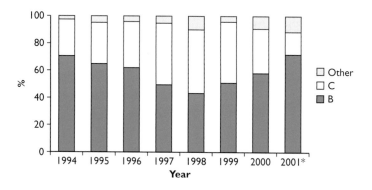

Figure 34.2 Meningococcal serogroups in Scotland, 1994–2001 (source: SCIEH).

Maiden and Stuart, 2002; Richmond *et al.*, 1999). Even so, there are still hundreds of cases of meningococcal disease each year in the UK alone. A rapid diagnosis of meningococcal disease is therefore still required clinically, with follow-up confirmation and typing performed in the laboratory (Diggle *et al.*, 2001). Due to the use of antibiotics, often before the patient has been admitted to hospital, laboratory confirmation of the disease has become less straightforward (Cartwright *et al.*, 1992). This has important implications because, traditionally, isolation of the infecting organism

provides the most typing information, which is used for public health management of cases and their contacts, particularly during case clusters (Anon, 2002). Non-culture diagnosis has therefore become important, using techniques such as latex agglutination, the polymerase chain reaction (PCR) and antibody detection (Borrow *et al.*, 1997; Diggle *et al.*, 2001; Gray *et al.*, 1999; Guiver *et al.*, 2000). Nucleotide sequencing methods now complement other non-culture methods to provide more typing information (Clarke, 2002; Clarke *et al.*, 2001; Clarke *et al.*, 2002). Extensive genetic studies have been and continue to be performed on the meningococcus. Genome sequences have been published in recent years, and new vaccines are being sought that protect against all of the serogroups commonly associated with meningococcal disease (Jodar *et al.*, 2002; Pollard and Moxon, 2002). A century after the first isolation of the meningococcus, it could be said that its demise as a human pathogen may now, at last, be imminent.

REFERENCES

Anon (2002). Guidelines for public health management of meningococcal disease in the UK. *Commun Dis Public Health* **5**, 187–204.

Borrow, R., Claus, H., Guiver, M., *et al.* (1997). Non-culture diagnosis and serogroup determination of meningococcal B and C infection by a sialyltransferase (siaD) PCR ELISA. *Epidemiol Infect* **118**, 111–17.

Cartwright, K., Reilly, S., White, D. and Stuart, J. (1992). Early treatment with parenteral penicillin in meningococcal disease. *Br Med J* **305**, 143–7.

Clarke, S.C. (2002). Nucleotide sequence-based typing of bacteria and the impact of automation. *Bioessays* **24**, 858–62.

Clarke, S.C., Diggle, M.A. and Edwards, G.F. (2001). Semiautomation of multilocus sequence typing for the characterisation of clinical isolates of *Neisseria meningitidis*. *J Clin Microbiol* **39**, 3066–71.

Clarke, S.C., Diggle, M.A. and Edwards, G.F. (2002). Multilocus sequence typing and porA gene sequencing differentiates strains of *Neisseria meningitidis* during case clusters. *Br J Biomed Sci* **59**, 160–62.

Diggle, M.A., Edwards, G.F. and Clarke, S.C. (2001). Developments in the diagnosis of meningococcal disease and the characterization of *Neisseria meningitidis*. *Rev Med Microbiol* **12**, 211–17.

Finn, A. and Lakshman, R. (2002). Meningococcal serogroup C conjugate vaccine. *Expert Opin Biol Ther* **2**, 87–96.

Gray, S.J., Sobanski, M.A., Kaczmarski, E.B., *et al.* (1999). Ultrasound-enhanced latex immunoagglutination and PCR as complementary methods for non-culture-based confirmation of meningococcal disease. *J Clin Microbiol* **37**, 1797–801.

Guiver, M., Borrow, R., Marsh, J., *et al.* (2000). Evaluation of the Applied Biosystems automated Taqman polymerase chain reaction system for the detection of meningococcal DNA. *FEMS Immunol Med Microbiol* **28**, 173–9.

Jodar, L., Feavers, I.M., Salisbury, D. and Granoff, D.M. (2002). Development of vaccines against meningococcal disease. *Lancet* **359**, 1499–508.

Maiden, M.C. and Stuart, J.M. (2002). Carriage of serogroup C meningococci 1 year after meningococcal C conjugate polysaccharide vaccination. *Lancet* **359**, 1829–31.

Pollard, A.J. and Moxon, E.R. (2002). The meningococcus tamed? *Arch Dis Child* **87**, 13–17.

Richmond, P., Borrow, R., Miller, E., *et al.* (1999). Meningococcal serogroup C conjugate vaccine is immunogenic in infancy and primes for memory. *J Infect Dis* **179**, 1569–72.

Tapsall, J.W., Shultz, T., Limnios, E., *et al.* (2001). Surveillance of antibiotic resistance in invasive isolates of *Neisseria meningitidis* in Australia 1994–1999. *Pathology* **33**, 359–61.

Vogel, U., Claus, H., Frosch, M. and Caugant, D.A. (2000). Molecular basis for distinction of the ET-15 clone within the ET-37 complex of *Neisseria meningitidis*. *J Clin Microbiol* **38**, 941–2.

Wang, J.F., Caugant, D.A., Morelli, G., Koumare, B. and Achtman, M. (1993). Antigenic and epidemiologic properties of the ET-37 complex of *Neisseria meningitidis*. *J Infect Dis* **167**, 1320–29.

35

Pneumococcal disease

Streptococcus pneumoniae is a Gram-positive coccus. It is one of the disease-causing members of a large genus of streptococci. It is an important human pathogen, causing a number of different diseases. Disease attributable to this organism is worldwide and affects all age groups and social classes (Diez-Domingo *et al.*, 2002; Ip *et al.*, 2001; Jette *et al.*, 2001; Kyaw *et al.*, 2002b; McGee *et al.*, 2001; Petrosillo *et al.*, 2002; Robinson *et al.*, 2001; Sleeman *et al.*, 2001). There are over 80 serotypes of *S. pneumoniae* based on the antigenic differences of capsular polysaccharide between each type. Infection with the organism results in a good antibody response. Immunoglobulin G (IgG) is the class of antibody responsible for immunity to pneumococci. The antibody reacts with cell-wall polysaccharides, leading to phagocytosis of the bacterium. Serotyping was clinically relevant in the earlier parts of the twentieth century, when antiserum was used as treatment. Today, however, the serotype is of little relevance in medicine, except for epidemiological purposes.

Nearly all infants are colonized on at least one occasion in the first two years of life. Although there is generally a good antibody response, colonization with pneumococci continues throughout life, probably due to the large number of serotypes. In adults, the average duration of colonization is six weeks. Serious pneumococcal infection is most common in the young and the old, when the immune system is at its poorest and is unable to combat infection. Generally, incidence of infection is greatest in infants under the age of two years, is low among older children and young adults, increases in older adults, and continues to increase to a high level in individuals over retirement age.

The pneumococcus is associated with four main infections:

- pneumonia
- meningitis
- septicaemia
- otitis media.

Pneumonia is a common problem worldwide and is the sixth leading cause of death in the USA (Puli and Clarke, 2002). It is associated with high overall treatment costs due to therapy, hospitalization and work absence. In the 1930s, almost all cases of pneumonia were caused by *S. pneumoniae*; nowadays, half the cases are of unknown aetiology, although some of these may actually be pneumococcal in origin but with no confirmatory diagnosis. *S. pneumoniae* still remains the most common bacterial cause of community-acquired pneumonia (CAP), although the proportion of cases of CAP attributable to the organism has varied from 15% to 76% in various studies (El-Solh *et al.*, 2001; Marrie, 2000; Woodhead, 1994). Pneumonia may occur after colonization of the nasopharynx following inhalation of pneumococci. It results in distinctive symptoms of cough, sputum production and fever; pleuritic chest pain, headaches and neck stiffness may also occur. Very old patients may not present with some of these symptoms, due to the lack of a satisfactory immune response. The absence of fever is often associated with increased morbidity and mortality. Pneumonia is more common in people with bronchopulmonary disease or other underlying conditions that result in a reduction in immunity due to the lack of adequate clearing of mucous from the lungs. Viral infections also predispose individuals to pneumococcal pneumonia. Conditions associated with reduced IgG immunity also result in a predisposition to pneumonia. Heavy smoking and alcoholism result in a predisposition to infection, the former because of inadequate lung mucous clearance and the latter due to a general decrease in immunity. Individuals who have had a splenectomy risk fulminating bacteraemia either during or preceding pneumonia; death may be as soon as 12–18 hours after initial symptoms. Blood cultures are positive in 15–30% of pneumococcal pneumonia cases. Bacteraemia may follow CAP or may also occur without an apparent source of infection and can lead to pneumococcal empyema, endocarditis and pericarditis. Septic arthritis, osteomyelitis, peritonitis and brain abscesses occur rarely.

Laboratory diagnosis of pneumococcal pneumonia can be straightforward. A Gram-stained sputum sample shows large numbers of polymorphonuclear lymphocytes and Gram-positive coccobacilli without the appearance of any or many other bacteria. This may be confirmed by culture on horse blood agar. Colony morphology may indicate draughtsman-shaped colonies, although not all isolates produce this morphology; furthermore, other commensal streptococci may also show this morphology. Bile solubility and optochin sensitivity or commercial kits may be used for confirmatory identification. However, such diagnosis relies heavily on a good-quality sputum sample. If a good sample is not taken, then contaminating commensal bacteria from squamous epithelial cells and saliva will be found in the sputum. If the individual cannot produce an expectorated sample, then nasotracheal suction or, in some cases, bronchoscopy may provide a good sputum sample.

S. pneumoniae is also the most common cause in adults and the second most common cause in young children of bacterial meningitis, except when there is an epidemic of meningococcal disease (Meli *et al.*, 2002). Diagnosis, like pneumococcal pneumonia, is by Gram stain and culture, but additionally capsular antigen may be detected using commercially available assays. These assays are particularly useful in individuals who have received antibiotics before the cerebrospinal fluid (CSF) sample being taken and where Gram stain and culture may be negative. Blood cultures are very useful in diagnosis because they are positive in nearly all cases of pneumococcal meningitis. Molecular methods such as the polymerase chain reaction (PCR) may also be used (Corless *et al.*, 2001; Dominguez *et al.*, 2001; Friedland *et al.*, 1994; Rintamaki *et al.*, 2002). Finally, pneumococci are also the most commonly isolated bacterial pathogens from cases of otitis media and acute sinusitis (Faden, 2001; Turner *et al.*, 2002). Such infections often occur due to predisposition following viral infection but do not usually lead to complications.

The treatment of pneumococcal disease has relied upon penicillin for the past 50 years, and the antibiotic is still used successfully today. Over this time, *S. pneumoniae* has become slightly resistant to the antibiotic; a few highly resistant strains have been isolated, which have probably originated due to horizontal gene transfer (Cunha, 2002; Greenberg *et al.*, 2002; Kyaw *et al.*, 2002a). Resistance to penicillin, chloramphenicol, erythromycin and clindamycin has been noted. However, other antibiotics can be used; amoxicillin is a good alternative to penicillin for the treatment of pneumococcal pneumonia, and for parenteral treatment a first-generation cephalosporin is a good alternative to penicillin. Erythromycin is widely used blindly to treat pneumococcal infection, but increasing resistance to this antibiotic is being noted.

The virulence determinants of *S. pneumoniae* are becoming increasingly understood (Brown *et al.*, 2001; Hava and Camilli, 2002; Lau *et al.*, 2001; Wizemann *et al.*, 2001). Research continues to determine the virulence mechanisms of the organism and whether toxin production is a feature of infection. Complication-free vaccines are available for the prevention of pneumococcal infection and are useful in epidemic settings, in people undergoing splenectomy, and in older individuals; such vaccination should be repeated at five-year intervals. However, it has yet to be determined whether all individuals, with the exception of healthy young adults, should be vaccinated. The question remaining is probably whether the benefits of vaccination are greater than the costs of vaccination. Conjugate vaccines are now becoming available; a seven-valent pneumococcal conjugate vaccine has been licensed in a number of countries and has been used in the USA since 2000 (Darkes and Plosker, 2002; Zimmerman, 2001). Further vaccines are also undergoing development (Obaro and Adegbola, 2002). Due to the availability of pneumococcal genome sequence data, the understanding of pneumococcal virulence is improving (Hava and Camilli, 2002; Lau *et al.*, 2001; Tettelin *et al.*, 2001; Wizemann *et al.*, 2001). This may also lead to improved therapies and vaccines.

REFERENCES

Brown, J.S., Gilliland, S.M. and Holden, D.W. (2001). A *Streptococcus pneumoniae* pathogenicity island encoding an ABC transporter involved in iron uptake and virulence. *Mol Microbiol* 40, 572–85.

Corless, C.E., Guiver, M., Borrow, R., Edwards-Jones, V., Fox, A.J. and Kaczmarski, E.B. (2001). Simultaneous detection of *Neisseria meningitidis*, *Haemophilus influenzae*, and *Streptococcus pneumoniae* in suspected cases of meningitis and septicemia using real-time PCR. *J Clin Microbiol* 39, 1553–8.

Cunha, B.A. (2002). Clinical relevance of penicillin-resistant *Streptococcus pneumoniae*. *Semin Respir Infect* 17, 204–14.

Darkes, M.J. and Plosker, G.L. (2002). Pneumococcal conjugate vaccine (Prevnar trade mark; PNCRM7): a review of its use in the prevention of *Streptococcus pneumoniae* infection. *Paediatr Drugs* 4, 609–30.

Diez-Domingo, J., Pereiro, I., Morant, A., *et al.* (2002). Epidemiology of invasive *Streptococcus pneumoniae* infections in children in Spain, 1996–1998. *J Infect* 45, 139–43.

Dominguez, J., Gali, N., Matas, L., *et al.* (2001). PCR detection of *Streptococcus pneumoniae* DNA in serum samples for pneumococcal pneumonia diagnosis. *Clin Microbiol Infect* 7, 164–6.

El-Solh, A.A., Sikka, P., Ramadan, F. and Davies, J. (2001). Etiology of severe pneumonia in the very elderly. *Am J Respir Crit Care Med* 163, 645–51.

Faden, H. (2001). The microbiologic and immunologic basis for recurrent otitis media in children. *Eur J Pediatr* 160, 407–13.

Friedland, L.R., Menon, A.G., Reising, S.F., Ruddy, R.M. and Hassett, D.J. (1994). Development of a polymerase chain reaction assay to detect the presence of *Streptococcus pneumoniae* DNA. *Diagn Microbiol Infect Dis* 20, 187–93.

Greenberg, D., Speert, D.P., Mahenthiralingam, E., Henry, D.A., Campbell, M.E. and Scheifele, D.W. (2002). Emergence of penicillin-nonsusceptible *Streptococcus pneumoniae* invasive clones in Canada. *J Clin Microbiol* 40, 68–74.

Hava, D. and Camilli, A. (2002). Large-scale identification of serotype 4 *Streptococcus pneumoniae* virulence factors. *Mol Microbiol* 45, 1389–406.

Ip, M., Lyon, D.J. and Cheng, A.F. (2001). Patterns of antibiotic resistance, serotype distribution, and patient demographics of *Streptococcus pneumoniae* in Hong Kong. *Chemotherapy* 47, 110–16.

Jette, L.P., Delage, G., Ringuette, L., *et al.* (2001). Surveillance of invasive *Streptococcus pneumoniae* infection in the province of Quebec, Canada, from 1996 to 1998: serotype distribution, antimicrobial susceptibility, and clinical characteristics. *J Clin Microbiol* 39, 733–7.

Kyaw, M.H., Jones, I.G. and Campbell, H. (2002a). Prevalence of penicillin non-susceptible invasive pneumococcal disease in the elderly in Scotland, 1992–99. *Scand J Infect Dis* 34, 559–63.

Kyaw, M.H., Clarke, S., Jones, I.G. and Campbell, H. (2002b). Incidence of invasive pneumococcal disease in Scotland, 1988–99. *Epidemiol Infect* 128, 139–47.

Lau, G.W., Haataja, S., Lonetto, M., *et al.* (2001). A functional genomic analysis of type 3 *Streptococcus pneumoniae* virulence. *Mol Microbiol* 40, 555–71.

Marrie, T.J. (2000). Community-acquired pneumonia in the elderly. *Clin Infect Dis* 31, 1066–78.

McGee, L., Wang, H., Wasas, A., Huebner, R., Chen, M. and Klugman, K.P. (2001). Prevalence of serotypes and molecular epidemiology of *Streptococcus* pneumoniae strains isolated from children in Beijing, China: identification of two novel multiply-resistant clones. *Microb Drug Resist* **7**, 55–63.

Meli, D.N., Christen, S., Leib, S.L. and Tauber, M.G. (2002). Current concepts in the pathogenesis of meningitis caused by *Streptococcus pneumoniae*. *Curr Opin Infect Dis* **15**, 253–7.

Obaro, S. and Adegbola, R. (2002). The pneumococcus: carriage, disease and conjugate vaccines. *J Med Microbiol* **51**, 98–104.

Petrosillo, N., Pantosti, A., Bordi, E., *et al*. (2002). Prevalence, determinants, and molecular epidemiology of *Streptococcus pneumoniae* isolates colonizing the nasopharynx of healthy children in Rome. *Eur J Clin Microbiol Infect Dis* **21**, 181–8.

Puli, V. and Clarke, S.C. (2002). Clinical aspects of pneumonia. *Br J Biomed Sci* **59**, 170–72.

Rintamaki, S., Saukkoriipi, A., Salo, P., Takala, A. and Leinonen, M. (2002). Detection of *Streptococcus pneumoniae* DNA by using polymerase chain reaction and microwell hybridization with Europium-labelled probes. *J Microbiol Methods* **50**, 313–18.

Robinson, K.A., Baughman, W., Rothrock, G., *et al*. (2001). Epidemiology of invasive *Streptococcus*

pneumoniae infections in the United States, 1995–1998: opportunities for prevention in the conjugate vaccine era. *JAMA* **285**, 1729–35.

Sleeman, K., Knox, K., George, R., *et al*. (2001). Invasive pneumococcal disease in England and Wales: vaccination implications. *J Infect Dis* **183**, 239–46.

Tettelin, H., Nelson, K.E., Paulsen, I.T., *et al*. (2001). Complete genome sequence of a virulent isolate of *Streptococcus pneumoniae*. *Science* **293**, 498–506.

Turner, D., Leibovitz, E., Aran, A., *et al*. (2002). Acute otitis media in infants younger than two months of age: microbiology, clinical presentation and therapeutic approach. *Pediatr Infect Dis J* **21**, 669–74.

Wizemann, T.M., Heinrichs, J.H., Adamou, J.E., *et al*. (2001). Use of a whole genome approach to identify vaccine molecules affording protection against *Streptococcus pneumoniae* infection. *Infect Immun* **69**, 1593–8.

Woodhead, M. (1994). Pneumonia in the elderly. *J Antimicrob Chemother* **34** (suppl A), 85–92.

Zimmerman, R.K. (2001). Pneumococcal conjugate vaccine for young children. *Am Fam Physician* **63**, 1991–8.

36

Haemophilus influenzae

The family *Pasteurellaceae* contains three genera: *Haemophilus*, *Actinobacillus* and *Pasteurella*. There are a number of *Haemophilus* species, some of which are pathogens of humans:

- *H. influenzae*
- *H. aegyptius*
- *H. haemolyticus*
- *H. haemoglobinophilus*
- *H. ducreyi*
- *H. aphrophilus*
- *H. parainfluenzae*
- *H. parahaemolyticus*
- *H. paraphrophilus*
- *H. segnis*
- *H. parasius*
- *H. paragallinarum*
- *H. avium*
- *H. paracuniculus*

H. influenzae is the type species and the main human pathogen within the genus. A number of species are pathogenic, although individuals may also be asymptomatic carriers, except for *H. ducreyi* which is found only in unhealthy individuals and is the cause of chancroid (Al-Tawfiq and Spinola, 2002). *H. influenzae* is an important cause of meningitis worldwide; before the introduction of an effective vaccine, it accounted for one-third of all cases of meningitis in the UK. The bacterium was first described by Pfeiffer in 1892. It is a Gram-negative coccobacillus or rod and requires X (haemin) and V (coenzyme I or II) factors for growth; it also requires carbon dioxide. There are six serotypes of *H. influenzae*, named a–f, based on the scheme developed by Pittman in 1931. The serotypes are denoted by antigenic differences between capsular types. Type b is associated most commonly with disease (Burns and Zimmerman, 2000). Non-encapsulated strains also exist and are usually associated with respiratory infections. Serotyping may be performed by latex agglutination, co-agglutination, counter-current immunoelectrophoresis (CIE), enzyme-linked immunosorbent assay (ELISA), and the polymerase chain reaction (PCR). Serotypes are based on capsule antigen. *H. influenzae* may also be divided into eight biotypes, denoted I–VIII.

H. influenzae has been used extensively for bacterial genetic studies. It was the second example of a naturally transformable bacterium, and it was the first bacterium to have its genome sequenced, in 1995. The non-pathogenic strain, Rd, was sequenced, which has a genome of 1.83 Mb. However, vaccines were developed before the advent of the genome sequence. The genome sequence is also helping researchers to unravel the virulence mechanisms of *H. influenzae*, which are now better understood. Polysaccharide vaccines against *H. influenzae* became available in the 1970s, but these were not immunogenic in children under two years. A conjugate *H. influenzae* type b (Hib) vaccine was later developed and introduced in 1992. This vaccine has an efficacy of 95%, is immunogenic in children under two years, and has a protective lifespan of more than a decade. It has led successfully to the control of Hib in many countries (Almuneef *et al.*, 2001; Heath and McVernon, 2002; Rosenstein and Perkins, 2000), although globally it has had little impact because it has not been introduced in a number of developing countries (Anon, 2002; Peltola, 2000).

H. influenzae is a common commensal: about a fifth of all children carry the organism before they are one year old, and half carry it by the time they are six years old. Each strain may be carried for weeks or even months before it is lost and then another strain may be acquired. Non-typeable strains are associated with non-invasive infections, particularly those involving respiratory system (Murphy, 2000). Non-typeable strains cause up to 30% of all episodes of acute otitis media and 40% of chronic otitis media (St Geme, 2000). Invasive cases of *H. influenzae* present as meningitis (60%), epiglottitis (15%) and septicaemia (10%). The case fatality rate is around 5%. *H. influenzae* meningitis was common in childhood before the introduction of the Hib vaccine in the UK, although it was rare in those aged under two months or over six years. Even so, the overall incidence of invasive disease in those under five years of age was 34/100 000. Nasopharyngeal carriage was also common, aiding in the spread of the bacterium, although only a small percentage of carried *H. influenzae* were serotype b.

Due to the lack of ready access to all required growth supplements, *H. influenzae* does not grow well on standard blood agar. However, heated blood agar (chocolate agar) releases the X and V factors required for growth. On this medium, *H. influenzae* forms grey, smooth colonies that have a characteristic pungent smell due to the production of indole. Basic identification is attained by X and V factor utilization on a basic medium, although biochemical utilization tests are more accurate. *H. influenzae* is catalase- and oxidase-positive, and ferments glucose, galactose and xylose. Strains are usually susceptible to most common antibiotics, including ampicillin, tetracycline, chloramphenicol, rifampicin and trimethoprim. However, more than 10% of strains are now resistant to ampicillin. Infection can also be confirmed using the PCR. Although the total number of cases confirmed by this method are relatively low, because most are confirmed by culture, they help in the surveillance of disease alongside meningitis and septicaemia caused by the meningococcus and pneumococcus.

Good typing methods now exist for the characterization of *H. influenzae*, and multi-locus sequence typing (MLST) has been described recently. This is timely, as the incidence of b and non-b serotypes is changing slightly in the UK, and surveillance centres are monitoring the situation closely. It is thought that the immunity of some individuals immunized with Hib vaccine a decade ago could be decreasing and that 'breakthrough' is occurring with certain serotypes. Techniques such as MLST will also help to determine whether this is the case.

REFERENCES

Almuneef, M., Alshaalan, M., Memish, Z. and Alalola, S. (2001). Bacterial meningitis in Saudi Arabia: the impact of *Haemophilus influenzae* type b vaccination. *J Chemother* **13** (suppl 1), 34–9.

Al-Tawfiq, J.A. and Spinola, S.M. (2002). *Haemophilus ducreyi*: clinical disease and pathogenesis. *Curr Opin Infect Dis* **15**, 43–7.

Anon (2002). Are *Haemophilus influenzae* infections a significant problem in India? A prospective study and review. *Clin Infect Dis* **34**, 949–57.

Burns, I.T. and Zimmerman, R.K. (2000). *Haemophilus influenzae* type B disease, vaccines, and care of exposed individuals. *J Fam Pract* **49**, S7–13, quiz S14.

Heath, P.T. and McVernon, J. (2002). The UK Hib vaccine experience. *Arch Dis Child* **86**, 396–9.

Murphy, T.F. (2000). *Haemophilus influenzae* in chronic bronchitis. *Semin Respir Infect* **15**, 41–51.

Peltola, H. (2000). Worldwide *Haemophilus influenzae* type b disease at the beginning of the 21st century: global analysis of the disease burden 25 years after the use of the polysaccharide vaccine and a decade after the advent of conjugates. *Clin Microbiol Rev* **13**, 302–17.

Rosenstein, N.E. and Perkins, B.A. (2000). Update on *Haemophilus influenzae* serotype b and meningococcal vaccines. *Pediatr Clin North Am* **47**, 337–52, vi.

St Geme, J.W., 3rd (2000). The pathogenesis of nontypable *Haemophilus influenzae* otitis media. *Vaccine* **19** (suppl 1), S41–50.

37

Lyme disease

Lyme disease occurs worldwide and is considered a public health problem in North America, where it is endemic, with problem areas in the north-east, Great Lakes and Pacific north-west areas (Marques, 2001). The disease is caused by infection with the spirochaete *Borrelia burgdorferi*, named after its discoverer, and is transmitted by ticks that inhabit wooded areas and low-lying grassland. In the USA, Lyme disease is the most common vector-borne disease among children. Its incidence is greater in children than in adults. The disease is named after the town of Old Lyme, CT, USA, after a cluster of arthritis cases occurred there in the 1970s and were later found to be due to spirochaete infection.

In Europe, the main species of tick that transmits infection is *Ixodes ricinus*. In the USA, the most common tick vector is *Ixodes scapularis* (deer tick), although other species, including *Amblyomma americanum* (lone star tick) and *Ixodes pacificus*, have been reported. It is estimated that between 1 and 90% of ticks can be infected with spirochaete, depending on the geographic location. Summer is typically the tick season, although Lyme disease can occur all year. Ticks become inactive at temperatures below about 5 °C, and therefore they are more active between April and October, leading to an increase in cases of Lyme disease at this time. Ticks cannot tolerate dry conditions. They have a two-year lifecycle consisting of three developmental stages. At each stage, the tick must feed. In the larval stage, the tick is very small (about the size of a pinhead) and feeds on the blood of small mammals, from which it may pick up the spirochaete. During the nymph stage, the tick is larger and feeds on the blood of larger mammals, such as cats and dogs.

Adult ticks feed on the blood of cattle, deer, dogs and humans.

In the USA, Lyme disease has been reported in 48 states. Its incidence varies from 8/100 000 population to as high as 1000/100 000 population. This dramatic variation in incidence is dependent wholly on the location within the USA. Generally, Lyme disease is more common in the eastern half of the USA, with increased incidence around Wisconsin and the north-eastern coast. In 1997, provisional data indicated that over 12 500 cases of Lyme disease were reported in the USA. There has been a 25-fold annual increase in reported cases since 1982. Compared with the USA, Lyme disease is uncommon in the UK, but there are around 50 cases per year. The New Forest area of England has been a focus for Lyme disease due to the habitat of this area and its relatively mild climate compared with other areas of the country. Lyme disease can also be found in low numbers throughout Europe (Hercogova and Brzonova, 2001).

Lyme disease is difficult to diagnose clinically because it mimics many other diseases. A rash, known as erythema migrans, typically occurs several days after infection, although in some patients there may be no rash (Montiel *et al.*, 2002). The rash can be small or very large in skin surface area and lasts from hours to several weeks. The rash occurs in about 85% of cases and can be characteristic of the disease; it was first described a century ago and begins as red macules or papules of erythema. Erythema migrans must be distinguished from other similar rashes caused by various cellulitis and dermatitis conditions. Flu-like symptoms often develop several days or weeks after infection, symptoms that are again similar to those of many other diseases. Other symptoms of Lyme disease are wide-ranging and may affect any organ of the body (Donta, 2002; Huppertz, 2001; Marques, 2001; Pinto, 2002) (Table 37.1). In addition, infection during pregnancy can lead to premature birth or miscarriage.

The gold standard for the laboratory diagnosis of Lyme disease is culture, although the most practical approach is by antibody detection (Bunikis and Barbour, 2002; van Dam, 2001). Although culture can be performed on blood, urine or cerebrospinal fluid (CSF), it lacks clinical sensitivity. However, false-positives with other flagellated organisms may occur, and cross-reactions are possible in the presence of rheumatoid factor or antinuclear antibodies. The humoral response is slow, but infected individuals display a good immunoglobulin M (IgM) and increased immunoglobulin G (IgG) levels about six weeks after initial infection. Although a polymerase chain reaction (PCR) test is available, false-positive results may occur (Dumler, 2001; van Dam, 2001).

Most ticks are not infected with spirochaete, and therefore prophylactic treatment after a tick bite is not necessary (Hu and Klempner, 2001; Ravishankar and Lutwick, 2001). Most infections are mild and do not warrant antibiotic therapy. Lyme disease is treatable using standard antibiotics for a recommended period of four to six weeks. Typical choices are penicillin, tetracycline, cefuroxime and erythromycin. No vaccine against Lyme

disease is licensed for use in humans in the UK. However, a vaccine has recently been licensed by the Food and Drug Administration (FDA) for use in the USA. The vaccine consists of an outer-membrane protein from *B. burgdorferi* and is given by intramuscular injection in three doses. It may be used in people aged between 15 and 70 years. It is not known how long the vaccine lasts and whether booster doses are required. A vaccine is also available for dogs, which reduces the possibility of transmission of Lyme disease to humans. The genome of *B. burgdorferi* has been sequenced, and research into its virulence mechanisms continues (Weis, 2002). Such research may lead to the development of additional therapies.

REFERENCES

Bunikis, J. and Barbour, A.G. (2002). Laboratory testing for suspected Lyme disease. *Med Clin North Am* 86, 311–40.

Donta, S.T. (2002). Late and chronic Lyme disease. *Med Clin North Am* 86, 341–9, vii.

Dumler, J.S. (2001). Molecular diagnosis of Lyme disease: review and meta-analysis. *Mol Diagn* 6, 1–11.

Hercogova, J. and Brzonova, I. (2001). Lyme disease in central Europe. *Curr Opin Infect Dis* 14, 133–7.

Hu, L.T. and Klempner, M.S. (2001). Update on the prevention, diagnosis, and treatment of Lyme disease. *Adv Intern Med* 46, 247–75.

Huppertz, H.I. (2001). Lyme disease in children. *Curr Opin Rheumatol* 13, 434–40.

Marques, A.R. (2001). Lyme disease: an update. *Curr Allergy Asthma Rep* 1, 541–9.

Montiel, N.J., Baumgarten, J.M. and Sinha, A.A. (2002). Lyme disease–part II: clinical features and treatment. *Cutis* 69, 443–8.

Pinto, D.S. (2002). Cardiac manifestations of Lyme disease. *Med Clin North Am* 86, 285–96.

Ravishankar, J. and Lutwick, L.I. (2001). Current and future treatment of Lyme disease. *Expert Opin Pharmacother* 2, 241–51.

Table 37.1 Some of the symptoms of Lyme disease

Rash (erythema migrans)

Respiratory infection

Pericarditis

Conjunctivitis

Lymphadenopathy

Meningitis

Abdominal cramps

Arthritis

Van Dam, A.P. (2001). Recent advances in the diagnosis of Lyme disease. *Expert Rev Mol Diagn* **1**, 413–27.

Weis, J.J. (2002). Host-pathogen interactions and the pathogenesis of murine Lyme disease. *Curr Opin Rheumatol* **14**, 399–403.

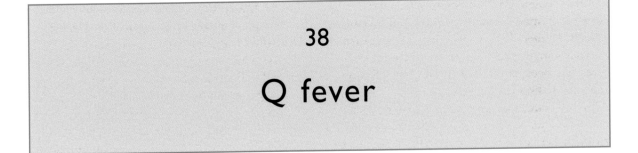

38

Q fever

Q fever (query fever) was first described in 1937 by Edward Derrick, after he investigated an outbreak of febrile illness that had occurred among abattoir workers in Queensland, Australia, in 1935. He was able to distinguish the disease from other abattoir fevers and typhus, although he did not know the identity of the causative organism. In 1937, researchers described the cause of Q fever after injecting blood or urine from Derrick's patients into guinea pigs. They isolated a fastidious intracellular bacterium that they called *Rickettsia burnetii*; the organism was later reclassified and named *Coxiella burnetii*. It was subsequently noted that Q fever is a zoonotic disease and is widespread throughout the world, except in New Zealand (Hellenbrand *et al.*, 2001; Maurin and Raoult, 1999; Serbezov *et al.*, 1999). It presents as either an acute or chronic disease. Endocarditis is its most serious form, occurring in 1–11% of cases.

Q fever is responsible for a wide range of clinical symptoms. Due to the absence of a specific clinical syndrome, the true incidence of the disease is not known. It is probably underreported at present, and it is therefore difficult to assess the impact that this disease has on the world population. Seroprevalence studies in Europe have indicated that between 5 and 30% of the general population have antibodies to *C. burnetii*. Lower figures are seen in urban areas, and higher figures occur in rural zones. *C. burnetii* has been isolated from a number of mammals, birds and ticks, and therefore the potential sources for zoonotic infection are widespread (Maltezou and Raoult, 2002). Ticks are thought to be the important vector for transmission to humans. However, pets have been associated with urban outbreaks of disease in humans.

C. burnetii is a fastidious intracellular Gram-negative bacterium. It is the only member of the genus *Coxiella*. The organism lives and multiplies within the lysosomes of infected cells. It has a spore-like cycle, which enables it to survive in the environment; it is also able to resist heat and disinfection. The disease is spread most commonly by inhalation or ingestion of the causative organism; it has an incubation period of one to four weeks (Norlander, 2000). The disease may be acute or chronic, and the clinical symptoms vary widely.

Acute Q fever is normally self-limiting, and many cases occur with seroconversion but no symptoms. However, acute infection may present with high fever accompanied by muscle pain and severe headache, usually lasting between one and two weeks, although recovery may be delayed in individuals with hepatitis or pneumonia. About 20% of individuals develop a maculopapular rash on the trunk. During pregnancy, Q fever infection may cause abortion or stillbirth (Jover-Diaz *et al.*, 2001; Raoult *et al.*, 2002). Up to 15% of patients develop post-Q fever chronic fatigue syndrome, which may last many months.

Chronic Q fever, which often presents as culture-negative endocarditis, is difficult to treat and can be fatal. Q fever endocarditis has been recognized for over 20 years and occurs in 5% of patients (Marrie and Raoult, 2002). Interestingly, most patients with Q fever endocarditis have pre-existing heart valve abnormalities for congenital, rheumatic, degenerative or syphilitic reasons. Although children can develop Q fever endocarditis, around 75% of patients are over the age of 40 and male. As the symptoms are non-specific and generally not indicative of endocarditis, diagnosis may take some time. More recently, Q fever has been implicated in chronic infection of the liver, known as granulomatous hepatitis. Although rare, this may be misdiagnosed if it is associated with endocarditis, but it is important to diagnose correctly as it can lead to cirrhosis. Chronic Q fever has also been associated with vascular infection and bone and joint infection.

Clinical diagnosis is based on the initial presenting symptoms and aided by epidemiological links (Table 38.1). A chest X-ray is the only imaging study likely to be useful. An atypical pneumonia pattern similar to that seen with mycoplasma, chlamydia, *Legionella* and viral pneumonia may be seen. Standard haematology and biochemistry tests are not usually diagnostic. The white blood cell count is most often normal, but the platelet count can be low initially, with a reactive thrombocytosis during the convalescence stage. Laboratory diagnosis is proven by serological testing (Hindiyeh and Carroll, 2000; Scola, 2002). Determination of antibodies to *C. burnetii* can be achieved by using complement fixation, indirect immunofluorescent antibodies (IFA) and enzyme-linked immunosorbent assay (ELISA) tests. No polymerase chain reaction (PCR) test has been developed.

Prompt treatment is important to ensure that the development of chronic infection is avoided. Antibiotic therapy is indicated for acute and chronic disease due to Q fever (Gikas *et al.*, 2001). Such treatment should continue for at least five days after the fever stops. Unfortunately, most patients with post-Q fever chronic fatigue do not respond to such therapy. Most infected individuals will improve without treatment, but antibiotic therapy is necessary to prevent progression to chronic disease, which is far more resistant to treatment. It is suggested that treatment should be prolonged for Q fever endocarditis (Calza *et al.*, 2002). Surgical therapy, such as valve replacement, is sometimes necessary, although prosthetic valves are a common locus for *C. burnetii* infection and subsequent endocarditis.

Table 38.1 Differential diagnosis of Q fever

Bacterial pneumonia
Hepatitis
Legionnaires' disease
Myocarditis
Viral pneumonia
Other tick diseases

REFERENCES

Calza, L., Attard, L., Manfredi, R. and Chiodo, F. (2002). Doxycycline and chloroquine as treatment for chronic Q fever endocarditis. *J Infect* 45, 127–9.

Gikas, A., Kofteridis, D.P., Manios, A., Pediaditis, J. and Tselentis, Y. (2001). Newer macrolides as empiric treatment for acute Q fever infection. *Antimicrob Agents Chemother* 45, 3644–6.

Hellenbrand, W., Breuer, T. and Petersen, L. (2001). Changing epidemiology of Q fever in Germany, 1947–1999. *Emerg Infect Dis* 7, 789–96.

Hindiyeh, M. and Carroll, K.C. (2000). Laboratory diagnosis of atypical pneumonia. *Semin Respir Infect* 15, 101–13.

Jover-Diaz, F., Robert-Gates, J., Andreu-Gimenez, L. and Merino-Sanchez, J. (2001). Q fever during pregnancy: an emerging cause of prematurity and abortion. *Infect Dis Obstet Gynecol* 9, 47–9.

Maltezou, H.C. and Raoult, D. (2002). Q fever in children. *Lancet Infect Dis* 2, 686–91.

Marrie, T.J. and Raoult, D. (2002). Update on Q fever, including Q fever endocarditis. *Curr Clin Top Infect Dis* 22, 97–124.

Maurin, M. and Raoult, D. (1999). Q fever. *Clin Microbiol Rev* 12, 518–53.

Norlander, L. (2000). Q fever epidemiology and pathogenesis. *Microbes Infect* 2, 417–24.

Raoult, D., Fenollar, F. and Stein, A. (2002). Q fever during pregnancy: diagnosis, treatment, and follow-up. *Arch Intern Med* **162**, 701–4.

Scola, B.L. (2002). Current laboratory diagnosis of Q fever. *Semin Pediatr Infect Dis* **13**, 257–62.

Serbezov, V.S., Kazar, J., Novkirishki, V., Gatcheva, N., Kovacova, E. and Voynova, V. (1999). Q fever in Bulgaria and Slovakia. *Emerg Infect Dis* **5**, 388–94.

39

Leptospirosis (Weil's disease)

Leptospirosis (or Weil's disease) is a bacterial disease that affects both humans and animals (Vinetz, 2001). It is caused by one of a number of genera of *Leptospira*. The disease was first described fully in 1887 by Goldsmidt for a syndrome of severe febrile illness with jaundice and renal abnormalities that had been described by Adolph Weil the previous year.

The family *Leptospiraceae* comprises helical, motile organisms. There are two genera, *Leptospira* and *Leptonema*, the latter of which is not of medical importance and therefore will not be discussed here. The genera *Leptospira* contains three species, namely *L. interrogans*, *L. biflexa* and *L. parva*. The former includes 23 serogroups (Table 39.1) and more than 200 serotypes and is the principal cause of leptospirosis in humans and animals. Traditionally, serotypes were identified by agglutination tests with polyclonal sera and, more recently, monoclonal antibodies. Increasingly, however, genetic studies are identifying new serotypes or subtypes. For example, serotype *hardjo* is now divided into two subtypes, *hardjo-prajitno* and *hardjo-bovis*. Serotype classification has shown that the disease is basically the same regardless of the serotype of infection; although certain serotypes were once thought to be responsible for specific symptoms, this is now known not to be the case.

Every year in the USA, between 100 and 200 cases of leptospirosis are identified. Interestingly, about half of these occur in Hawaii. A similar proportion of cases is thought to occur in the UK each year. Although the incidence of leptospirosis is relatively low in the USA and the UK, the disease is considered by many to be the most widespread

Table 39.1 Serogroups of Leptospira interrogans

Australis
Autumnalis
Ballum
Bataviae
Canicola
Celledoni
Cynopteri
Djasiman
Grippotyphosa
Hebdomadis
Icterohaemorrhagiae
Javanica
Lousiana
Manhoa
Mini
Panama
Pomona
Pyrogenes
Ranarum
Sarmin
Sejroe
Shermani
Tarrasovi

zoonotic disease worldwide (Bishara *et al.*, 2002; Chandrasekaran, 1999; Lomar *et al.*, 2000; Thornley *et al.*, 2002). Leptospirosis occurs worldwide but is most common in temperate and tropical climates. It is an occupational hazard for many people who work outdoors or with animals, such as farmers, sewer workers and vets. It is also a recreational hazard for campers and those who participate in water sports.

Various animals may be infected by *Leptospira*; they may or may not become symptomatic. These animals can act as potential sources for human infection. *Leptospira* have been isolated from cattle, pigs, horses, dogs, rodents and other wild animals (Hartskeerl and Terpstra, 1996). Infections in pets, such as cats and dogs, provide additional risks for zoonotic infection. Various serotypes of *L. interrogans* are normally found in animals. However, the introduction of animal vaccines against leptospirosis has led to a reduction in associated human cases. For example, a dramatic fall in the number of notified cases of this disease in humans coincided in Australia with the introduction of a bivalent animal vaccine against serotypes *pomona* and *hardjobovis*. The vaccine was introduced at the end of 1979, and the notifications of human infection dropped from 677 to 325 in two years. Humans may become infected through contact with water, food or soil contaminated with urine from infected animals. This may happen by swallowing contaminated food or water, or through skin contact, especially via mucosal surfaces, such as the eyes or nose, or via broken skin. The disease is not thought to spread by person-to-person contact.

In humans, leptospirosis presents with a wide range of symptoms. After infection, the onset period is between two days and four weeks. Symptoms usually begin abruptly, with fever accompanied by chills, headache, muscle aches, vomiting and diarrhoea (Rajajee *et al.*, 2002). Such unspecific symptoms may not point towards leptospirosis. The course of infection may occur in two phases. After the initial phase, the individual may recover before becoming ill again. The second phase is also called Weil's disease and is more severe than the first. The symptoms may include respiratory failure, kidney or liver failure, and meningitis (Vieira and Brauner, 2002; Yang *et al.*, 2001). The illness can last from a few days to more than three weeks, and recovery can take many months if left untreated. Leptospirosis causes death only rarely.

Many of the symptoms of leptospirosis can be mistaken for other diseases. Therefore, clinical suspicion must be raised followed by a supportive laboratory diagnosis. Infection with the organism can be demonstrated by antigen detection, strain isolation and serological tests. Antigen detection and strain isolation can be performed on blood or urine samples. Serological tests are probably most useful for the laboratory confirmation of leptospirosis and, in theory, can be performed in any clinical laboratory. Tests include enzyme-linked immunosorbent assay (ELISA), complement fixation test (CFT) and immunofluorescence (Field *et al.*, 2002). Polymerase chain reaction (PCR) tests are now also being developed (Smythe *et al.*, 2002).

Leptospirosis is treated with antibiotics, which should be given early in the course of the disease (Guidugli *et al.*, 2000). Apart from chloramphenicol, most other commonly used antibiotics can also be used to treat leptospirosis. Intravenous antibiotics may be required for patients with more severe symptoms. As immune protection is generally serotype-specific, vaccination is not a realistic option unless prepared from a local strain. However, molecular research is providing information that may lead to the development of new vaccines (Zuerner *et al.*, 2000). The scientific community also awaits with anticipation the leptospiral genome sequence (Vinetz, 2001).

REFERENCES

Bishara, J., Amitay, E., Barnea, A., Yitzhaki, S. and Pitlik, S. (2002). Epidemiological and clinical features of leptospirosis in Israel. *Eur J Clin Microbiol Infect Dis* **21**, 50–52.

Chandrasekaran, S. (1999). Review on human leptospirosis. *Indian J Med Sci* **53**, 291–8.

Field, P.R., Santiago, A., Chan, S.W., *et al.* (2002). Evaluation of a novel commercial enzyme-linked immunosorbent assay detecting *Coxiella burnetii*-

specific immunoglobulin G for Q fever prevaccination screening and diagnosis. *J Clin Microbiol* **40**, 3526–9.

Guidugli, F., Castro, A.A. and Atallah, A.N. (2000). Antibiotics for preventing leptospirosis. *Cochrane Database Syst Rev*, CD001305.

Hartskeerl, R.A. and Terpstra, W.J. (1996). Leptospirosis in wild animals. *Vet Q* **18** (suppl 3), S149–50.

Lomar, A.V., Diament, D. and Torres, J.R. (2000). Leptospirosis in Latin America. *Infect Dis Clin North Am* **14**, 23–39, vii–viii.

Rajajee, S., Shankar, J. and Dhattatri, L. (2002). Pediatric presentations of leptospirosis. *Indian J Pediatr* **69**, 851–3.

Smythe, L.D., Smith, I.L., Smith, G.A., *et al.* (2002). A quantitative PCR (TaqMan) assay for pathogenic *Leptospira* spp. *BMC Infect Dis* **2**, 13.

Thornley, C.N., Baker, M.G., Weinstein, P. and Maas, E.W. (2002). Changing epidemiology of human leptospirosis in New Zealand. *Epidemiol Infect* **128**, 29–36.

Vieira, S.R. and Brauner, J.S. (2002). Leptospirosis as a cause of acute respiratory failure: clinical features and outcome in 35 critical care patients. *Braz J Infect Dis* **6**, 135–9.

Vinetz, J.M. (2001). Leptospirosis. *Curr Opin Infect Dis* **14**, 527–38.

Yang, C.W., Wu, M.S. and Pan, M.J. (2001). Leptospirosis renal disease. *Nephrol Dial Transplant* **16** (suppl 5), 73–7.

Zuerner, R., Haake, D., Adler, B. and Segers, R. (2000). Technological advances in the molecular biology of *Leptospira. J Mol Microbiol Biotechnol* **2**, 455–62.

40

Brucellosis

Brucellosis, also known as undulant fever and Bang's disease, is a disease that affects cattle worldwide and can be spread among various wildlife species. Although the spread from wildlife to humans is thought to be slight, the spread from cattle and other domestic animals to humans remains a public health problem. The disease is a zoonosis both of public health and economic significance in many developing countries. It has been brought under control in developed countries, leading to a decrease in human cases. However, where an animal reservoir exists, human cases still occur.

Brucellae are small, non-motile, non-sporing, Gram-negative coccobacilli. They grow aerobically but poorly on standard laboratory media; they require blood or serum for improved growth. There are several species (Table 40.1). Species are associated within certain animal species, hence their species names. Each species is divided further into biogroups based on the A and M antigen determinants within the lipopolysaccharide cell envelope. The type species, *B. melitensis*, was first isolated in 1887 by Bruce (hence the genera name)

Table 40.1 Common species of *Brucella*

B. abortus
B. melitensis
B. suis
B. canis
B. ovis
B. neotomae

from the spleen of a patient who had died of Malta fever.

Brucellosis is a systemic infection (Sauret and Vilissova, 2002). *B. abortus* is the species associated most commonly with host animal and human disease. The incubation period is usually one to three weeks but may be as much as several months The symptoms of human brucellosis are highly variable; they include fever, night sweats, fatigue, anorexia, weight loss, headache and arthralgia. During the acute phase, which occurs less than eight weeks after onset of symptoms, non-specific signs are common and resemble a flu-like condition. During the undulant phase, which occurs less than one year after onset, symptoms include a characteristic undulant fever and arthritis. In the chronic phase, which occurs more than one year after onset, symptoms include chronic fatigue syndrome and depression. Sequelae may include granulomatous hepatitis, peripheral arthritis, anaemia, meningitis, uveitis and endocarditis (Delahaye *et al.*, 2002). Human disease is normally associated with the consumption of raw milk and cheeses made with raw milk. Risk of human infection is increased in farmers and animal health professionals due to direct exposure with infected animals or exposure with needlesticks after giving immunizations. Laboratory workers are also at risk, as the organism is highly transmissible.

The geographical distribution of human cases of brucellosis is related directly to the distribution of animal brucellosis. Most human cases are caused by *B. melitensis*. Previously, *B. abortus* was most common in Europe, until bovine brucellosis was brought under control. Brucellosis is a widespread disease, with millions of individuals at risk of the disease worldwide, especially in developing countries, where a significant animal reservoir exists (Bandara and Mahipala, 2002; Baumgarten, 2002; Deqiu *et al.*, 2002; Dobrean *et al.*, 2002; Godfroid and Kasbohrer, 2002; Luna-Martinez and Mejia-Teran, 2002; McDermott and Arimi, 2002; Moreno, 2002; Poester *et al.*, 2002; Refai, 2002; Renukaradhya *et al.*, 2002; Rivera *et al.*, 2002; Samartino, 2002; Taleski *et al.*, 2002; Vargas, 2002). In these countries, milk pasteurization is not routine and the consumption of raw milk products is common. In the USA, there are fewer than 0.5 cases per 100 000 population, with most cases being reported from California, Florida, Texas and Virginia. In many countries, brucellosis is a notifiable disease.

The clinical diagnosis of brucellosis is difficult due to the occurrence of subclinical and atypical infections, and because of the wide range of presenting symptoms. Therefore, laboratory confirmation is often essential in order to gain a diagnosis. However, even laboratory confirmation is difficult. *Brucellae* may be isolated from blood culture or other clinical samples, but this is dependent on the presence of live organisms. As such, blood cultures may be negative if antibiotics have been administered in advance. The organisms may also be demonstrated by direct or indirect immunofluorescence in clinical samples. Serological confirmation can be ascertained by a four-fold or greater rise in *Brucella* agglutination titre between acute and convalescent phase sera (Morata *et al.*, 2003; Nielsen, 2002; Ozturk *et al.*, 2002). Polymerase chain reaction (PCR) assays are now also becoming available (Bricker, 2002; Richtzenhain *et al.*, 2002). *Brucella* is susceptible to many antibiotics, but since the organism is localized intracellularly treatment requires the use of more than one antibiotic for several weeks. The most effective antibiotics against *Brucella* are the tetracyclines. Rifampicin is also effective, but the *Brucella* strain used in the animal vaccine is resistant to this antibiotic. Rifampicin must be used with caution in people with a possible occupational exposure to brucellosis.

Programmes to control brucellosis have been based on various strategies, including vaccination and slaughter of infected animals. These programmes have been successful in controlling the disease in animals in several countries and have therefore reduced the number of cases of disease in humans. Pasteurization of milk and milk products is also essential in the prevention of human brucellosis. However, customs in some countries do not allow for such treatment. The Brucellosis Eradication Program was established to eradicate the disease in the USA. Between 1956 and 1998, the number of herds infected with *Brucella* was reduced from 124 000 to 15. However, bison and elk in the northern Rocky Mountain states remain infected with *Brucella* and could act as reservoirs for the reintroduction of brucellosis into domestic livestock herds. The World Health Organization (WHO) has also been involved in the control of brucellosis for many years because of the human and economic concerns.

The virulence mechanisms of *Brucella* are becoming better understood (DelVecchio *et al.*, 2002b; Ko and Splitter, 2003). It is now known that they possess type IV secretion mechanisms, similar to other bacterial pathogens (Boschiroli *et al.*, 2002; Christie and Vogel, 2000). *Brucella* genome sequences, including those of *B. melitensis*, *B. suis* and *B. abortus*, are now also becoming available (DelVecchio *et al.*, 2002a; Michaux-Charachon *et al.*, 2002), which may lead to the development of vaccines that would be particularly useful for use in domestic animals (Schurig *et al.*, 2002).

REFERENCES

Bandara, A.B. and Mahipala, M.B. (2002). Incidence of brucellosis in Sri Lanka: an overview. *Vet Microbiol* 90, 197–207.

Baumgarten, D. (2002). Brucellosis: a short review of the disease situation in Paraguay. *Vet Microbiol* 90, 63–9.

Boschiroli, M.L., Ouahrani-Bettache, S., Foulongne, V., *et al.* (2002). Type IV secretion and *Brucella* virulence. *Vet Microbiol* 90, 341–8.

Bricker, B.J. (2002). PCR as a diagnostic tool for brucellosis. *Vet Microbiol* **90**, 435–46.

Christie, P.J. and Vogel, J.P. (2000). Bacterial type IV secretion: conjugation systems adapted to deliver effector molecules to host cells. *Trends Microbiol* **8**, 354–60.

Delahaye, F., Hoen, B., McFadden, E., Roth, O. and de Gevigney, G. (2002). Treatment and prevention of infective endocarditis. *Expert Opin Pharmacother* **3**, 131–45.

DelVecchio, V.G., Kapatral, V., Elzer, P., Patra, G. and Mujer, C.V. (2002a). The genome of *Brucella melitensis*. *Vet Microbiol* **90**, 587–92.

DelVecchio, V.G., Wagner, M.A., Eschenbrenner, M., *et al.* (2002b). *Brucella* proteomes – a review. *Vet Microbiol* **90**, 593–603.

Deqiu, S., Donglou, X. and Jiming, Y. (2002). Epidemiology and control of brucellosis in China. *Vet Microbiol* **90**, 165–82.

Dobrean, V., Opris, A. and Daraban, S. (2002). An epidemiological and surveillance overview of brucellosis in Romania. *Vet Microbiol* **90**, 157–63.

Godfroid, J. and Kasbohrer, A. (2002). Brucellosis in the European Union and Norway at the turn of the twenty-first century. *Vet Microbiol* **90**, 135–45.

Ko, J. and Splitter, G.A. (2003). Molecular host-pathogen interaction in brucellosis: current understanding and future approaches to vaccine development for mice and humans. *Clin Microbiol Rev* **16**, 65–78.

Luna-Martinez, J.E. and Mejia-Teran, C. (2002). Brucellosis in Mexico: current status and trends. *Vet Microbiol* **90**, 19–30.

McDermott, J.J. and Arimi, S.M. (2002). Brucellosis in sub-Saharan Africa: epidemiology, control and impact. *Vet Microbiol* **90**, 111–34.

Michaux-Charachon, S., Jumas-Bilak, E., Allardet-Servent, A., *et al.* (2002). The *Brucella* genome at the beginning of the post-genomic era. *Vet Microbiol* **90**, 581–5.

Morata, P., Queipo-Ortuno, M.I., Reguera, J.M., Garcia-Ordonez, M.A., Cardenas, A. and Colmenero, J.D. (2003). Development and evaluation of a pcr-enzyme-linked immunosorbent assay for diagnosis of human brucellosis. *J Clin Microbiol* **41**, 144–8.

Moreno, E. (2002). Brucellosis in central America. *Vet Microbiol* **90**, 31–8.

Nielsen, K. (2002). Diagnosis of brucellosis by serology. *Vet Microbiol* **90**, 447–59.

Ozturk, R., Mert, A., Kocak, F., *et al.* (2002). The diagnosis of brucellosis by use of BACTEC 9240 blood culture system. *Diagn Microbiol Infect Dis* **44**, 133–5.

Poester, F.P., Goncalves, V.S. and Lage, A.P. (2002). Brucellosis in Brazil. *Vet Microbiol* **90**, 55–62.

Refai, M. (2002). Incidence and control of brucellosis in the Near East region. *Vet Microbiol* **90**, 81–110.

Renukaradhya, G.J., Isloor, S. and Rajasekhar, M. (2002). Epidemiology, zoonotic aspects, vaccination and control/eradication of brucellosis in India. *Vet Microbiol* **90**, 183–95.

Richtzenhain, L.J., Cortez, A., Heinemann, M.B., *et al.* (2002). A multiplex PCR for the detection of *Brucella* spp. and *Leptospira* spp. DNA from aborted bovine fetuses. *Vet Microbiol* **87**, 139–47.

Rivera, S.A., Ramirez, M.C. and Lopetegui, I.P. (2002). Eradication of bovine brucellosis in the 10th Region de Los Lagos, Chile. *Vet Microbiol* **90**, 45–53.

Samartino, L.E. (2002). Brucellosis in Argentina. *Vet Microbiol* **90**, 71–80.

Sauret, J.M. and Vilissova, N. (2002). Human brucellosis. *J Am Board Fam Pract* **15**, 401–6.

Schurig, G.G., Sriranganathan, N. and Corbel, M.J. (2002). Brucellosis vaccines: past, present and future. *Vet Microbiol* **90**, 479–96.

Taleski, V., Zerva, L., Kantardjiev, T., *et al.* (2002). An overview of the epidemiology and epizootology of brucellosis in selected countries of Central and Southeast Europe. *Vet Microbiol* **90**, 147–55.

Vargas, O.F. (2002). Brucellosis in Venezuela. *Vet Microbiol* **90**, 39–44.

41

Mycoplasma infection

Mycoplasma is a little publicized organism that is a pathogen of almost 200 different species of plants and animals. The organism infects humans and can cause a whole range of infections, some of which are of disputed aetiology. *Mycoplasma*, and the related *Ureaplasma* and *Acholeplasma*, are common organisms found mainly in the mouth and respiratory tract of humans and animals. There are over 80 species within these three genera, although the majority are of the genus *Mycoplasma*. Many of the species are host-specific. Some cause serious diseases, while others are non-pathogenic.

Mycoplasma were first given their name in 1929 by Nowak to describe the group of wall-less organisms. Human infection was described in 1938 by Reimann, who observed cases of atypical pneumonia. The name *Mycoplasma* was re-proposed in the 1950s. *Mycoplasma* belong to the order *Mycoplasmatales*. They are pleomorphic organisms that have a triple-layered membrane instead of a cell wall. *Mycoplasma* do not stain well by most methods; however, they are Gram-negative and they do stain by the Giemsa method. The microscopic morphology of *Mycoplasma* varies widely, according to the species and growth conditions. Their usual size is between 0.3 and 0.4 μm in width and 100 μm in length. *Mycoplasma* require rich media for growth due to their limited biosynthetic capabilities. *Mycoplasma* are thought to be the closest to the most minimal organism that can still self-replicate. Only a dozen mycoplasma species have been isolated from humans, 10 of which were of the genus *Mycoplasma*. The majority are isolated from the oropharynx and are not normally associated with disease. Only *M. pneumoniae* has

been implicated in serious human disease, although *M. genitalium* is emerging as an important cause of genital disease and has also been recovered from respiratory secretions (Deguchi and Maeda, 2002; Herrmann and Reiner, 1998). Other *Mycoplasma* have also been related to various clinical conditions (Fernandez Guerrero *et al.*, 1999; Uuskula and Kohl, 2002).

M. pneumoniae is a common cause of community-acquired pneumonia (CAP) (Andersen, 1998; Principi and Esposito, 2001). The organism occurs worldwide and causes endemic infection in many countries. In temperate climates, infection is most common during the late summer and early autumn months. The incubation period is approximately three weeks. In the USA, an infection rate of around 6% is thought to occur, but most infections are mild, presenting as subclinical or mild upper-respiratory tract infection, while others are completely asymptomatic (Cimolai, 1998). However, a small number of infections can lead to pneumonia and other complications (Chan *et al.*, 1999; Chian and Chang, 1999; Paz and Potasman, 2002). Although person-to-person spread occurs, it is slow and requires repeated contact. Infection is more common in children than in adults; pneumonia is more common in younger children but becomes more severe in older children. Disease is usually limited to the respiratory tract and results in a range of symptoms, including fever, malaise, dry cough, headache and sore throat. Serious complications are uncommon, although extrapulmonary infections do occur sometimes during or after respiratory tract infection (Table 41.1). *M. pneumoniae* has two properties that result in the pathology seen during infection: the organism has

Table 41.1 Sites of *Mycoplasma pneumoniae* infection

Site	Frequency
Cardiovascular	<5%
Dermatological	5%
Gastrointestinal	Up to 50%
Haematological	Up to 50%
Musculoskeletal	Up to 50%
Neurological	5%
Pulmonary	>80%
Urogenital	<1%

an affinity for respiratory epithelial cells, and it produces hydrogen peroxide, which causes cell damage.

A definitive diagnosis based on symptoms is not usually possible. The differential diagnosis includes many other viral illnesses, so a laboratory confirmation is required. This may be achieved by culture and serological testing. Edward medium is often used for the isolation of the organism, although in the absence of other organisms *Mycoplasma* can be grown on standard blood agar medium. Growth is slow, taking between one and three weeks. Identification of *M. pneumoniae* after culture is achieved with the use of antisera, using various methods, including disc susceptibility and immunofluorescence. The polymerase chain reaction (PCR) may also be used for the detection of *M. pneumoniae* from throat or nasopharyngeal swabs and can be 100–1000-fold more sensitive than culture (Honda *et al.*, 2000). Serological testing may be specific or non-specific, depending on the type of test used, but is useful in the absence of a positive culture or negative PCR result.

The tetracyclines are the most effective antibiotics against *Mycoplasma*, although erythromycin is also very effective against *M. pneumoniae*. Reinfection can occur, even in the presence of high antibody titres, and serum antibodies do not therefore normally confer full protection. No effective vaccine is available against *M. pneumoniae* infection. However, the genomes of *M. pneumoniae* and *M. genitalium* have been sequenced recently; therefore, the mechanisms involved during mycoplasma infection may be defined during the coming years, which may lead to the development of better drugs or even vaccines against the organism (Herrmann and Reiner, 1998).

REFERENCES

Andersen, P. (1998). Pathogenesis of lower respiratory tract infections due to *Chlamydia*, *Mycoplasma*, *Legionella* and viruses. *Thorax* **53**, 302–7.

Chan, E.D., Kalayanamit, T., Lynch, D.A., *et al.* (1999). *Mycoplasma pneumoniae*-associated bronchiolitis causing severe restrictive lung disease in adults: report of three cases and literature review. *Chest* **115**, 1188–94.

Chian, C.F. and Chang, F.Y. (1999). Acute respiratory distress syndrome in *Mycoplasma* pneumonia: a case report and review. *J Microbiol Immunol Infect* **32**, 52–6.

Cimolai, N. (1998). *Mycoplasma pneumoniae* respiratory infection. *Pediatr Rev* **19**, 327–31, quiz 332.

Deguchi, T. and Maeda, S. (2002). *Mycoplasma genitalium*: another important pathogen of nongonococcal urethritis. *J Urol* **167**, 1210–17.

Fernandez Guerrero, M.L., Manuel Ramos, J. and Soriano, F. (1999). *Mycoplasma hominis* bacteraemia not associated with genital infections. *J Infect* **39**, 91–4.

Herrmann, R. and Reiner, B. (1998). *Mycoplasma pneumoniae* and *Mycoplasma genitalium*: a comparison of two closely related bacterial species. *Curr Opin Microbiol* **1**, 572–9.

Honda, J., Yano, T., Kusaba, M., *et al.* (2000). Clinical use of capillary PCR to diagnose *Mycoplasma* pneumonia. *J Clin Microbiol* **38**, 1382–4.

Paz, A. and Potasman, I. (2002). Mycoplasma-associated carditis. Case reports and review. *Cardiology* **97**, 83–8.

Principi, N. and Esposito, S. (2001). Emerging role of *Mycoplasma pneumoniae* and *Chlamydia pneumoniae* in paediatric respiratory-tract infections. *Lancet Infect Dis* **1**, 334–44.

Uuskula, A. and Kohl, P.K. (2002). Genital mycoplasmas, including *Mycoplasma genitalium*, as sexually transmitted agents. *Int J STD AIDS* **13**, 79–85.

42

Bacterial urinary tract infections

The urinary tract is the second most common site (after the respiratory tract) for bacterial infection. The majority of urinary tract infections (UTIs) occur in the bladder after migration of bacteria from the urethra or perineum. UTIs are much more common in females than in males, probably because of the difference in length of the urethra and other anatomical differences (Moore *et al.*, 2002). UTIs are also more common in elderly people of both sexes. Many UTIs are asymptomatic and do not result in any complications. In some circumstances, however, such as in pregnancy, asymptomatic UTIs must be diagnosed and treated to avoid renal scarring and complications with regard to the developing fetus.

Urine may be a good medium for bacterial growth. Unlike other body fluids, it does not contain significant levels of lysozyme or immunoglobulin, and any complement present is inactivated. Protection of the urinary tract against bacterial infection therefore relies strongly on the constant flow of urine and regular emptying of the bladder, although the interaction of mucosal surface defence mechanism also plays an important role. Only a limited number of bacteria are able to initiate infection in the normal urinary tract. Infecting bacteria usually originate from the patient's own faecal flora. In uncomplicated infections, the bacteria may include *Escherichia coli*, *Proteus mirabilis* and *Klebsiella* spp. Other bacteria, however, including some Gram-positive species, may also be implicated. Complicated infections, such as those involving the upper urinary tract, may be caused by the bacteria listed above, but *Enterobacter* spp., *Pseudomonas aeruginosa* and *Citrobacter* spp. may also be causative organisms. Most Gram-negative bacteria

involved in UTIs possess one or more virulence factors that enable them to persist in the urinary tract and cause infection. These may include O-antigens, K-antigens, flagella, haemolysins, siderophores and fimbriae (Hacker, 1992; Oelschlaeger *et al.*, 2002). These factors enable the bacteria to evade the host response and multiply in the urinary tract. The presence or absence of these factors may also affect the severity of clinical symptoms.

E. coli are the most common cause of UTIs, accounting for about 90% of acute uncomplicated infections and 50% of hospital-acquired infections (Ronald, 2002). Members of a small number of *E. coli* O-serogroups cause most episodes of UTIs, and it has been suggested that some serogroups may have a special nephropathogenic potential. However, these serogroups appear to predominate in the faecal flora of both infected and non-infected patients. *Proteus* spp. is the second most common cause of UTIs, accounting for up to 10% of all uncomplicated acute UTIs. *Proteus* spp. UTIs are common in elderly males and females and in young boys, although the mechanisms involved in the latter are not known. *P. mirabilis* is the most common *Proteus* cause of UTIs. *Proteus* spp. may cause chronic UTIs in hospital patients in association with obstruction or use of instruments. It may also lead to serious complications, such as acute pyelonephritis and bacteraemia.

The diagnosis of UTIs relies on isolation of the infecting organisms from fresh urine. The best sample is a midstream urine sample, which ensures that bacteria in the urethral flora do not contaminate the urine sample. Most bacteria that cause UTIs can be isolated on cysteine lysine electrolyte deoxycholate (CLED) or similar medium and distinguished by their morphology. Further identification can be performed as for other bacterial pathogens, such as sugar utilization. Urinary tract pathogens have varying susceptibility to antibiotics, and therefore susceptibility testing is necessary (Mazzulli, 2002; Nicolle, 2002).

REFERENCES

Hacker, J. (1992). Role of fimbrial adhesins in the pathogenesis of *Escherichia coli* infections. *Can J Microbiol* **38**, 720–27.

Mazzulli, T. (2002). Resistance trends in urinary tract pathogens and impact on management. *J Urol* **168**, 1720–22.

Moore, K.N., Day, R.A. and Albers, M. (2002). Pathogenesis of urinary tract infections: a review. *J Clin Nurs* **11**, 568–74.

Nicolle, L.E. (2002). Resistant pathogens in urinary tract infections. *J Am Geriatr Soc* **50**, S230–35.

Oelschlaeger, T.A., Dobrindt, U. and Hacker, J. (2002). Virulence factors of uropathogens. *Curr Opin Urol* **12**, 33–8.

Ronald, A. (2002). The etiology of urinary tract infection: traditional and emerging pathogens. *Am J Med* **113** (suppl 1A), 14–19S.

43

Cyanobacteria

Cyanobacteria are the oldest organisms known to man, with fossils dating back 3.5 billion years. They are also one of the most widespread life forms on earth (Garcia-Pichel, 1998; Kaiser, 2001; Knoll, 1979). Fossil records can be found today, the oldest being the Archaean rocks in Australia. They are thought to be one of the oldest forms of life ever to exist on earth, as they are almost as old as the oldest known rocks (3.8 billion years old). Cyanobacterial fossils are the easiest microfossils to recognize, as their morphology has remained the same over time and they often leave behind a chemical imprint that can be analysed by electron microscopy. Cyanobacteria have been important organisms in evolutionary terms for a number of reasons, including their ancient history. There is strong evidence to suggest that cyanobacteria provided the oxygen in the atmosphere during the Archaean and Proterozoic eras. Before this time, the chemical composition of the atmosphere was different and was unable to support life as it is known today.

Cyanobacteria may be found in almost every habitat around the world, including fresh water, salt water, rock surfaces and soil (Mur, 1983). They are responsible for the 'earthy' smell detected in soil and some waters, and for the green slime that grows in moist areas. Cyanobacteria may exist as single cells and as colonies. Depending on the species and environmental conditions, they may form filaments or sheets. They are responsible for the colour of the Red Sea due to the occasional bloom growth of a red genus known as *Oscillatoria*. Cyanobacteria form blooms on the surface of brackish or marine waters, particularly during hot weather (Atkins *et al.*, 2001). In temperate climates, such as that of the UK, the formation of cyanobacterial blooms is not usually a problem as growth below 10 °C is very slow.

Cyanobacteria are bacteria of the class Photobacteria, which means that they are autotrophic organisms and able to provide their own nourishment by photosynthesis. They were previously classified as blue–green algae because of their resemblance to eukaryotic green algae. However, cyanobacteria lack internal organelles and a discrete nucleus, and therefore they are classified as eubacteria. Although they are prokaryotic, cyanobacteria possess a highly organized system of internal membranes that are responsible for functional photosynthesis. Chlorophyll and several other pigments are contained within these membranes, thereby causing the variable colours of cyanobacteria. Cyanobacteria are known to be yellow, red, violet, green, deep blue and blue–green. As part of their growth, they are also able to convert inert atmospheric nitrogen into organic forms, such as nitrate and ammonia. Such chemical conversion is important to other plants, as nitrogen fixation (conversion from gas to organic form) is required for plant growth and must be obtained from the soil. However, nitrogen fixation cannot occur in the presence of oxygen. Therefore, cyanobacteria possess specialized cells known as heterocysts in which the atmosphere is anaerobic, thereby permitting nitrogen fixation to occur. Many plants, particularly the legumes, have developed a symbiotic relationship with nitrogen-fixing cyanobacteria so a supply of organic nitrogen can be guaranteed. Such symbiosis has been used to commercial advantage in rice cultivation, where the floating fern, *Azolla*, is spread over rice paddies. The fern contains colonies of the genus *Anabaena* within its leaves, so the fern indirectly provides an inexpensive fertilizer by providing a fixed nitrogen source to the rice plants.

Some cyanobacteria have been valued as food sources. For example, in tropical countries, the genus *Spirulina* can be cultivated easily and may be an important part of the diet. It was eaten regularly by the Aztecs, and it is also served today in several Oriental dishes. In the USA, *Spirulina* is considered a health food and is sold as a dried powder or in tablet form.

However, some species of cyanobacteria may also produce potent toxins, and they are a potential public health problem worldwide (Carmichael *et al.*, 2001; Chorus *et al.*, 2000). Although not publicized widely, there are a number of reported deaths in humans and animals each year (Codd, 1984; Hunter, 1992). The first scientific account of cyanobacteria toxin production was in *Nature* in 1878. This reported that cattle deaths had occurred as a result of drinking water from a bloom-infested lake in Australia. The organism identified was *Nodularia spumigena* and the toxin, nodularin, has since been characterized. Over 40 other cyanobacterial genera and their toxins have been described, some of which are shown in Table 43.1 (Codd, 1984). One group of toxins produced by cyanobacteria are the microcystins. These are produced most commonly by the widespread genus *Microcystis*, from which the toxins take their name.

Blooms on the surface of ponds and lakes have continued to be associated with poisoning of cattle and dogs. Descriptions of blooms occurring on water surfaces go back as far as the twelfth century, although their association with animal and human health is more recent. Occasional poisoning of humans occurs, usually as a result of swimming in such waters, and there has been at least one report of a suspected outbreak due to cyanobacterial poisoning. Apart from poisoning, skin irritation may occur with some species. Climate change is a public health concern with regards to cyanobacterial poisoning. Temperature regions, such as the UK, which have few reported cases of cyanobacterial poisoning, may see a slow increase in the number of reported cases in the future. However, the numbers should remain low as long as drinking waters are not contaminated.

Table 43.1 Some of the cyanobacteria known to produce toxins

Anabaena
Cylindrospermum
Microcystis
Nodularia
Nostoc
Oscillatoria

REFERENCES

Atkins, R., Rose, T., Brown, R.S. and Robb, M. (2001). The *Microcystis* cyanobacteria bloom in the Swan River – February 2000. *Water Sci Technol* **43**, 107–14.

Carmichael, W.W., Azevedo, S.M., An, J.S., *et al.* (2001). Human fatalities from cyanobacteria: chemical and biological evidence for cyanotoxins. *Environ Health Perspect* **109**, 663–8.

Chorus, I., Falconer, I.R., Salas, H.J. and Bartram, J. (2000). Health risks caused by freshwater cyanobacteria in recreational waters. *J Toxicol Environ Health B Crit Rev* **3**, 323–47.

Codd, G.A. (1984). Toxins of freshwater cyanobacteria. *Microbiol Sci* **1**, 48–52.

Garcia-Pichel, F. (1998). Solar ultraviolet and the evolutionary history of cyanobacteria. *Orig Life Evol Biosph* **28**, 321–47.

Hunter, P.R. (1992). Cyanobacteria and human health. *J Med Microbiol* **36**, 301–2.

Kaiser, D. (2001). Building a multicellular organism. *Annu Rev Genet* **35**, 103–23.

Knoll, A.H. (1979). Archean photoautotrophy: some alternatives and limits. *Orig Life* **9**, 313–27.

Mur, L.R. (1983). Some aspects of the ecophysiology of cyanobacteria. *Ann Microbiol (Paris)* **134B**, 61–72.

PART III

Virology

44

Viral hepatitis

Hepatitis may be caused by a variety of agents, including viruses, non-viral infectious agents, parasites, autoimmune mechanisms, drugs and neoplasia. This chapter describes the main causes of viral hepatitis. At least five viruses are recognized as causes of hepatitis in humans, namely hepatitis A virus (HAV), hepatitis B virus (HBV), hepatitis C virus (HCV), hepatitis D virus (HDV) and hepatitis E virus (HEV). Historically, hepatitis was thought to be due to two viruses, HAV and HBV, but research over the past few decades has determined that at least three further viruses, namely HCV, HDV and HEV, are structurally, biologically and epidemiologically distinct.

HAV is an enterovirus that is spread from person to person by the faecal–oral route. It is endemic in developing countries, and outbreaks may occur due to faecal contamination of a common source. Foodborne outbreaks also occur, caused most commonly by the ingestion of raw or improperly cooked molluscs cultivated in polluted waters. The largest ever outbreak occurred in Shanghai in 1988, affecting more than 290 000 people. HAV infection is otherwise known as infective jaundice. After infection, the incubation period is between two and six weeks. Clinical presentation of infection with the virus is wide-ranging, from asymptomatic to acute icteric disease and occasionally fulminant hepatitis. However, HAV is not thought to cause chronic liver disease. The incidence of HAV has reduced drastically in developed countries. However, in areas where sanitary standards are low, HAV remains an important cause of disease. HAV vaccination is available and is recommended for individuals travelling to developing areas. The diagnosis of viral hepatitis is usually by detection of immunoglobulin M (IgM) antibody. HAV IgM may persist for 10 weeks, whilst immunoglobulin G (IgG), although appearing slowly, lasts for many years, thereby conferring immunity. HAV antibodies may also be detected in the urine and saliva of infected individuals. Some general properties of the hepatitis viruses are shown in Table 44.1.

HBV has been well studied in terms of its morphology and genomic structure (Figure 44.1). It is a DNA virus and therefore differs from the other hepatitis viruses. During infection, the virus secretes a high level of antigen into the host's circulation, which is useful for diagnostic purposes.

Table 44.1 General properties of hepatitis viruses

	HAV	HBV	HCV	HDV	HEV
Transmission	Faecal–oral	Blood	Blood	Blood	Faecal–oral
Nucleic acid	RNA	DNA	RNA	RNA	RNA
Vaccine?	Yes	Yes	No	No	No

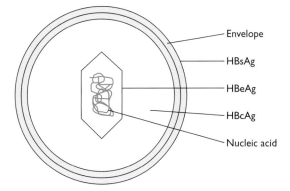

Figure 44.1 Diagrammatic representation of hepatitis B virus.

HBV is excreted in most body fluids, including blood, saliva, semen, vaginal fluid and breast milk. This is of particular importance because activities such as kissing and sexual intercourse between infected and non-infected individuals can lead to virus transmission. Transmission can also occur in the laboratory via aerosol contact or accidental inoculation. The incubation period is approximately three months. Asymptomatic infection is not uncommon, but fulminant hepatitis is rare. Most individuals recover uneventfully, although a small number remain HBV surface antigen (HBsAg) positive. Some of these individuals develop chronic hepatitis or cirrhosis. In terms of laboratory diagnosis, there are a number of serological markers and antibodies that may be detected and used as markers to determine the stage of infection and whether the patient is a carrier of hepatitis B (Table 44.2). The polymerase chain reaction (PCR) may also be used to detect the

virus in infected individuals (Balderas-Renteria *et al.*, 2002). Hepatitis B can be treated effectively with antiviral agents (Esteban, 2002).

The diagnosis of HBV infection is determined by testing for the presence of HBsAg and hepatitis B core antibody (HBcAb) IgM (acute phase) or anti-hepatitis B core (anti-HBc) or anti-hepatitis B surface (anti-HBs) (convalescent phase) in serum. Although the serological profile is not always straightforward, HBsAg and anti-HBc IgG are almost always detectable. HBV immunoglobulin may be given to individuals exposed to HBV. An HBV vaccine is used extensively in healthcare professionals, but it is not generally given to the public or as part of the childhood vaccination programme. Blood screening has been adopted in developed countries to ensure that post-transfusion hepatitis is a rare occurrence. Some developing countries screen all blood, some are selective depending upon geography, and others do not screen at all.

HCV is related to the flaviviruses and is shed into the circulation of infected individuals in low concentrations. Bloodborne transmission is well documented, but the reasons for the persistence of HCV in the community are poorly understood. Sexual transmission does not appear to be important. The incubation period after initial infection is between six and eight weeks. Acute infection is milder, with only 5–10% of cases showing symptoms of acute hepatitis compared with hepatitis A or B; infection may therefore pass unrecognized. HCV is not associated with fulminant hepatitis. However, 20–50% of acute infections progress to chronic liver disease. HCV has therefore become an important disease in recent years due to its potential chronicity and distribution in the community. The diagnosis of hepatitis C infection depends on the demonstration of anti-HCV IgG in serum. This is also performed on transfusion blood and has led to an important decrease in post-transfusion non-A, non-B hepatitis. Infected individuals can be treated with antiviral agents (Bruchfeld *et al.*, 2002).

HDV, otherwise known as delta agent, infection is common in areas where the prevalence of

Table 44.2 Serological markers of hepatitis B

HBsAg	Hepatitis B surface antigen
HBeAg	Hepatitis B envelope antigen
HBcAb	Hepatitis B core antibody (IgM + IgG)
HBeAb	Hepatitis B envelope antibody (IgM + IgG)
HBsAb	Hepatitis B surface antibody (IgM + IgG)

HBV infection is also high, such as Eastern Europe, the Middle East, Africa and South America. HDV possesses an RNA genome. It is different from the other hepatitis viruses in that it requires the help of HBV for transmission (Karayiannis, 1998; Rizzetto, 2000). Two types of HDV infection are known: (i) co-infection with HDV and HBV and (ii) chronic HBV infection followed by superinfection with HDV. In both types of infection, acute hepatitis or chronic liver disease is more severe than in HBV infection alone. HDV exists as an RNA genome associated with delta antigen and is surrounded by an HBsAg envelope (Figure 44.2).

HDV infection is unable to persist without HBV infection. However, the absence of demonstrable HBsAg should not be used for excluding HDV infection. Diagnosis relies on the demonstration of hepatitis D antigen (HDAg) in liver biopsies or serum. Anti-HDV status may also be determined to ascertain whether infection is acute or chronic. Transmission occurs via blood. There is no treatment for HDV, and the prevention of transmission relies on the screening of blood products and the education of those at risk, such as intravenous drug abusers. Vaccination with HBV vaccine is effective against HDV, as the HBsAg envelope is the target.

HEV is a non-enveloped, single-stranded RNA virus that is similar to calicivirus. It is responsible for sporadic and epidemic non-A, non-B hepatitis in the Indian subcontinent and areas of Africa, Central Asia and Mexico. Hepatitis E, like hepatitis A, is spread primarily through food and water contaminated by faeces from an infected person (Kurstak et al., 1996; Slavkin, 1996). The incubation period for the virus is approximately 40 days. HEV is transmitted from person to person less commonly than HAV, and adequate sanitary measures are sufficient to prevent or control HEV outbreaks. The diagnosis of HEV is by exclusion, although the virus may be demonstrated in faeces by electron microscopy during acute infection. Attack rates are highest in young adults, but mortality rates are greatest in pregnant women, in whom they may be as high as 20%. Sequencing of the HEV genome has now made it possible to diagnose infection using PCR on blood and faeces or enzyme-linked immunosorbent assay (ELISA) on serum (for IgM or IgG). There is no specific treatment and no vaccine for HEV.

Hepatitis F and hepatitis G viruses have been described recently in post-blood-transfusion patients and haemophiliacs, respectively (Alonso-Rubiano et al., 2003; Tepper and Gully, 1997). Hepatitis F has not been confirmed in the scientific literature, but hepatitis G has been accepted by the scientific and medical community.

REFERENCES

Alonso-Rubiano, E., Gerber, M., Friedman, P., Hodges, S. and Leissinger, C. (2003). Hepatitis G virus in clotting factor concentrates. *Haemophilia* 9, 110–15.

Balderas-Renteria, I., Munoz-Espinosa, L.E., Dector-Carrillo, M.A., Martinez-Martinez, F.J. and Barrera-Saldana, H.A. (2002). Detection of hepatitis B virus in seropositive and seronegative patients with chronic liver disease using DNA amplification by PCR. *Arch Med Res* 33, 566–71.

Bruchfeld, A., Lindahl, K., Schvarcz, R. and Stahle, L. (2002). Dosage of ribavirin in patients with hepatitis C should be based on renal function: a population pharmacokinetic analysis. *Ther Drug Monit* 24, 701–8.

Esteban, R. (2002). Management of chronic hepatitis B: an overview. *Semin Liver Dis* 22 (suppl 1), 1–6.

Karayiannis, P. (1998). Hepatitis D virus. *Rev Med Virol* 8, 13–24.

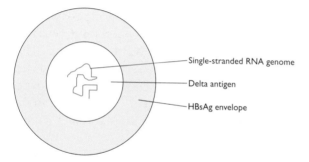

Figure 44.2 Diagrammatic representation of hepatitis D virus.

Single-stranded RNA genome

Delta antigen

HBsAg envelope

Kurstak, E., Hossain, A. and Kurstak, C. (1996). Progress in diagnosis of viral hepatitis A, B, C, D and E. *Acta Virol* **40**, 107–15.

Rizzetto, M. (2000). Hepatitis D: virology, clinical and epidemiological aspects. *Acta Gastroenterol Belg* **63**, 221–4.

Slavkin, H.C. (1996). The A, B, C, D and E of viral hepatitis. *J Am Dent Assoc* **127**, 1667–70.

Tepper, M.I. and Gully, P.R. (1997). Viral hepatitis: know your D, E, F and Gs. *CMAJ* **156**, 1735–8.

45

The common cold

The common cold is probably the most common infectious disease to affect humans, and everyone can relate to it from personal experience (Gwaltney, 2002; Monto, 2002). On average, adults have two to five colds a year, although the exact number depends on how the illness is defined. Children are generally more susceptible and therefore experience more colds each year. In the UK, the Common Cold Unit (CCU) was set up in the 1940s and provided much of the information now known about the disease. At that time it was thought that the cold was an important disease with economic implications and that it could precipitate serious problems in patients with underlying complications, such as heart disease. Today, however, it is widely thought that colds are no longer a threat and research on the illness has declined, although it still has economic importance due to absence from work (Takkouche et al., 2001). The CCU operated until 1990.

The common cold is more common in spring and autumn, although there is no correlation with extremes of weather. Spread is fairly rapid within close groups such as families, and it is known to occur by both aerosol transmission and fomite contact (Goldmann, 2000). Hand contact is the most common mode of transmission. After an incubation period of two to three days, the cold presents as a mild upper respiratory tract infection (URTI). The duration of symptoms is also two to three days; symptoms include rhinitis, coughing, sneezing and mild pharyngitis. Fever is rare. More severe colds are seen in smokers and asthmatics, and might result in secondary bacterial complications (Corne et al., 2002; Skoner, 2002). Some evidence supports the theory that stressed or tired people are more likely to get a cold, and research at the CCU found that stressed individuals developed more colds mostly because they were readily infected (Takkouche et al., 2001). The reasons, whether physiological or immunological, are still unknown.

The causative micro-organisms of the common cold have been identified as viruses (Greenberg, 2002). The structure and molecular biology of replications has been studied in detail, and the genome sequence of several of the viruses has been determined. The rhinoviruses and coronaviruses cause about 50% and 15%, respectively, of common colds. The remainder are caused by other viruses such as Epstein–Barr virus, influenza and parainfluenza. More than 100 different serotypes of rhinovirus exist, which explains why common colds are so common. However, 10–40% of rhinovirus infections are subclinical. It is thought, therefore, that there might be differences in the pathogenicity of different serotypes of the virus. Rhinoviruses are very temperature-sensitive and have an optimum growth temperature of 33 °C. They therefore most commonly infect the upper respiratory tract, where the human body temperature is lower than elsewhere in the body. When it does occur, lower respiratory tract infection is characterized by decreased lung function in adults and wheezing in children. Although rhinoviruses are not implicated as a significant cause of adult pneumonia, rhinovirus infection has been associated with up to 40% of exacerbations in patients with chronic bronchitis. These patients have also been found to be more susceptible to infection with rhinovirus.

Infection with coronavirus is similar to that of rhinovirus. The main differences are that the nasal discharge tends to be greater and virus shedding is prolonged.

Infection with any of the viruses that may cause the common cold is initiated after a virus attaches and penetrates the mucosa of the respiratory tract. The virus replicates and infiltrates the surrounding cells, causing cilia stasis and cell destruction. The release of bradykinin occurs, resulting in local oedema, and a cellular immune response is activated. There is always the possibility of secondary bacterial infection. A humoral response is essential in the resistance of infection but takes time to develop. This provides protection against future challenges with the same serotype of the causative virus. It is estimated that up to two-thirds of the viruses that might cause colds are prevented from doing so by the presence of virus-neutralizing antibodies.

Although diagnosis of a common cold is rarely necessary, it can be performed by organ culture. Some limited prophylaxis is available; certain compounds have been discovered that bind to rhinoviruses, and one of these drugs has been shown to be effective chemotherapy against rhinoviruses. However, these compounds are not effective against coronaviruses. The use of interferon alfa protects against virus infection, but its use has been shown to produce local inflammation because of its cytotoxicity. Further development of the interferon was therefore abandoned. Facial steam baths are also effective because they raise the temperature of the upper respiratory tract. Vaccines have not yet been developed, probably because of the large number of different serotypes and the complexity of the immune response. Although further research is probably required to develop effective vaccines for the prevention of common colds, it is debatable whether they would be of any real value.

REFERENCES

Corne, J.M., Marshall, C., Smith, S., *et al.* (2002). Frequency, severity, and duration of rhinovirus infections in asthmatic and non-asthmatic individuals: a longitudinal cohort study. *Lancet* **359**, 831–4.

Goldmann, D.A. (2000). Transmission of viral respiratory infections in the home. *Pediatr Infect Dis J* **19**, S97–102.

Greenberg, S.B. (2002). Respiratory viral infections in adults. *Curr Opin Pulm Med* **8**, 201–8.

Gwaltney, J.M. (2002). Clinical significance and pathogenesis of viral respiratory infections. *Am J Med* **112** (suppl 6A), 13–18S.

Monto, A.S. (2002). Epidemiology of viral respiratory infections. *Am J Med* **112** (suppl 6A), 4–12S.

Skoner, D.P. (2002). Viral infection and allergy: lower airway. *Allergy Asthma Proc* **23**, 229–32.

Takkouche, B., Regueira, C. and Gestal-Otero, J.J. (2001). A cohort study of stress and the common cold. *Epidemiology* **12**, 345–9.

46

Respiratory syncytial virus

The respiratory syncytial virus (RSV) causes acute childhood bronchiolitis, particularly in infants under the age of 18 months. It is a helical RNA virus and a member of the paramyxoviruses. There are two recognized serotypes, A and B. They appear to circulate concomitantly, but one usually predominates during a given season. Serotype A predominates more commonly and appears to be associated with more severe disease. About 80–90% of children possess serum neutralizing antibodies by the age of four years, but these do not protect fully against further exposure, and no life-long immunity is established. Re-infection is very common throughout life. Symptoms are usually comparatively mild, except in elderly people (Falsey and Walsh, 2000). Infection may also take place in the presence of maternal antibody. The major modes of transmission appear to be through hand-to-nose and hand-to-eye contact, but the virus may also be transmitted through fomites or large particle aerosols. Its spread is slower than that of other viruses, such as influenza, which may be transmitted rapidly by droplet nuclei.

RSV infection results from multiplication of the virus in the epithelium of the upper respiratory tract. It infects boys and girls equally, but hospitalization is more common in boys. Symptoms are of sudden onset, usually within 24 hours of infection. The initial disease presentation is similar to that of a common cold, such as nasal discharge, cough and poor feeding, and is usually accompanied by rapid, distressed breathing (Collins and Pollard, 2002). The general illness may include fever, but cyanosis and chest distension are more common. Chest radiographs show a clear translucent picture at this stage. The patient usually improves within several days, and complete recovery from the infection is seen in most cases, usually in three to four days. However, more serious infection is not uncommon if the conditions are favourable for the virus and the lower respiratory tract (LRT) is involved. The most frequent feature of the infection before LRT involvement is a cough, which may be paroxysmal and may be associated with vomiting. Infection of the LRT usually presents as bronchiolitis. This is because the bronchioles of young infants have such a fine bore that if the epithelial lining becomes inflamed due to infection, then the passage of air may be blocked. Bronchiolitis results in necrosis, which causes the partial blocking of surrounding bronchioles. This leads to both collapse and over-inflammation in the alveoli beyond. Peribronchial infiltration also occurs; this may spread, producing widespread interstitial pneumonia. There is also good reason to implicate antibody-mediated hyper-sensitivity in the disease. It seems likely that the local formation of immunoglobulin G (IgG) virus complexes in the lung exacerbates inflammation. Pneumonitis may also coexist with bronchiolitis, and viraemia may occur. The long-term outlook for children who recover from severe infection is good. By the age of eight years, any defect in respiratory efficiency due to severe RSV infection in infancy is minimal.

In severe cases of RSV infection, hospitalization is often necessary. In the UK, RSV is the most frequent cause of hospitalization for respiratory tract infection during the first two years of life. It is also a common cause of nosocomial infection in paediatric wards, although good screening procedures upon hospital admission and isolation of RSV-positive children have reduced the spread of

RSV in wards (Mlinaric-Galinovic and Varda-Brkic, 2000). RSV infection may be life-threatening in a few cases, but mortality is generally low. Patients who develop severe, life-threatening RSV are those with underlying cardiopulmonary disease or immunosuppression or who were born prematurely. A mortality rate as high as 73% has been reported in infants with congenital heart disease and pulmonary hypertension. In the USA, RSV infection is the leading primary diagnosis in infant hospitalization (Leader and Kohlhase, 2002). It is responsible for 40–50% of hospitalizations for bronchiolitis and 25% of hospitalizations for pneumonia. This total of over 90 000 admissions has been estimated to cost $300 million each year.

Uncommon manifestations of RSV infection include disease of the central nervous system, myocarditis and exanthema. Patients with these manifestations are still at significant risk of death and morbidity, despite the absence of LRT infection in most cases. In disease affecting the central nervous system, illness is characterized by drowsiness and near-coma for a few days. Respiratory symptoms may then appear. This clinical picture is seen most commonly in neonates, particularly those born prematurely. Complications may also occur with RSV infection. They occur most frequently in young infants and include apnoea, respiratory failure and secondary bacterial infection. RSV has also been associated with sudden infant death syndrome.

RSV infection may occur at any time of year, but the epidemic peak of RSV infection occurs in the winter or the rainy season. In the UK, the typical outbreak begins in the autumn and takes two to three months to reach its peak between February and March. In other countries, the peak may be between November and December. The diagnosis of RSV infection is based on clinical characteristics and microbiological testing. The latter may be achieved by virus isolation in cell culture, by the complement fixation test using paired sera, or by direct antigen immunofluorescence. The latter method is the best for a rapid diagnosis.

There is no specific treatment for RSV infection, although drugs are available that relieve symptoms of the disease. Supportive therapy, such as oxygen and intravenous hydration, remain the mainstays of therapy (Staat, 2002). For high-risk infants, however, the administration of high doses of RSV immunoglobulin has proven to be a safe and effective method of preventing LRT infection caused by the virus. Ribavirin, an antiviral agent administered by aerosol, is also useful in severe infections (Randolph and Wang, 2000). There is no known associated toxin with RSV infection, and therefore vaccines must be based on the virus itself rather than its products. The development of a safe and effective vaccine is a priority. Identification of the major immunogenic glycoproteins has been completed, and a number of vaccines have undergone clinical trials (Kneyber and Kimpen, 2002). A greater understanding of RSV biology and genetics may lead to the identification of further therapeutic targets (Cane, 2001; Collins and Murphy, 2002; Sullender, 2000).

REFERENCES

Cane, P.A. (2001). Molecular epidemiology of respiratory syncytial virus. *Rev Med Virol* **11**, 103–16.

Collins, P.L. and Murphy, B.R. (2002). Respiratory syncytial virus: reverse genetics and vaccine strategies. *Virology* **296**, 204–11.

Collins, C.L. and Pollard, A.J. (2002). Respiratory syncytial virus infections in children and adults. *J Infect* **45**, 10–17.

Falsey, A.R. and Walsh, E.E. (2000). Respiratory syncytial virus infection in adults. *Clin Microbiol Rev* **13**, 371–84.

Kneyber, M.C. and Kimpen, J.L. (2002). Current concepts on active immunization against respiratory syncytial virus for infants and young children. *Pediatr Infect Dis J* **21**, 685–96.

Leader, S. and Kohlhase, K. (2002). Respiratory syncytial virus-coded pediatric hospitalizations, 1997 to 1999. *Pediatr Infect Dis J* **21**, 629–32.

Mlinaric-Galinovic, G. and Varda-Brkic, D. (2000). Nosocomial respiratory syncytial virus infections in children's wards. *Diagn Microbiol Infect Dis* **37**, 237–46.

Randolph, A.G. and Wang, E.E. (2000). Ribavirin for respiratory syncytial virus infection of the lower respiratory tract. *Cochrane Database Syst Rev*, CD000181.

Staat, M.A. (2002). Respiratory syncytial virus infections in children. *Semin Respir Infect* **17**, 15–20.

Sullender, W.M. (2000). Respiratory syncytial virus genetic and antigenic diversity. *Clin Microbiol Rev* **13**, 1–15.

47

Rubella

Rubella was first described by two German physicians in 1752. At the time, the disease was known by the German name *Röteln* and was subsequently called German measles. For many years, it was confused with measles and scarlet fever because of some similarities in their symptoms; it was not accepted as a distinct disease until 1881. Little attention was drawn to rubella until the early 1940s, when it was recognized that there was an association between rubella in pregnancy and congenital defects in the fetus.

The causative agent of rubella, the rubella virus, was discovered in 1938. It is a single-stranded RNA virus of the genus Rubivirus and the family Togaviridae. It has a worldwide distribution, and outbreaks occur frequently among schoolchildren and young adults. Outbreaks are more common in spring and summer in temperate climates. The transmission of rubella is by respiratory secretions. Upon entering the respiratory tract, the virus replicates in the nasopharyngeal epithelium before causing viraemia. The incubation period is one to two weeks, after which the characteristic features of the disease develop. Symptoms may include rash, pharyngitis and lymphadenopathy, but some cases are asymptomatic. Fever and malaise may also present a few days before the appearance of the rash. In young children, this occurs one to two days before the rash appears, but in older children and adults it may be three to four days. The clinical diagnosis of rubella infection may be difficult due to the symptoms being mild or atypical. Infection with other viruses, such as enterovirus and parvovirus B19, may cause similar clinical features.

Complications associated with rubella infection are rare but can include encephalitis, thrombocytopenia and joint problems (Lee and Bowden, 2000). Encephalitis is estimated to occur in one in 10 000 cases, but the prognosis is good. Thrombocytopenia is rare but may result in purpuric rash, epistaxis, haematuria and gastrointestinal bleeding. More common are joint problems, which are often acquired postnatally and may occur in up to 60% of post-pubertal females. The symptoms develop after the rash subsides in natural infection or after the administration of rubella vaccine and vary in their severity from mild stiffness to arthritis. However, the problems are temporary, usually lasting only about three days, and they are not associated with any sequelae.

The rubella virus is one of the few microorganisms that is able to cross the placenta and cause congenital disease (Coulter *et al.*, 1999; Gilbert, 2002). This is a particular problem during the first three months of pregnancy. The fetus is most at risk during maternal viraemia, when placental infection may take place. However, infection can also occur through direct contact because the rubella virus may also be excreted via the cervix or may persist in the genital tract. Infection of the fetus may result in multisystem disease arising from virus-associated retardation of cell division or tissue necrosis. This can result in spontaneous abortion of the fetus in up to 20% of cases, occurring most commonly during the first eight weeks of pregnancy. Numerous transient, developmental and permanent congenital defects may be present if the developing fetus survives. Transient features may include a low birth weight, hepatosplenomegaly and lesions in the long bones. Developmental features include deafness and mental retardation. Permanent features include cataract and diabetes mellitus. These defects are known collectively as the congenital rubella syndrome. Laboratory testing is therefore essential in determining immune status and for the diagnosis of rubella infection.

A number of tests may be used in the laboratory for the detection of immunity to rubella (Cradock-Watson, 1991; Dwyer *et al.*, 2001). The most commonly used test is single radial haemolysis (SRH), but others include enzyme immunoassay (EIA), radioimmunoassay (RIA) and latex agglutination. None of these tests, however, should be used to diagnose rubella infection. Diagnosis of rubella infection is attained by detecting the presence of immunoglobulin M (IgM) antibody using enzyme-linked immunosorbent assay (ELISA) or immunofluorescence. Active rubella may also be diagnosed by detecting a rising titre of immunoglobulin G (IgG) antibody by haemagglutination inhibition (HAI). The virus may be isolated in tissue culture, but this is used only for the diagnosis of congenital rubella in the fetus. This method may take up to six weeks for confirmation.

Exposure to the rubella virus provides long-lasting immunity against reinfection. However, not all females are exposed to the virus before childbearing age, and therefore effective vaccination programmes are essential for the prevention of congenital rubella and extensive epidemics. Effective rubella vaccines have been licensed for use in the UK since 1970, and since then the number of cases in immunized individuals has decreased substantially (Figure 47.1). An immune response is induced in approximately 95% of susceptible vaccinees, providing about 18 years' protection. Rubella vaccination is given to preschool children as part of the combined MMR (measles, mumps, rubella) vaccine. Although public concern has been associated with this vaccine in recent years, the vaccine is considered to be safe (Afzal *et al.*, 2000). Rubella vaccination is also given to schoolgirls aged 10–14 years and to seronegative adult women. Vaccination is contraindicated during pregnancy and in immunocompromised people. Cases can be common in males attending colleges and universities, however, because they have not been immunized. Rubella elimination may be possible in the

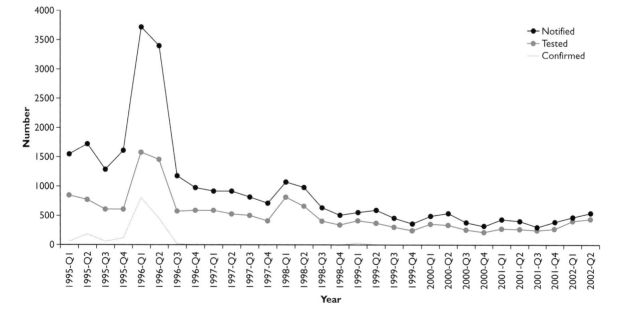

Figure 47.1 Notifications and confirmations of rubella in England and Wales, 1995–2002* (source: HPA CDSC).
*2002 data are provisional.

USA in the future (Reef *et al.*, 2000); there were only 176 cases reported during the year 2000 (source: US CDC). However, rubella vaccine is not given worldwide, and therefore the disease remains a problem in developing nations (Hinman *et al.*, 2002; Plotkin, 2001).

REFERENCES

Afzal, M.A., Minor, P.D. and Schild, G.C. (2000). Clinical safety issues of measles, mumps and rubella vaccines. *Bull World Health Organ* **78**, 199–204.

Coulter, C., Wood, R. and Robson, J. (1999). Rubella infection in pregnancy. *Commun Dis Intell* **23**, 93–6.

Cradock-Watson, J.E. (1991). Laboratory diagnosis of rubella: past, present and future. *Epidemiol Infect* **107**, 1–15.

Dwyer, D.E., Robertson, P.W. and Field, P.R. (2001). Broadsheet: clinical and laboratory features of rubella. *Pathology* **33**, 322–8.

Gilbert, G.L. (2002). 1: Infections in pregnant women. *Med J Aust* **176**, 229–36.

Hinman, A.R., Irons, B., Lewis, M. and Kandola, K. (2002). Economic analyses of rubella and rubella vaccines: a global review. *Bull World Health Organ* **80**, 264–70.

Lee, J.Y. and Bowden, D.S. (2000). Rubella virus replication and links to teratogenicity. *Clin Microbiol Rev* **13**, 571–87.

Plotkin, S.A. (2001). Rubella eradication. *Vaccine* **19**, 3311–19.

Reef, S.E., Plotkin, S., Cordero, J.F., *et al.* (2000). Preparing for elimination of congenital rubella syndrome (CRS): summary of a workshop on CRS elimination in the United States. *Clin Infect Dis* **31**, 85–95.

48

Filoviruses

There has been increased concern among infectious disease experts over the possibility of 'new' viruses causing disease in humans (Borchert *et al.*, 2000; Lee and Henderson, 2001). Clusters or outbreaks of previously unknown or rare diseases are becoming more frequent. Of course, these diseases are not completely new, but they have remained in remote areas, such as in deep jungles, until now. Human civilization and exploration, and the ease with which we now travel, have disturbed the ecological balance between humans and nature, thereby creating vehicles for transmission of these viruses. Most of the emerging viruses are zoonotic and appear to originate from Africa or Asia. Epidemics of 'new' viruses have occurred throughout history after their introduction to a previously unexposed population. For example, smallpox was introduced from the Old World to the New World, aiding the Spanish in the conquest of South America. One group of 'new' viruses that is of particular interest is the filoviruses (Feldmann *et al.*, 1996). These are commonly known as the cause of viral haemorrhagic fevers and are of interest because they are thought to be relatively new as human pathogens. They are associated mostly with rare but devastating disease, with mortalities ranging from around 5% to 90%. There are numerous viral haemorrhagic fevers caused by a number of different viruses that affect humans (Table 48.1).

The family Filoviridae, in the order Mononegavirales, contains a number of extremely pathogenic viruses that cause fulminating, febrile haemorrhagic disease (Peters and Khan, 1999). They are characteristic threadlike viruses about 790 nm in length and 80 nm in width, hence their name (*filo* is Latin for filament). The family

Table 48.1 Viral haemorrhagic fevers of humans

Marburg virus
Rift Valley fever
Dengue fever
Yellow fever
Lassa fever
Ebola virus
Hantavirus
Chikungunya
Omsk haemorrhagic fever
Argentinian haemorrhagic fever
Bolivian haemorrhagic fever
Kyasanur Forest disease
Crimean-Congo haemorrhagic fever

includes the Marburg virus, which is thought to be of a single species, and Ebola virus, of which there are three known subtypes: Sudan, Zaire and Reston. Although other important viruses are contained within the filovirus family, only Ebola and Marburg will be described in this chapter.

Marburg virus was first described in 1967 after simultaneous outbreaks occurred in Germany and Yugoslavia (Dowdle, 1976; Slenczka, 1999). The index cases were laboratory workers who were thought to have been infected by direct contact with African green monkeys from Uganda. The disease spread from the 25 index cases to six other close contacts, including patients, nurses and doctors; there were seven deaths. The mortality of Marburg virus is approximately 25%. Further cases were not reported until 1980, when a French engineer working in western Kenya developed Marburg virus disease and subsequently infected one close contact. In 1987, one sporadic case occurred, which resulted in the death of the individual. An outbreak also occurred recently in the Democratic Republic of Congo (Borchert *et al.*, 2000).

Ebola virus was first identified in 1976, when simultaneous outbreaks occurred in Sudan and Zaire (Streether, 1999). The outbreaks were unrelated and resulted in mortalities of 53% and 88%, respectively. A sporadic case occurred in northwestern Zaire in 1977. Another outbreak occurred in Sudan in 1979, this time with a lower mortality of 65%. An outbreak of Ebola-related filovirus disease in 1989 involved cynomolgus monkeys imported from the Philippines (DeMarcus *et al.*, 1999). The monkeys were being maintained at Reston, VA, USA. There were no human cases, although antibodies were demonstrated in some of the animal handlers without any history of disease. The virus was shown to be sufficiently different from the Ebola viruses isolated in the African outbreaks and is therefore referred to as Ebola Reston. It was the first incident in which a filovirus was isolated from a non-human primate without deliberate infection, which raised the possibility of animal reservoirs. Outbreaks of Ebola virus have occurred in Africa in recent years (Khan *et al.*, 1999; Okware *et al.*, 2002). During these outbreaks, over 100 cases have been reported by the World Health Organization (WHO), although they have remained confined to a relatively small geographic area. Ebola fever has a usual incubation period of 5–10 days, with a range up to three weeks. The disease presents with rapid onset of fever accompanied by diarrhoea, myalgia and headache. Chest pain, rash, photophobia and jaundice may also be common. As disease progresses, haemorrhagic features manifest, including bloody diarrhoea, haemoptysis, haematemesis and haemorrhaging of the mucous membranes. Patients who survive infection excrete the virus for a period of days or weeks after the fever resolves.

Marburg virus differs from Ebola virus in many ways at the molecular level. When more is known about these viruses, it may be proposed that there should be two genera within the family. Little is known about their natural history, and the natural reservoir is not known. To date, disease is known to have occurred only in primates. Human spread of filoviruses is by direct contact with body fluids or contaminated needles. There is little epidemiological evidence to suggest that filoviruses are transmitted by aerosol. Secondary and tertiary cases of filovirus infections appear to have a lower mortality, thereby suggesting that the viruses are attenuated by human passage. Primates are not thought to be natural reservoirs of the filoviruses, although no other animal reservoir has yet been found. A number of animal reservoirs have been suspected during outbreak investigations, including spiders, soft ticks, bats and monkeys. It has also been suggested that Ebola is a plant virus. There is no treatment and no vaccine for filovirus infection. Animal experiments have shown that there is nothing to be gained from the use of interferon or immunoglobulin. Supportive therapy is all that can be done for the patient. Trauma should be kept to a minimum, and fluid rehydration should be maintained.

Future sporadic cases or outbreaks will hopefully lead to definition of the natural reservoir for these filovirus infections and the development of a good treatment or vaccine. The emergence of viral infections with a high mortality should not surprise us. To date, serious filovirus outbreaks have not been easily transmissible between humans and have therefore remained confined geographically, although they remain a hazard for travellers (Isaacson, 2001). We must therefore hope that a filovirus does not emerge that is spread by aerosols, has a high mortality, and is readily transmissible from human to human without any decrease in virulence. In addition, we must be aware of the potential of the use of filoviruses as agents of bioterrorism (Broussard, 2001; Cunha, 2002).

REFERENCES

Borchert, M., Boelaert, M., Sleurs, H., *et al.* (2000). Viewpoint: filovirus haemorrhagic fever outbreaks:

much ado about nothing? *Trop Med Int Health* 5, 318–24.

Broussard, L.A. (2001). Biological agents: weapons of warfare and bioterrorism. *Mol Diagn* 6, 323–33.

Cunha, B.A. (2002). Anthrax, tularemia, plague, ebola or smallpox as agents of bioterrorism: recognition in the emergency room. *Clin Microbiol Infect* 8, 489–503.

DeMarcus, T.A., Tipple, M.A. and Ostrowski, S.R. (1999). US policy for disease control among imported nonhuman primates. *J Infect Dis* 179 (suppl 1), S281–2.

Dowdle, W.R. (1976). Marburg virus. *Bull Pan Am Health Organ* 10, 333–4.

Feldmann, H., Slenczka, W. and Klenk, H.D. (1996). Emerging and reemerging of filoviruses. *Arch Virol Suppl* 11, 77–100.

Isaacson, M. (2001). Viral hemorrhagic fever hazards for travelers in Africa. *Clin Infect Dis* 33, 1707–12.

Khan, A.S., Tshioko, F.K., Heymann, D.L., *et al.* (1999). The reemergence of Ebola hemorrhagic fever, Democratic Republic of the Congo, 1995. Commission de Lutte contre les Epidemies a Kikwit. *J Infect Dis* 179 (suppl 1), S76–6.

Lee, L.M. and Henderson, D.K. (2001). Emerging viral infections. *Curr Opin Infect Dis* 14, 467–80.

Okware, S.I., Omaswa, F.G., Zaramba, S., *et al.* (2002). An outbreak of Ebola in Uganda. *Trop Med Int Health* 7, 1068–75.

Peters, C.J. and Khan, A.S. (1999). Filovirus diseases. *Curr Top Microbiol Immunol* 235, 85–95.

Slenczka, W.G. (1999). The Marburg virus outbreak of 1967 and subsequent episodes. *Curr Top Microbiol Immunol* 235, 49–75.

Streether, L.A. (1999). Ebola virus. *Br J Biomed Sci* 56, 280–84.

49

Smallpox

Smallpox is one of the most famous human diseases, due to its historical importance and current interest (Fenner, 1993). It has been of major significance to humans for thousands of years, perhaps since the time of Rameses V in 1160 BC. Human civilization led to the domestication of a number of animals, which have been the source of many diseases, possibly including smallpox. Smallpox was a devastating worldwide disease until only relatively recently. It has an incubation period of about 10 days, after which fever, headache, prostration, nausea and vomiting develop (Breman and Henderson, 2002; Ellner, 1998). Two to three days later a rash appears, with the previous symptoms persisting. The rash begins with small macules, which progress over the course of a week to form vesicles and then pustules. After this time, scabs form and then fall off, leaving depigmented areas. Individuals surviving the disease may therefore be left badly scarred. The case fatality rate was difficult to establish until organized outbreak investigations took place in the 1960s and 1970s; during this time, the case fatality rate ranged from 0.2 to 20%.

The need for a cure had been recognized for centuries, and various African countries, China and India had tried a form of vaccination called variolation. This involved inoculating susceptible individuals with live smallpox virus. However, people who had been variolated could pass on smallpox to susceptible individuals, which resulted in many outbreaks during its use. It was not until the latter half of the eighteenth century that Edward Jenner devised the smallpox vaccine. There are also a few accounts of farmers vaccinating their families with cowpox to protect themselves from smallpox before the introduction of Jenner's vaccine. Jenner gave his first immunization to James Phipps on 14 May 1796. The origin of the virus preparation is not known, but the virus used in the preparation was vaccinia virus, which replicates and produces a subclinical or mild infection in the immunised individual. Vaccinia immunization may therefore be regarded as similar to a live, attenuated vaccination.

The wonders of Jenner's vaccine were acknowledged, and vaccination was made available to the public (Baxby, 1996; Willis, 1997). Smallpox vaccination of infants was made compulsory in the UK in 1853. However, this still did not halt classical (variola major) smallpox epidemics, the last of which occurred between 1902 and 1903. In 1907, the Vaccination Act allowed parents to oppose vaccination of their children. This was probably because smallpox epidemics had ceased to occur and because there was greater public awareness of possible vaccination complications. Smallpox continued to affect virtually every country in the world. Even in the UK, more than 10 000 cases were reported each year between 1926 and 1930, although the majority of these were probably non-classical smallpox (a milder strain called variola minor), and no further epidemics had occurred. After 1930 the number of reports declined, and by the middle of the twentieth century smallpox was no longer endemic in the UK, North America and many other Western countries. The Vaccination Act was repealed in 1946, upon the introduction of the National Health Service (NHS), and vaccination was provided free on a voluntary basis. As imported cases of smallpox were still not uncommon, other public health measures, including quarantine, surveillance and ring vaccination, were introduced. Ring vaccination was of particular importance in stopping further spread of smallpox. This involved vaccination of close contacts of index cases, thereby limiting the potential for spread. There were also many known routes of infection, such as corpses, insect vectors, clothing, bedding and other fomites with which contact was controlled both in endemic and non-endemic areas. Furthermore, people entering non-endemic countries after visiting or living in endemic areas such as Africa and Asia were required to present a valid certificate showing proof of vaccination within the preceding three years. This was due to an increase of travel of various populations because of pilgrimage, civil unrest and tourism.

Smallpox eradication was considered for a number of years because of the continuous burden the disease had on government resources and medical services. Smallpox was considered to be a good candidate for eradication for many reasons: it is an easily recognized disease, it is not very communicable, it has a long incubation period, there is no carrier state, and there is no known animal reservoir. However, smallpox eradication required an international effort and pooling of resources. This was first discussed in 1959 in the report of the Director General of the World Health Organization (WHO) and eventually came into reality in the mid-1960s. In 1966, the World Health Assembly decided to intensify smallpox control. An Expert Committee of Smallpox was set up in the following year by the WHO in Geneva, Switzerland. It was decided that smallpox vaccination should cover at least 80% of the population within two or three years. However, the cost of the programme far exceeded the WHO's total annual smallpox budget. Fortunately, donations totalling $18 million were received from 26 countries. Progress in the programme was slow in some countries but rapid in others. In 1967 endemic smallpox was present in 42 countries, but by 1973 the WHO had succeeded in reducing this number to four. A country was certified as being smallpox-free after it was shown that no cases were reported in the two years following the last known case and after commission members had conducted

field studies to confirm this. The last known case of naturally acquired smallpox occurred in October 1977 in Merka village near Mogadishu, Somalia. In the two years after this last case, extensive house-to-house searches were carried out in India and Bangladesh, the last two endemic areas in the world. No further cases of naturally acquired smallpox were reported in these areas, or from any other country, and therefore the world was declared smallpox-free in October 1979.

Although vaccination provided very good protection against infection with smallpox, it was not, however, without its drawbacks: immunity was not lifelong and therefore revaccination was recommended every three years, and complications of primary vaccination were not uncommon, resulting in about one complication per thousand and one death per million vaccinees. A number of serious complications may occur, including autoinoculation, generalized vaccinia, post-vaccination encephalitis, progressive vaccinia, abortion and eczema vaccinatum (Goldstein *et al.*, 1975).

In 1971, the vaccination of children in the UK and the USA was stopped because the risk of smallpox had become less than the risk of complications from the vaccine. Discontinuation of the vaccine in the USA saved an estimated $3 billion. The worldwide savings in terms of vaccine discontinuation, morbidity and mortality are enormous and could never be estimated in real terms. The need for vaccination of those handling vaccinia and other related orthopoxviruses for research purposes is still uncertain. UK authorities no longer recommend vaccination but US authorities recommend it. From 1963, methisazone, which prevented smallpox developing if given in the incubation period, had also been available. This drug was perhaps a little late because the worldwide incidence of smallpox had fallen dramatically by then. No drug was ever developed that was able to cure smallpox once the illness had started, i.e. after the incubation period.

The virus used for smallpox vaccine was, until 1976, produced in the skins of calves, sheep and buffaloes. Interestingly, WHO regulations at the time stated that the vaccine should not contain more than 500 bacteria per millilitre; this would not be tolerated in a new vaccine today. Early preparations of the vaccine were frozen or lyophilized preparations that lost their infectivity when used in the tropics or when being rehydrated, respectively. Therefore, a dried vaccine preparation was developed in France and Germany. This was a paste substance that was dispensed into a three-pronged hollow needle that could then be stored without refrigeration until the time of vaccination. This preparation was used for mass vaccination programmes. In 1967, at the start of the WHO programme, 64 laboratories in 62 countries were producing freeze-dried vaccine.

Although smallpox has been eradicated, a number of valid questions are still being asked. Most of these are in connection with related pox viruses. Some pox viruses are able to cause diseases in humans that are clinically very similar to smallpox itself. However, at present, these viruses are not readily transmissible between humans. Another concern is whether smallpox can lie dormant in vaccinated individuals until such a time that the immune levels fall enough for the virus to become reactivated. However, there is no evidence that this will happen and it is often disputed. The most important and recent concern is the use of smallpox as a biological weapon, particularly after the use of anthrax as a bioterrorism agent in letters sent through the US postal system in late 2001 (Atlas, 2002; Clarke, 2002). Two batches of smallpox have been retained in the former USSR and in the USA, and for some years debate continued as to whether the stocks should be destroyed. It has now been agreed that they should not be destroyed, in particular because we do not know whether small amounts of smallpox exist elsewhere. Intense research has now started on smallpox in order to develop improved vaccines and detection methods. A number of Western countries are now producing policy relating to smallpox immunization for healthcare workers; this is controversial (Benjamin, 2002; Bicknell, 2002; Bozzette et al., 2003), even though new cell-culture-based vaccination is now available (Bicknell and James, 2003; Mortimer, 2003). In addition, improved awareness and renewed education of medical staff and the public are required to understand the implications of smallpox infection (Blendon et al., 2003; Breman and Henderson, 2002).

REFERENCES

Atlas, R.M. (2002). Bioterrorism: from threat to reality. *Annu Rev Microbiol* **56**, 167–85.

Baxby, D. (1996). The Jenner bicentenary: the introduction and early distribution of smallpox vaccine. *FEMS Immunol Med Microbiol* **16**, 1–10.

Benjamin, G.C. (2002). Smallpox vaccine policy: the national debate. *Physician Exec* **28**, 64–6.

Bicknell, W.J. (2002). The case for voluntary smallpox vaccination. *N Engl J Med* **346**, 1323–5.

Bicknell, W. and James, K. (2003). The new cell culture smallpox vaccine should be offered to the general population. *Rev Med Virol* **13**, 5–15.

Blendon, R.J., DesRoches, C.M., Benson, J.M., Herrmann, M.J., Taylor-Clark, K. and Weldon, K.J. (2003). The public and the smallpox threat. *N Engl J Med* **348**, 426–32.

Bozzette, S.A., Boer, R., Bhatnagar, V., *et al.* (2003). A model for a smallpox-vaccination policy. *N Engl J Med* **348**, 416–25.

Breman, J.G. and Henderson, D.A. (2002). Diagnosis and management of smallpox. *N Engl J Med* **346**, 1300–1308.

Clarke, S.C. (2002). Bioterrorism: an overview. *Br J Biomed Sci* **59**, 232–4.

Ellner, P.D. (1998). Smallpox: gone but not forgotten. *Infection* **26**, 263–9.

Fenner, F. (1993). Smallpox: emergence, global spread, and eradication. *Hist Philos Life Sci* **15**, 397–420.

Goldstein, J.A., Neff, J.M., Lane, J.M. and Koplan, J.P. (1975). Smallpox vaccination reactions, prophylaxis, and therapy of complications. *Pediatrics* **55**, 342–7.

Mortimer, P.P. (2003). The new cell culture smallpox vaccine should not be offered to the general population. *Rev Med Virol* **13**, 17–20.

Willis, N.J. (1997). Edward Jenner and the eradication of smallpox. *Scott Med J* **42**, 118–21.

50

Influenza

Respiratory viruses remain a significant cause of morbidity and mortality worldwide, especially in children. One of the most important viral diseases of humans, in terms of morbidity and mortality, is influenza. Outbreaks of influenza have occurred since ancient times (Ghendon, 1994; Potter, 2001). The disease has a characteristic epidemiology, whereby unpredictable epidemics occur, usually annually, with periodic pandemics often occurring every decade. There were four pandemics in the twentieth century, the last being in 1977. In the 1918–19 pandemic, 200 000 deaths were recorded in England and Wales, with about 20 million deaths worldwide (Kuszewski and Brydak, 2000; Reid *et al.*, 2001). Since the early 1990s, between 1500 and 3200 cases of influenza have been reported each year (source: HPA CDSC). Depending on the year, these are split between influenza A and influenza B; few cases are due to non-groupable influenza. Mortality due to pneumonia-associated influenza is still high and increases with age. Epidemics of influenza occur due to antigenic drift of two viral proteins, haemagglutinin and neuraminidase, whereas pandemics are caused by antigenic shift of these proteins. Many different animal species may carry influenza virus, and evidence suggests that different strains of the virus may mix, resulting in subsequent genetic rearrangement. This process has been confirmed loosely by farming practices in South-East Asia, where ducks, pigs and humans mix closely; it is in this geographical area that many epidemics and pandemics begin (Alexander, 1982; Alexander, 2000; Lopez and Woods, 1984).

Until the middle of the twentieth century, there was no effective prophylaxis or therapy against influenza. Therefore, preventive methods were the only way of reducing the incidence of infection. In the 1940s, there was a great deal of research into such methods, resulting in ideas including the creation of antiseptic vapours in buildings by the use of ultraviolet light and the wearing of antiseptic-laden masks. The latter method was not entirely new because cotton-gauze face masks, some treated with antiseptics, had been used extensively during the 1918–19 pandemic in a number of countries.

There are three strategies for the prevention of influenza: (i) increasing herd immunity through vaccination or the use of drugs; (ii) preventive measures, i.e. to stop the spread of the virus; and (iii) stopping the emergence of pandemics. Of course, this philosophy is true for the control of many diseases. However, due to the antigenic properties of the influenza virus and the continuous antigenic drift, no vaccine has been produced that protects against all strains of the virus. Vaccines have been available since 1945 that protect against single subtypes, although these also often give limited protection against other subtypes. The early vaccines were of the whole-virus killed type and had many side effects. Modern vaccines are of the subunit type and are associated with few side effects. These vaccines also result in a good serological immune response. The management of influenza includes relief of symptoms, treatment of any complications, and specific antiviral therapy. Most individuals with uncomplicated infection require only symptomatic treatment.

Commercial influenza subunit vaccines are usually trivalent and contain two influenza A subtypes and influenza B (Belyavin, 1975; Palese and Garcia-Sastre, 2002). The actual antigenic composition of the vaccine is reviewed annually and is dependent upon the strains of influenza circulating in the community and on any information relating to a potential epidemic or pandemic. The efficacy of the vaccines can be as high as 70–90%, but this depends strongly on the antigenic homology between the vaccine and the circulating strain of virus and also on many factors associated with the vaccinee. Use of influenza vaccine, although not providing protection against all strains of influenza, has been shown to be of particular value in certain populations, such as elderly people and other people who may be at risk from influenza-related complications, and residents of nursing homes, old people's homes and other long-stay facilities. Vaccination is associated with a significant reduction in the severity of disease, incidence of complications such as bronchopneumonia, rate of hospital admission, and mortality. However, protective immunization usually lasts only a few months, and therefore revaccination is required each winter. Since the advent of influenza vaccines, the control of the disease has remained fairly constant. The only changes have been in the vaccination recommendations and in the use of the newer antiviral drugs. Live vaccines have been used extensively with apparent success and are administered by nasal sprays or drops, inducing a secretory immunoglobulin A (IgA) immune response (Bradshaw and Wright, 2002; Fiers et al., 2001; Glueck, 2001). However, Western opinions differ over their value. Future approaches to influenza vaccine include recombinant proteins and liposome carrier systems.

Communicable disease surveillance centres monitor the incidence and spread of influenza throughout the world and are prepared to respond when a pandemic occurs. These include the World Health Organization (WHO) Influenza Surveillance Centres stationed in 50 countries, which are able to detect new subtypes of influenza so that new vaccines can be defined at early stage. Such collaboration represents an important measure in the global control of influenza.

Three antiviral drugs have been developed for influenza therapy. The first is amantadine, which inhibits all subtypes of influenza A but is of little value against influenza B or C. Amantadine therapy leads to a reduction in virus shedding and shortens the duration of symptoms if the drug is started promptly. As well as good prophylactic efficacy, it is also of some therapeutic benefit. The use of amantadine, like most drugs, is contraindicated in some individuals. It should not be used in patients with cardiovascular or cerebral disorders, and it should be avoided during pregnancy. Rimantadine has a similar efficacy to amantadine but is not currently licensed for use in the UK. Ribavirin is effective against both influenza A and B and has been used with success by aerosol inhalation. Clinical trials of interferon, the human antiviral protein, have failed to show any significant therapeutic value; however, research is continuing into its potential benefits.

Due to the antigenic properties of influenza and the presence of animal reservoirs, it is unlikely that eradication is possible. Therefore, vaccination remains the only real solution to infection. However, as research continues, improved antiviral treatment may become available.

REFERENCES

Alexander, D.J. (1982). Ecological aspects of influenza A viruses in animals and their relationship to human influenza: a review. *J R Soc Med* 75, 799–811.

Alexander, D.J. (2000). A review of avian influenza in different bird species. *Vet Microbiol* 74, 3–13.

Belyavin, G. (1975). Experience in the control of influenza by vaccination. A brief review. *J Antimicrob Chemother* 1, 27–33.

Bradshaw, J. and Wright, P.F. (2002). Cold-adapted influenza vaccines. *Curr Opin Pediatr* 14, 95–8.

Fiers, W., Neirynck, S., Deroo, T., Saelens, X. and Jou, W.M. (2001). Soluble recombinant influenza vaccines. *Philos Trans R Soc Lond B Biol Sci* 356, 1961–3.

Ghendon, Y. (1994). Introduction to pandemic influenza through history. *Eur J Epidemiol* 10, 451–3.

Glueck, R. (2001). Review of intranasal influenza vaccine. *Adv Drug Deliv Rev* 51, 203–11.

Kuszewski, K. and Brydak, L. (2000). The epidemiology and history of influenza. *Biomed Pharmacother* **54**, 188–95.

Lopez, J.W. and Woods, G.T. (1984). Influenza virus in ruminants: a review. *Res Commun Chem Pathol Pharmacol* **45**, 445–62.

Palese, P. and Garcia-Sastre, A. (2002). Influenza vaccines: present and future. *J Clin Invest* **110**, 9–13.

Potter, C.W. (2001). A history of influenza. *J Appl Microbiol* **91**, 572–9.

Reid, A.H., Taubenberger, J.K. and Fanning, T.G. (2001). The 1918 Spanish influenza: integrating history and biology. *Microbes Infect* **3**, 81–7.

51

Epstein–Barr virus

Epstein–Barr virus (EBV) is a member of the herpes virus group. The virus was first visualized in 1964 by Epstein, Achong and Barr in tissue cultures of biopsies from individuals with Burkitt's lymphoma. The virions are 180–200 nm in diameter and appear under electron microscopy as enveloped hexagonal nucleocapsids. Like all herpes viruses, EBV DNA is double-stranded, although structurally the DNA is unique among the herpes viruses.

EBV infection is common and has a worldwide distribution (Faulkner *et al.*, 2000; Rickinson, 2002). Infections are common during childhood, but most are mild or asymptomatic. In the UK and the USA, EBV seroconversion occurs before the age of five years in approximately 50% of the population. Seroconversion occurs in another large percentage of the population during the teenage years. However, adolescent primary infection is more severe and carries a 50% risk of developing glandular fever (infectious mononucleosis). The incubation period of glandular fever is between four and seven weeks, after which time the patient presents with general symptoms of sore throat, lymphadenopathy, malaise and fever. The latter is present in more than 90% of patients with glandular fever. A rash may also be present in a small number of patients. The symptoms are therefore similar to those of other viral infections. The acute phase of EBV infection may persist for a number of weeks, causing a fairly debilitating illness in some people. Relapses may occur. Complications include hepatic necrosis, tracheal obstruction, Guillain–Barré syndrome and splenic rupture (Murray and Young, 2002). Death due to EBV infection, normally as a result of complications, has been

reported but is very rare. In immunocompromised people, infection is often significant due to reactivation of previous infection. Reactivation of EBV may result in the production of B-cell lymphomas, and in acquired immune deficiency syndrome (AIDS) patients hairy leukoplakia may develop (Cesarman, 2002; Markoulatos *et al.*, 2001).

EBV may also be oncogenic and may be associated with Burkitt's lymphoma or nasopharyngeal carcinoma. Burkitt's lymphoma is a disease seen in young children. It presents at multiple sites and often involves the jaw, orbital cavities and gastrointestinal tract. Although progression of the disease is rapid, it responds to anti-tumour chemotherapy. Burkitt's lymphoma occurs in equatorial Africa and New Guinea, where malaria is hyperendemic. Malaria may act as a cofactor for the lymphoma for a number of reasons, including immunosuppression. Nasopharyngeal carcinoma, however, often does not respond to chemotherapy. This is because the primary tumour, which develops in the epithelial cells of the postnasal space, is usually inconspicuous and patients do not present until the carcinoma has spread to the regional lymph nodes in the neck. The disease is restricted mainly to areas of southern China and to people of southern Chinese descent. Genetic predisposition is therefore thought to be important. Overpowering EBV infection, known as X-linked lymphoproliferative syndrome or Duncan syndrome, can occur. Seen in boys who have been otherwise healthy, this results in a clinically severe form of glandular fever, lymphoma or hypogammaglobulinaemia.

EBV has a limited host range, although it is fairly well adapted to those that it can infect. In vitro cultivation has been described only in B-lymphocytes of humans and some higher primates. Data suggest that the spread of infection is by salivary transmission via intimate contact between susceptible and infected symptomatic or asymptomatic individuals. In common with other herpes viruses, EBV persists in the body following primary infection; the virus has been shown to persist in the oropharynx of individuals up to 18 months after clinical recovery. The virus can also be transmitted via blood transfusion, but the significance of this is thought to be low because recipients may already have seroconverted and because the donor blood may contain neutralizing antibody.

The clinical diagnosis of glandular fever is often straightforward. About 70% of individuals have a mononuclear lymphocytosis. However, it must be remembered that other infectious diseases, such as rubella, cytomegalovirus and mumps, may also result in an atypical lymphocytosis. The presence of lymphocytosis, general symptoms and a positive Paul–Bunnell–Davidsohn test (see below) may establish the diagnosis of glandular fever. Difficulties arise when the general symptoms are mild or when the Paul–Bunnell–Davidsohn test is negative.

The majority of EBV infections are diagnosed in the laboratory by serological testing (Brengel-Pesce *et al.*, 2002; Debyser *et al.*, 1997; Gulley, 2001; Tsuchiya, 2002). Modern molecular techniques, such as the polymerase chain reaction (PCR), may also be used (Barkholt *et al.*, 1998; Gulley, 2001; Hausler *et al.*, 2003; Markoulatos *et al.*, 2001). Acute infection may be determined by detecting immunoglobulin M (IgM) against EBV virus capsid antigen or by performing acute and convalescent serology for the presence of antibodies against virus nuclear antigen. These tests are useful for confirming the diagnosis of Burkitt's lymphoma or nasopharyngeal carcinoma. Serological diagnosis of glandular fever may be achieved by using the Paul–Bunnell–Davidsohn test. This permits the detection of heterophile antibodies after differential absorbance of the serum. However, the test may be falsely negative in children and elderly people undergoing primary infec-

tion. The test can also be falsely positive. Active infection is ideally diagnosed by the detection of the actual virus. This may be achieved in lymphocyte culture or, more recently, by DNA hybridization. The presence of EBV in tumour biopsies may be determined by staining with specific antibodies.

There is currently no treatment for EBV infection. A number of vaccines have been developed based on a 340-kDa surface glycoprotein, and others are undergoing clinical trials (Morgan, 1992). A satisfactory animal model has not yet been found, which therefore hinders the production of a suitable treatment or vaccine. EBV infection in primates does not lead to glandular fever but results instead in inapparent infection or neoplasia. Aciclovir in low concentrations may be useful because it has been shown to inhibit EBV replication, although clinical studies have been disappointing. Ganciclovir and bromovinyldeoxyuridine have also been shown to inhibit EBV replication.

REFERENCES

Barkholt, L., Reinholt, F.P., Teramoto, N., Enbom, M., Dahl, H. and Linde, A. (1998). Polymerase chain reaction and in situ hybridization of Epstein–Barr virus in liver biopsy specimens facilitate the diagnosis of EBV hepatitis after liver transplantation. *Transpl Int* **11**, 336–44.

Brengel-Pesce, K., Morand, P., Schmuck, A., *et al.* (2002). Routine use of real-time quantitative PCR for laboratory diagnosis of Epstein–Barr virus infections. *J Med Virol* **66**, 360–69.

Cesarman, E. (2002). Epstein–Barr virus (EBV) and lymphomagenesis. *Front Biosci* **7**, e58–65.

Debyser, Z., Reynders, M., Goubau, P. and Desmyter, J. (1997). Comparative evaluation of three ELISA techniques and an indirect immunofluorescence assay for the serological diagnosis of Epstein–Barr virus infection. *Clin Diagn Virol* **8**, 71–81.

Faulkner, G.C., Krajewski, A.S. and Crawford, D.H. (2000). The ins and outs of EBV infection. *Trends Microbiol* **8**, 185–9.

Gulley, M.L. (2001). Molecular diagnosis of Epstein–Barr virus-related diseases. *J Mol Diagn* **3**, 1–10.

Hausler, M., Scheithauer, S., Ritter, K. and Kleines, M. (2003). Molecular diagnosis of Epstein–Barr virus. *Expert Rev Mol Diagn* **3**, 81–92.

Markoulatos, P., Georgopoulou, A., Siafakas, N., Plakokefalos, E., Tzanakaki, G. and Kourea-Kremastinou, J. (2001). Laboratory diagnosis of common herpesvirus infections of the central nervous system by a multiplex PCR assay. *J Clin Microbiol* **39**, 4426–32.

Morgan, A.J. (1992). Epstein–Barr virus vaccines. *Vaccine* **10**, 563–71.

Murray, P.G. and Young, L.S. (2002). The role of the Epstein–Barr virus in human disease. *Front Biosci* **7**, d519–40.

Rickinson, A. (2002). Epstein–Barr virus. *Virus Res* **82**, 109–13.

Tsuchiya, S. (2002). Diagnosis of Epstein–Barr virus-associated diseases. *Crit Rev Oncol Hematol* **44**, 227–38.

52

Rabies

The rabies virus is a member of the Rhabdovirus family. Rabies is an ancient disease (Dreesen, 1997): it was first recognized in 2300 BC, but it was not until AD 1 that the association between bites and saliva was first made. The virus is able to infect and survive in all warm-blooded animals, and it has a worldwide distribution. Cases of human rabies reported to the World Health Organization (WHO) suggest that over 35 000 deaths are attributable to rabies each year.

The symptoms of rabies are very similar in all infected animals. However, there are three types of rabies: urban rabies occurs in dogs and foxes in the developing world; sylvatic rabies occurs in foxes, skunks and bats in North America and Europe (Baevsky and Bartfield, 1993); and vampire bat rabies occurs in South America, where it is a particular problem. Over three-quarters of vampire bats may carry rabies, and large numbers of cattle are lost after being bitten by these creatures. Cases of human rabies have occurred worldwide, except in Australia and the Atlantic islands. Although a number of countries are now rabies-free, the disease is still endemic in many developing countries (Turner, 1976). Rabies is almost always contracted as a result of a bite from a rabid animal; transmission occurs via saliva. However, rarely rabies may be contracted via urine or even aerosols if concentrations of virus are great enough; this may occur, for example, in caves inhabited by large numbers of rabies-infected bats. Over 90% of the total number of human rabies cases are contracted after being bitten by a rabid dog or cat. However, in countries where domestic animal rabies is controlled, dogs account for less than 5% of rabies cases in humans. There are a number of factors affecting the suscep-

tibility of clinical disease, including the quantity and site of the bite, the age of the animal, and the strain of virus. About 75% of human rabies cases result in dumb rabies; the other 25% result in furious rabies. Although the total number of deaths from rabies in developed countries and the associated mortality rate is low, a large amount of money is spent on vaccinating people after being bitten by potentially rabid dogs and cats; for example, in France around £5 million is spent each year.

The symptoms of rabies are similar in both humans and animals. During the incubation period, the patient is well except for any symptoms relating to the bite wound. The incubation period is usually between 20 and 90 days, but it may range from days to months to years; reports have been made of incubation periods as short as four days and as long as 19 years. The incubation period is at its longest when the bite is at the extremities, and at its shortest when the bite is on the head. The virus is excreted in the saliva before the onset of clinically apparent disease throughout the symptomatic stage. Symptoms begin when the rabies virus enters the central nervous system. There is a prodromal stage, during which symptoms are non-specific and include malaise, fatigue, anorexia and fever. This stage lasts up to 10 days, after which the acute neurological stage develops. At this point, central nervous stage signs are apparent and may include hyperactivity, disorientation, hallucinations and paralysis. In many cases, hyperactivity is marked, and the disease is known as 'furious rabies' (Goswami et al., 1984). Patients may die during this stage due to respiratory obstruction or cardiac arrest. Coma occurs after the acute neurological stage. This varies in length, depending on the availability of supportive therapy. Complications may follow during the coma phase, which usually result in death. Although most infected animals die, rabies is able to survive as a disease and persist in animal populations by self-sustaining enzootics in many animals, such as dogs, foxes, skunks and bats.

The main European source of rabies is the fox. Urban foxes are extremely sociable and are particularly common in the UK. Therefore, if an outbreak should occur, rabies is able to spread quickly through the fox population. Since 1989, vaccine baits have been distributed in parts of Europe. This has been an effective method of reducing the number of cases. In 1977, the number of cases was 11 000; by 1992, this had fallen to 1300. Rabies can be controlled in dog populations by a few simple measures (Wandeler *et al.*, 1993). In rabies-free areas, quarantine and vaccination are sufficient. In rabies-endemic areas, surveillance, immunization, dog control and public education may reduce the number of rabies cases.

Diagnosis of rabies is based upon clinical findings, epidemiology or ante-mortem diagnosis. Laboratory diagnosis may be achieved by a number of methods. Cell culture and fluorescence tests were developed in the late 1950s. Other methods include enzyme-linked immunosorbent assay (ELISA), the mouse inoculation test, reverse transcriptase polymerase chain reaction (RT-PCR), and histopathology (Turner, 1982; Wacharapluesadee and Hemachudha, 2001; Wacharapluesadee and Hemachudha, 2002; Warner *et al.*, 1999). In humans, the rabies virus may be isolated from saliva, brain tissue, cerebrospinal fluid and urine. Before the advent of vaccination, cauterization of the animal bite was the treatment of choice. The first human rabies vaccine was introduced by Pasteur in 1885, but hyperimmune serum was not developed until 1954 (Dreesen, 1997). Antiviral treatment is not thought to be effective. In humans, if there is a known potential risk of acquiring rabies, then pre-exposure vaccination is available. Post-exposure vaccination is also available for both unvaccinated and previously vaccinated individuals. Hyperimmune serum can be used only in unvaccinated individuals. The protection gained from cell culture vaccines is virtually 100% (Dreesen, 1997; Turner, 1982).

REFERENCES

Baevsky, R.H. and Bartfield, J.M. (1993). Human rabies: a review. *Am J Emerg Med* 11, 279–86.

Dreesen, D.W. (1997). A global review of rabies vaccines for human use. *Vaccine* 15 (suppl), S2–6.

Goswami, U., Shankar, S.K., Channabasavanna, S.M. and Chattopadhyay, A. (1984). Psychiatric presentations in rabies. A clinico-pathologic report from South India with a review of literature. *Trop Geogr Med* 36, 77–81.

Turner, G.S. (1976). A review of the world epidemiology of rabies. *Trans R Soc Trop Med Hyg* 70, 175–8.

Turner, G.S. (1982). Brief review of diagnosis, management and immunotherapy of rabies. *Trop Doct* 12, 204–7.

Wacharapluesadee, S. and Hemachudha, T. (2001). Nucleic-acid sequence based amplification in the rapid diagnosis of rabies. *Lancet* 358, 892–3.

Wacharapluesadee, S. and Hemachudha, T. (2002). Urine samples for rabies RNA detection in the diagnosis of rabies in humans. *Clin Infect Dis* 34, 874–5.

Wandeler, A.I., Matter, H.C., Kappeler, A. and Budde, A. (1993). The ecology of dogs and canine rabies: a selective review. *Rev Sci Tech* 12, 51–71.

Warner, C.K., Zaki, S.R., Shieh, W.J., *et al.* (1999). Laboratory investigation of human deaths from vampire bat rabies in Peru. *Am J Trop Med Hyg* 60, 502–7.

53

HIV and AIDS

In the mid to late 1970s, young gay men in the USA started presenting to their doctors with unexplained swollen glands, fever and fatigue. No treatment given to these individuals was effective. At the same time, a number of cases of Kaposi's sarcoma, a rare skin tumour, appeared in young men (Cotter and Robertson, 2002). There was also an outbreak of *Pneumocystis carinii* pneumonia (PCP), a condition usually seen in immunocompromised patients such as those undergoing cancer therapy, in the summer of 1981 in Los Angeles. This was accompanied by a general increase in the number of cases of PCP. It was soon discovered that these individuals, who were previously healthy, had poor immune systems and were therefore susceptible to diseases that would normally not affect healthy young adults. The first case of this new syndrome in the UK was in December 1981, and by this time there were almost 200 reported cases in the USA. By the end of the following year, this had increased to over 500 cases in the USA, with another 200 cases reported in a total of 14 countries.

By September 1983, 2259 cases had been reported in the USA, resulting in 917 deaths. Approximately 70% of these were in homosexuals, which led to the syndrome initially being called gay-related immune deficiency (GRID). The majority of the early cases were seen only in gay men, but then cases in intravenous drug users came to light. A few cases were also seen in women and in haemophiliacs. A link between the syndrome and blood was established, the term GRID was dropped, and a new term – acquired immunedeficiency syndrome (AIDS) – was coined. The transmission of the causative agent to haemophiliacs and transfusion recipients became a great concern

before the aetiological agent was known and before any diagnostic or screening test was available. Thousands of AIDS cases were reported in haemophiliacs and transfusion recipients in the USA, but the problem was not as great in the UK. Meanwhile, the total number of cases worldwide was rising, and interest in the causative agent increased.

The aetiological agent of AIDS was soon found to be a virus. The initial suspicion that a retrovirus was the cause of AIDS came from Luc Montagnier's laboratory at the Institut Pasteur in Paris (Montagnier, 2002; Shampo amd Kyle, 2002). They isolated a reverse transcriptase-containing virus from the lymph node of a man with persistent lymphadenopathy. Possession of the enzyme reverse transcriptase is a known feature of retroviruses, while persistent lymphadenopathy is known to be a symptom of seroconversion in AIDS, although this symptom may also be seen in other viral infections. At the same time, Robert Gallo's laboratory at the National Institutes of Health (NIH) in the USA reported the isolation of a human T-cell leukaemia virus (HTLV) from individuals with AIDS. However, there were doubts of an HTLV being the cause of AIDS. Further studies by Montagnier's group showed that their virus had properties that were distinct from HTLV, and so they named it lymphadenopathy-associated virus (LAV). Soon after, Gallo's laboratory reported the isolation of a human retrovirus that was distinct from HTLV, which they named human T-cell leukaemia virus type III (HTLV-III). Another group also reported the identification of retroviruses from individuals with AIDS, and named them AIDS-associated retroviruses (ARVs). The three viruses,

LAV, HTLV-III and ARV, were soon recognized as being lentiviruses, a genus within the retrovirus group, and in 1986 they were collectively recommended the name human immunodeficiency virus (HIV) by the International Committee on Taxonomy of Viruses. HIV was therefore the name given to the causative agent of AIDS. By this time, over 24 000 individuals in the USA and over 2000 in Western Europe had died of AIDS.

The schematic structure of HIV is shown in Figure 53.1. HIV is a member of the lentiviruses, which are a genus of the family Retroviridae. Retroviruses are enveloped viruses between 90 and 120 nm in diameter and with a single-stranded RNA genome. There are many different known retroviruses, which mostly cause encephalopathy or immune deficiency; they occur in animals such as cows, cats, goats, horses and primates. All such retroviruses infect either macrophages or T-lymphocytes. There are two known subtypes of HIV. HIV-1 has a worldwide distribution and is not related closely to simian immunodeficiency virus (SIV) (Blankson et al., 2002); HIV-2, although originally restricted to west Africa, has spread to Asia and Europe and is related genetically to two species of SIV (Reeves and Doms, 2002).

The origin of HIV is unclear. There are reports of a sailor from Manchester, UK, who had an AIDS-like illness in 1959; HIV was found in preserved tissue from the man. He had travelled to Africa on a number of occasions and may have introduced HIV into the USA. However, this does not explain why the apparent spread of the virus was not noticed until the 1970s. It is more likely that multiple introductions of the virus occurred in the USA. The African origin is thought to be from monkeys; this forms the basis of another theory, which suggests that a monkey virus contaminated a polio vaccination programme. However, if HIV did originate from another animal, such as the monkey, then why did it not appear in humans until the 1970s? There are a number of possible answers to this, such as the host barrier effect, evolution in virulence, and various social factors.

By the mid-1980s, heterosexually transmitted AIDS was becoming a problem in Africa. The clinical picture was slightly different to that seen in individuals in the Western world. The main differing feature was the severe loss of weight, which led to the disease also being known in Africa as slim disease. Around three-quarters of all AIDS cases are thought to occur in sub-Saharan Africa. It is now thought that around 50 million people have been infected with HIV worldwide (Lears and Alwood, 2000) and that as many as 13 million children have been orphaned due to their parents dying of AIDS. In the UK, there are over 41 000 people living with HIV, the majority of whom have been infected through sex between men (source: HPA CDSC). Around one-third of all infections are thought to be undiagnosed, and approximately 15 000 deaths are known to have occurred in the UK since the HIV epidemic began. In the USA, there were 774 467 cases of AIDS up to the end of 2000, resulting in 448 060 deaths (source: US CDC).

HIV may be transmitted through sexual intercourse, via infected body fluids, and before or during birth by the transmission of virus-infected cells or free virus particles. HIV transmission through heterosexual sex has been shown to occur more easily from infected males to uninfected females than from infected females to uninfected males. Any damage to or inflammation of the genital mucosa increases the risk of HIV transmission. Therefore, individuals who already have a sexually transmitted disease (STD) are more likely than those without an STD to become infected.

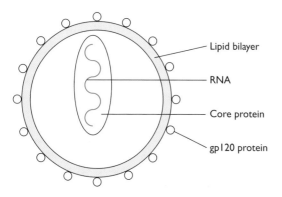

Lipid bilayer

RNA

Core protein

gp120 protein

Figure 53.1 Schematic diagram of the structure of HIV.

Following infection with HIV, replication of the virus occurs throughout the body in almost every organ, including the peripheral blood, bone marrow, lymph nodes and central nervous system (CNS). Infection results in the development of a strong response from both the humoral and cellular systems, usually within three months (Appay *et al.*, 2002; Aquaro *et al.*, 2002; Chinen and Shearer, 2002). Sometimes seroconversion takes longer, but an HIV antibody-negative status is extremely rare if true infection has occurred and even more so if the individual has AIDS. The antibody titre increases for approximately six months; once antibody production begins, it is maintained throughout life. Antibodies are produced against the envelope (env) and gag protein as well as other gene products. Infection of T-lymphocytes occurs by virus binding between the CD4 molecule of the lymphocyte and the envelope protein gp120 of HIV. After entry into the cell, the virus is able to integrate its own RNA genome into the host cell DNA chromosome. It does this by use of its enzyme reverse transcriptase. The genetic material of the virus remains dormant in the host cell until such a time that viral messaging occurs and translation of the viral genome takes place. This is followed by virion assembly and virus budding.

Seroconversion is associated with an acute illness in about half of HIV-infected individuals. Symptoms resemble those of aseptic meningitis and include oral and oesophageal ulceration, a maculopapular rash on the trunk, and generalized lymphadenopathy. After seroconversion, there is an asymptomatic period, although symptoms may occur in some patients. At a later stage, most HIV-infected individuals develop AIDS, although this may not occur for 10–12 years. In simple terms, AIDS develops due to a change in virus dynamics. It is now thought that the indicator of HIV infection and the likeliness of AIDS development is the viral load, and not the CD4-positive lymphocyte cell concentration. After seroconversion, the immune response is able to keep viral replication, and hence the viral load, in check. However, at some stage the immune system is no longer able to cope, the CD4-positive lymphocyte count falls, and opportunistic infections are able to occur. Not only do these infections occur, most of which would normally not take place in immunocompetent individuals, but the infections are also more severe. The CD4-positive lymphocyte count falls further and the CD8-positive lymphocyte count also begins to fall. Opportunistic infections are more significant, mild cytopenia occurs, and direct HIV infection of the CNS takes place.

There are many different infections and symptoms seen in AIDS, depending on previous exposure to micro-organisms, local infectious disease epidemiology, and the severity of the immunocompromised state. During late HIV and AIDS, infections may manifest in almost any part of the body and may be due to viruses, bacteria, fungi and parasites (Table 53.1). Many of the opportunistic infections seen in individuals with AIDS have preclinical phases, during which they can be diagnosed and treated. It is therefore beneficial to screen for such infections before symptoms are apparent.

Table 53.1 Some of the opportunistic infections that may be seen in individuals with HIV and AIDS

Pneumocystis carinii pneumonia
Cryptosporidiosis
Cytomegalovirus infection
Toxoplasma encephalitis
Herpes simplex infection
Microsporidiosis
Varicella-zoster virus infection
Bartonella infection
Tuberculosis
Candidiasis
Bacterial respiratory infections
Cryptococcosis
Bacterial enteric infections
Histoplasmosis
Mycobacterium avium complex (disseminated infection)
Coccidioidomycosis

Fungal diseases, which are difficult to treat in immunocompetent individuals, pose even more of a problem in people with AIDS and are a significant cause of morbidity. The most common fungal infection is candidiasis, which may occur on any mucosal surface. Others include cryptococcosis, histoplasmosis, blastomycosis and aspergillosis, although these infections occur infrequently. Mycobacterial infections are also important in AIDS. In the early phases of AIDS *Mycobacterium tuberculosis* may reactivate, while in the later phase disseminated *Mycobacterium avium* infection may occur.

Detection of HIV for diagnostic purposes may be achieved by cell culture or polymerase chain reaction (PCR). Additionally, antibodies to HIV may be detected using an antibody detection system such as enzyme-linked immunosorbent assay (ELISA) (Yilmaz, 2001). Antibody detection may be used for either diagnostic or screening purposes. The diagnosis of AIDS may be based on HIV seropositivity and clinical signs. Progress in the development of a therapy for HIV or AIDS has been slow, even though billions of pounds are spent on HIV and AIDS research each year. There is as yet no wholly effective therapy, mainly because HIV is able to mutate rapidly due to its fairly inefficient method of replication – reverse transcription – which leads to occasional changes in its structure when it multiplies. When therapies are used, they must be monitored closely (Telenti, 2002). As well as the two subtypes, there are many strains of HIV. Even in one individual the HIV population may be highly heterogeneous due to slight mutations, which may affect a number of features of the virus, such as cellular tropism, cytopathicity and replication.

The first AIDS therapy was azidothymidine (also know as zidovudine and AZT; commercial name Retrovir), which was introduced at an initial cost of $8000–10 000 per patient per year. This drug works by inhibiting the action of the enzyme reverse transcriptase. It was licensed in the USA in 1987 for the treatment of patients with AIDS. The cost of the drug led to intense opposition by AIDS activists, and the price was reduced. AZT initially provided hope for AIDS sufferers, but it soon became apparent that the drug's effects were only temporary and did not benefit all users. It was thought initially that AZT would delay the onset of AIDS, but in 1993 the Concorde trial showed that AZT does not significantly delay AIDS in those infected with HIV. However, it can prevent the transmission of HIV from mother to child. Other protease inhibitors are now also available (Bhana *et al.*, 2002; Hervey and Perry, 2000).

Another target for HIV therapy is the viral enzyme protease. This enzyme is essential for HIV replication: if the virus does not possess it, then immature virions that are unable to complete replication are produced, and therefore the viral load does not increase. The protease of HIV is sufficiently distinct from human proteases to make it an ideal target for a therapeutic agent. A number of protease inhibitors are now available, which, if given in combination with AZT, may be useful in reducing the viral load of HIV (Hermans, 2001). However, such therapies are very new and therefore long-term results in patients are awaited. They are very expensive, costing about $6000 per patient each year. These drugs may not be absorbed well, meaning that high doses have to be given. Drug resistance is also a problem due to the mutation rate of HIV (Aleman *et al.*, 2002; Andreoletti *et al.*, 2002; Condra *et al.*, 2002). Despite these negative points, HIV therapies have had a big impact on HIV in developed countries (Mwau and McMichael, 2003).

Now that HIV infection is so widespread, many countries, but not the UK, insist on HIV tests for long-term visitors, and it is a criminal offence in Australia and some states in the USA to fail to disclose HIV-positive status to a sexual partner. As effective therapies are unavailable to prevent HIV infection after transmission, other preventive measures must be followed. Such measures may be simple. Condoms should be used during heterosexual, anal and oral sex, clean needles should be used by intravenous drug users, and risk assessment can be used to avoid vertical transmission of HIV, such as from mother to child (Anon, 2001). Occupational transmission of HIV is very rare. Such occupations include medical laboratories, dental surgeries, surgical theatres and care institutions, where exposure to bodily fluids may be possible. It is estimated that the risk of acquiring HIV from blood in an occupational routine is less than 1%, although the cumulative lifetime risk depends on local HIV seroprevalence and the incidence of exposure. However, with due care and by following routine health and safety measures, any risk can be minimized greatly.

With the recent increases in the understanding of HIV viral dynamics in infected individuals and advances in therapies, the HIV pandemic has levelled out slowly. At present, however, preventive measures and public awareness are the main methods of reducing the transmission of HIV in both developed and developing countries until a suitable vaccine candidate is found (Mwau and McMichael, 2003).

REFERENCES

Aleman, S., Soderbarg, K., Visco-Comandini, U., Sitbon, G. and Sonnerborg, A. (2002). Drug resistance at low viraemia in HIV-1-infected patients with antiretroviral combination therapy. *Aids* **16**, 1039–44.

Andreoletti, L., Weiss, L., Si-Mohamed, A., *et al.* (2002). Multidrug-resistant HIV-1 RNA and proviral DNA variants harboring new dipeptide insertions in the reverse transcriptase pol gene. *J Acquir Immune Defic Syndr* **29**, 102-4.

Anon (2001). Special NIH review confirms condoms effective against transmission of HIV, gonorrhea. *FDA Consum* **35**, 7.

Appay, V., Papagno, L., Spina, C.A., *et al.* (2002). Dynamics of T cell responses in HIV infection. *J Immunol* **168**, 3660–66.

Aquaro, S., Calio, R., Balzarini, J., Bellocchi, M.C., Garaci, E. and Perno, C.F. (2002). Macrophages and HIV infection: therapeutical approaches toward this strategic virus reservoir. *Antiviral Res* **55**, 209–25.

Bhana, N., Ormrod, D., Perry, C.M. and Figgitt, D.P. (2002). Zidovudine: a review of its use in the management of vertically-acquired pediatric HIV infection. *Paediatr Drugs* **4**, 515–53.

Blankson, J.N., Persaud, D. and Siliciano, R.F. (2002). The challenge of viral reservoirs in HIV-1 infection. *Annu Rev Med* **53**, 557–93.

Chinen, J. and Shearer, W.T. (2002). Molecular virology and immunology of HIV infection. *J Allergy Clin Immunol* **110**, 189–98.

Condra, J.H., Miller, M.D., Hazuda, D.J. and Emini, E.A. (2002). Potential new therapies for the treatment of HIV-1 infection. *Annu Rev Med* **53**, 541–55.

Cotter, M.A., 2nd and Robertson, E.S. (2002). Molecular biology of Kaposi's sarcoma-associated herpesvirus. *Front Biosci* **7**, d358–75.

Hermans, P. (2001). Current review and clinical management of patients with primary HIV-1 infection: limits and perspectives. *Biomed Pharmacother* **55**, 301–7.

Hervey, P.S. and Perry, C.M. (2000). Abacavir: a review of its clinical potential in patients with HIV infection. *Drugs* **60**, 447–79.

Lears, M.K. and Alwood, K.S. (2000). The natural history, current status, and future trends of HIV infection. *Lippincotts Prim Care Pract* **4**, 1–19.

Montagnier, L. (2002). Historical essay. A history of HIV discovery. *Science* **298**, 1727–8.

Mwau, M. and McMichael, A.J. (2003). A review of vaccines for HIV prevention. *J Gene Med* **5**, 3–10.

Reeves, J.D. and Doms, R.W. (2002). Human immunodeficiency virus type 2. *J Gen Virol* **83**, 1253–65.

Shampo, M.A. and Kyle, R.A. (2002). Luc Montagnier – discoverer of the AIDS virus. *Mayo Clin Proc* **77**, 506.

Telenti, A. (2002). New developments in laboratory monitoring of HIV-1 infection. *Clin Microbiol Infect* **8**, 137–43.

Yilmaz, G. (2001). Diagnosis of HIV infection and laboratory monitoring of its therapy. *J Clin Virol* **21**, 187–96.

54

Herpes simplex viruses I and II

There are more than 80 herpes viruses, eight of which are known to affect humans. These include herpes simplex viruses I and II (HSV-I and HSV-II), cytomegalovirus (CMV), varicella zoster virus (VZV), Epstein–Barr virus (EBV) and three more recent additions, human herpes viruses 6, 7 and 8 (HHV-6, HHV-7 and HHV-8). This chapter will discuss only HSV-I and HSV-II. Of the herpes viruses known to affect humans, HSV-I and HSV-II are the most common causes of human disease (Taylor *et al.*, 2002). Infection with HSV-I may result in cold sores and genital infection, while HSV-II is associated solely with genital infection. HSV-II is by far the most common cause of genital herpes. HSV-I and HSV-II have a worldwide distribution, and humans are the sole reservoirs of infection. Infections caused by HSV have been documented for thousands of years, and the name herpes is derived from the Greek word meaning 'to crawl'. Infection is rarely fatal in otherwise healthy individuals, and asymptomatic excretion can occur. There is no seasonal variation associated with infection. Both HSV-I and HSV-II are double-stranded DNA viruses between 110 and 220 nm in diameter. Their characteristic pathology is ballooning of infected cells, with the presence of condensed chromatin within the nuclei of these cells and subsequent degeneration of cellular nuclei. Cells eventually lyse after being infected, leading to an intense inflammatory response. During infection, the virus replicates within cells and spreads from cell to cell. The virus also reaches the sacral ganglia, where it may enter latency.

Genital herpes is acquired through sexual contact, and seroprevalence correlates directly with the onset of sexual activity. The worldwide incidence of genital herpes continues to increase due to the lack of a widely available and effective vaccine. Epidemiological studies in the UK and the USA suggest that the prevalence of genital herpes exceeds that of all other major sexually transmitted diseases (STDs), with as many as one in 10 individuals being infected. In the UK, for example, almost 18 000 new cases of genital herpes were reported in 2001 (source: HPA CDSC); between 1972 and 2001, the number of diagnoses increased two-fold in men and nine-fold in women (Figure 54.1). The prevalence of herpes labialis, more commonly known as cold sores, is even greater. Infection results in a symptomatic stage lasting about three weeks, with the formation of macules and papules at the site of infection. During late infection, these turn to pustules and then ulcers. Virus is also excreted for three weeks, meaning that infection can be passed to other sexual partners during this time. In both sexes, the initial days of infection result in malaise, fever, headache and other flu-like symptoms. In females, herpetic lesions are bilateral and vulval, with the cervix often being involved. Urinary retention and aseptic meningitis are common. In males, lesions occur on the glans penis or penile shaft and also possibly on the thigh, buttock and perineum; urinary retention and aseptic meningitis may also occur.

Primary genital herpes in individuals with pre-existing antibodies from a previous exposure to herpes at another body site is less severe with regards to the severity of symptoms, the healing of ulcers, and the incidence of complications. Once genital infection with HSV has occurred, then recurrent mild infections may take place, which are of shorter duration (usually 7–10 days). Reactivation of infection may be due to a number of factors, such as stress, immunosuppression and

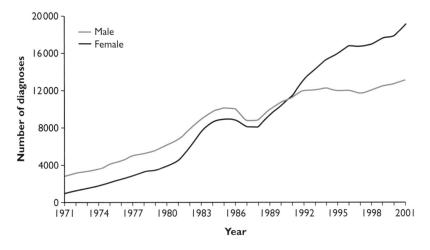

Figure 54.1   Diagnosis of genital herpes in England and Wales, 1971–81* (source: HPA CDSC).
*As Scotland and Northern Ireland data for 1971–2001 are incomplete, they have been excluded from this figure.

another infection (Wolff *et al.*, 2002). An average of four recurrences may occur in the first year after primary infection has taken place, although in some individuals there may be as many as 12 recurrences per year. As well as the obvious symptomatic effects of genital herpes, infection with HSV can also cause strain in sexual relationships and can lead to psychological disturbances. Therefore, counselling is sometimes required after primary infection and then throughout infection, particularly after reactivation.

The diagnosis of genital herpes is important due to the personal and social implications of infection. Diagnosis may be based upon the description of clinical symptoms, genital examination and laboratory testing. A number of laboratory tests are available, including cell culture, electron microscopy, enzyme-linked immunosorbent assay (ELISA) and polymerase chain reaction (PCR), depending on the clinical sample required for diagnosis (Aldea *et al.*, 2002; Druce *et al.*, 2002; Espy *et al.*, 2000; Wald and Ashley-Morrow, 2002). These tests may be used to detect live or dead virus, or to detect antibodies from an immune response in the infected individual. It is also important to differentiate between HSV-I and HSV-II (Diamond *et al.*, 1999). For most cases, fluid from vesicular lesions should be collected early in infection and used for analysis. Some methods of diagnosis are better than others, and some are better for the diagnosis of certain types of HSV infection.

Although there is no effective vaccine for HSV infection, the availability of the antiviral drug aciclovir has reduced the frequency and severity of recurrent genital herpes, thereby improving the lifestyle of many patients, both emotionally and psychologically. Aciclovir is a DNA polymerase inhibitor available in intravenous, topical and oral preparations. Few side effects have been reported. It is excreted in the urine. Aciclovir does not prevent infection, but when taken orally it has been shown to reduce the duration and severity of symptoms. In extremely recurrent cases, aciclovir can be given as a suppressive therapy to reduce the number of recurrent episodes.

Infection during pregnancy results rarely in disseminated infection (Eskild *et al.*, 2002). However, upon delivery, if infection is still occurring, then the neonate is at serious risk of infection, which can lead to death. Such infection may occur during delivery due to vaginal contact or after delivery due to cold sore exposure. Transmission depends on a number of factors, including the mother's antibody status, the amount of virus shedding, and the duration of contact with ruptured membranes. HSV infection during acquired immune deficiency syndrome (AIDS) is also serious; genital herpes results in severe recurrent infections, which are more extensive and last longer. Disseminated HSV may also occur, which involves the entire skin surface. The outcome of infection depends on the general condition of the individual and the success of aciclovir therapy.

HSV-I and HSV-II remain very important causes of viral STD, and HSV-I is a common cause of cold sores. Although there is effective therapy to reduce the duration and severity of infection, a vaccine is needed to prevent further spread of the virus and to diminish the current prevalence of these viruses (Whitley and Roizman, 2002).

REFERENCES

Aldea, C., Alvarez, C.P., Folgueira, L., Delgado, R. and Otero, J.R. (2002). Rapid detection of herpes simplex virus DNA in genital ulcers by real-time PCR using SYBR green I dye as the detection signal. *J Clin Microbiol* **40**, 1060–62.

Diamond, C., Selke, S., Ashley, R., Benedetti, J. and Corey, L. (1999). Clinical course of patients with serologic evidence of recurrent genital herpes presenting with signs and symptoms of first episode disease. *Sex Transm Dis* **26**, 221–5.

Druce, J., Catton, M., Chibo, D., *et al.* (2002). Utility of a multiplex PCR assay for detecting herpesvirus DNA in clinical samples. *J Clin Microbiol* **40**, 1728–32.

Eskild, A., Jeansson, S., Stray-Pedersen, B. and Jenum, P.A. (2002). Herpes simplex virus type-2 infection in pregnancy: no risk of fetal death: results from a nested case-control study within 35,940 women. *Bjog* **109**, 1030–35.

Espy, M.J., Uhl, J.R., Mitchell, P.S., *et al.* (2000). Diagnosis of herpes simplex virus infections in the clinical laboratory by LightCycler PCR. *J Clin Microbiol* **38**, 795–9.

Taylor, T.J., Brockman, M.A., McNamee, E.E. and Knipe, D.M. (2002). Herpes simplex virus. *Front Biosci* **7**, d752–64.

Wald, A. and Ashley-Morrow, R. (2002). Serological testing for herpes simplex virus (HSV)-1 and HSV-2 infection. *Clin Infect Dis* **35**, S173–82.

Whitley, R.J. and Roizman, B. (2002). Herpes simplex viruses: is a vaccine tenable? *J Clin Invest* **110**, 145–51.

Wolff, M.H., Schmitt, J., Rahaus, M., Dudda, H. and Hatzmann, W. (2002). Clinical and subclinical reactivation of genital herpes virus. *Intervirology* **45**, 20–23.

55

Dengue fever

Dengue fever and dengue haemorrhagic fever (DHF) are caused by the dengue virus, a member of the flaviviruses. There are four distinct serogroups, DEN-1, DEN-2, DEN-3 and DEN-4. The vector responsible for transmission of the dengue virus is the *Aedes aegypti* mosquito. Dengue is primarily an urban disease in the tropics. The mosquito vector prefers to feed on human blood, although it can also feed on animals. It is considered to be the most important mosquito-borne viral disease that affects humans. Its global distribution is comparable to that of malaria, but importantly it is not treatable. Dengue fever occurs about one week after infection with the virus, resulting in high fever, headache, body aches and a measles-like rash (Kautner *et al.*, 1997). Previous infection with another serotype does not protect against new infection, but infection with the same serotype does. Therefore, individuals living in dengue-endemic areas can have four episodes of dengue during their lifetime (one episode for each serogroup). The acute illness usually lasts for one week, but fatigue and depression may last for some weeks after. DHF occurs in individuals who have been infected with one strain of dengue virus and who are subsequently infected with a different strain. This results in high fever, abdominal pain and vomiting, and can progress to spontaneous bleeding, shock and death (Kabra *et al.*, 1999; Pelenkahu *et al.*, 1972).

The first epidemics of dengue fever were reported between 1779 and 1780 in Asia, Africa and North America. Over the past 200 years, there have been long intervals of 10–40 years between major epidemics, mainly because the viruses and their mosquito vector could be transported between population centres only by sailing vessels.

However, a global pandemic of dengue began in South-East Asia after the Second World War and has intensified during the last 20 years. Epidemics caused by multiple serotypes are now more frequent, and the geographic distribution of dengue viruses and their mosquito vectors has expanded. In South-East Asia, epidemic DHF first appeared in the 1950s, but by 1975 it had become a leading cause of hospitalization and death among children in many countries in that region. Epidemics have since occurred in Sri Lanka, India, the Maldives, Pakistan and Bangladesh (Agarwal *et al.*, 1999; Rahman *et al.*, 2002). In addition, although dengue fever was absent in Taiwan and the People's Republic of China for 35 years, epidemic dengue fever occurred again in both countries in the 1980s and has spread to Indonesia (Chairulfatah *et al.*, 1995; Chairulfatah *et al.*, 2001). A resurgence also occurred in Singapore between 1990 and 1994 after a successful control programme had prevented significant transmission for over 20 years (Chung and Pang, 2002), and epidemics have occurred in Malaysia (George, 1987). In Africa, epidemic dengue fever caused by all four serotypes has increased dramatically since 1980. Most activity has occurred in east Africa.

Today, dengue is prevalent in over 100 tropical and subtropical countries in areas including Africa, South-East Asia, the western Pacific and Latin America (Barbosa da Silva *et al.*, 2002). More than 2.5 billion people are at risk of dengue, and the annual incidence is estimated to be in the tens of millions. The case fatality rate of DHF in most countries is about 5%; most fatal cases are among children and young adults. The emergence of dengue fever and DHF as a major public health problem has been most dramatic in the American region. In an effort to prevent urban yellow fever, which is also transmitted by A. *aegypti*, the Pan American Health Organization organised a campaign that eradicated A. *aegypti* from most Central and South American countries during the 1950s and 1960s. This programme was officially discontinued in the USA in 1970, and the species began to re-infest countries from which it had been eradicated.

There is now a small but significant risk for dengue outbreaks in the continental USA. Two competent mosquito vectors, A. *aegypti* and A. *albopictus*, are present and could therefore transmit dengue viruses. This type of transmission has been detected a number of times over the past 20 years in south Texas (Rodriguez-Tan and Weir, 1998). Numerous viruses are introduced annually by travellers returning from tropical areas where dengue viruses are endemic. Over 2000 suspected cases of imported dengue were reported in the USA between the late 1970s and mid-1990s. Many more cases were probably unreported because surveillance is passive rather than active.

The reasons for this dramatic global emergence of dengue fever and DHF as a major public health problem are not well understood. However, several important factors can be identified. First, effective mosquito control is virtually non-existent in most dengue-endemic countries. Second, major global demographic changes have occurred, the most important of which have been uncontrolled urbanization and concurrent population growth, resulting in inadequate water, sewerage and waste-management systems. Third, increased air travel provides the ideal mechanism for transporting dengue viruses between populations in the tropics. Fourth, in many tropical countries, the public health infrastructure has deteriorated, resulting in emergency control methods in response to epidemics rather than developing programs to prevent epidemic transmission. This approach has been particularly detrimental to dengue control, because surveillance is inadequate. Finally, changes in global climate due to the El Niño phenomenon and the greenhouse effect are leading to increased land masses that are able to support dengue transmission.

Approximately 500 000 hospitalized cases of dengue occur each year, resulting in 24 000 deaths, 90% of which are in children under the age of 15 years. There is no treatment and no vaccine; therapy is merely symptomatic. In the short term, little can be done about the problem of dengue/DHF. Recently, attenuated candidate vaccine viruses have been developed in Thailand. These vaccines are safe and immunogenic when given in various formulations, including a quadrivalent vaccine for all four dengue virus serotypes. Efficacy trials in human volunteers have yet to be initiated. It is estimated that an effective dengue vaccine will be available in five to ten years. Continuing vector control by eliminating breeding sites of mosquitoes is therefore required in tropical and subtropical regions endemic for dengue. However, building development in endemic areas may allow for an increase in the number of breeding sites due to the presence of small areas of stagnant water. Also, such control programmes are expensive and are often slow, and in the past they have not been particularly effective. Nevertheless, it is hoped that eventually the incidence of dengue fever and DHF will be reduced drastically by a vaccine or vector control strategy. In the meantime, improved diagnostic methods must link with active, laboratory-based surveillance systems to provide early warning of an impending dengue epidemic (De Paula and Lopes da Fonseca, 2002; De Paula et al., 2002).

REFERENCES

Agarwal, R., Kapoor, S., Nagar, R., *et al.* (1999). A clinical study of the patients with dengue hemorrhagic fever during the epidemic of 1996 at Lucknow, India. *Southeast Asian J Trop Med Publ Health* **30**, 735–40.

Barbosa da Silva, J., Jr, Siqueira, J.B., Jr, Coelho, G.E., Vilarinhos, P.T. and Pimenta, F.G., Jr (2002). Dengue in Brazil: current situation and prevention and control activities. *Epidemiol Bull* **23**, 3–6.

Chairulfatah, A., Setiabudi, D., Ridad, A. and Colebunders, R. (1995). Clinical manifestations of dengue haemorrhagic fever in children in Bandung, Indonesia. *Ann Soc Belg Med Trop* **75**, 291–5.

Chairulfatah, A., Setiabudi, D., Agoes, R., van Sprundel, M. and Colebunders, R. (2001). Hospital based clinical surveillance for dengue haemorrhagic fever in Bandung, Indonesia 1994–1995. *Acta Trop* **80**, 111–15.

Chung, Y.K. and Pang, F.Y. (2002). Dengue virus infection rate in field populations of female *Aedes aegypti* and *Aedes albopictus* in Singapore. *Trop Med Int Health* **7**, 322–30.

De Paula, S.O. and Lopes da Fonseca, B.A. (2002). Optimizing dengue diagnosis by RT-PCR in IgM-positive samples: comparison of whole blood, buffy-coat and serum as clinical samples. *J Virol Methods* **102**, 113–17.

De Paula, S.O., Lima, D.M. and da Fonseca, B.A. (2002). Detection and identification of dengue-1 virus in clinical samples by a nested-PCR followed by restriction enzyme digestion of amplicons. *J Med Virol* **66**, 529–34.

George, R. (1987). Dengue haemorrhagic fever in Malaysia: a review. *Southeast Asian J Trop Med Publ Health* **18**, 278–83.

Kabra, S.K., Jain, Y., Singhal, T. and Ratageri, V.H. (1999). Dengue hemorrhagic fever: clinical manifestations and management. *Indian J Pediatr* **66**, 93–101.

Kautner, I., Robinson, M.J. and Kuhnle, U. (1997). Dengue virus infection: epidemiology, pathogenesis, clinical presentation, diagnosis, and prevention. *J Pediatr* **131**, 516–24.

Pelenkahu, T.B., Pudjiadi, S.H., Samsudin, Siahaan, C.M., *et al.* (1972). Dengue hemorrhagic fever (literature review and report of 14 cases). *Paediatr Indones* **12**, 21–30.

Rahman, M., Rahman, K., Siddque, A.K., *et al.* (2002). First outbreak of dengue hemorrhagic fever, Bangladesh. *Emerg Infect Dis* **8**, 738–40.

Rodriguez-Tan, R.S. and Weir, M.R. (1998). Dengue: a review. *Tex Med* **94**, 53–9.

56

Human papillomavirus infection

Warts and verrucas are caused by papillomaviruses, members of the Papovaviridae family. They possess a double-stranded DNA genome. Papillomaviruses are largely associated with benign epithelial tumours in both animals and humans, and in this respect they have been recognized for centuries. In humans, there are over 100 types of papillomaviruses, simply named sequentially (Munger, 2002). Almost half of the reported types of papillomavirus have been isolated from individuals with epidermodysplasia verruciformis (EPV), a rare, life-long condition associated with impaired immunity. In these individuals, papillomas are very common. Generally, the most common papillomaviruses to cause infection are types 1, 2, 3 and 4. These cause benign epithelial tumours, known as papillomas, warts or verrucas, which usually occur on the hands and feet during childhood and adolescence (Wiley et al., 2002). Most papillomas are exophytic lesions on cutaneous or mucosal epithelia and are benign. They are transmitted most commonly via close contact and by activities such as swimming. Many other types are transmitted during sexual intercourse, and it is estimated that 1% of the sexually active population in the USA possesses genital papillomas (Schneede, 2002; Wiley et al., 2002). Transmission to the fetus may occur during delivery if the mother is infected. Papillomaviruses replicate in the squamous epithelium of both mucosal and non-mucosal surfaces and are subsequently transmitted via shedding of infected squamous cells. Papillomas are described according to their site or clinical characteristics as follows:

- Papillomas on the genitalia or anus are known as *condylomata acuminata*.

- Papillomas of the larynx are known as *laryngeal papilloma*.

- Common warts are known as *verruca vulgaris*.

- Papillomas due to type 7 are known as butchers' warts, due to their association with butchers.

It has been known for many years that papillomaviruses possess oncogenic potential. This was first shown in 1935 by Rous and Beard, who performed experiments on rabbits to demonstrate oncogenesis. More recently, it has been shown that papillomaviruses can cause squamous cell carcinomas in humans (Munger, 2002). Further studies in Australia have shown that type 5 is also a cause of squamous cell carcinoma. Other types of papillomavirus are associated with genital oncogenic infections, and it is estimated that 50% of young sexually active women are infected with papillomaviruses that have oncogenic potential (Bosch and de Sanjose, 2002; Bosch et al., 2002). Although most malignancies will be controlled by an effective immune response, a proportion will proceed to carcinoma or cervical cancer (Woodworth, 2002). Types 6 and 11 have been associated with premalignant lesions of the cervix, vulva and penis, but these are often of low grade. Types 16 and 18 are associated with all grades of intraepithelial neoplasia and with malignant disease of the cervix and penis. Type 16 is the most common type in Europe, accounting for 70% of severe cervical intraepithelial neoplasia and up to 80% of invasive carcinoma of the cervix cases in some countries (Furumoto and Irahara, 2002). Another 15 types of papillomavirus infect and produce lesions in the genital region, although it is currently unclear what role these play in carcinomas. In total, over 90% of cervical cancers are caused by papilloma infection. The incidence of papillomavirus infections in developing countries is poorly understood. Furthermore, it is not known what interaction, if any, occurs between human immunodeficiency virus (HIV) and papillomaviruses. Some developing countries have a high incidence of HIV-positive individuals, and papillomavirus infection would seem to be a further serious problem with respect to spread via sexual intercourse and its oncogenic potential due to poor immune responses in HIV-positive individuals.

Most papillomavirus infections do not require laboratory diagnosis because the papillomas remain benign. However, as some are now known to be associated with carcinomas, there are some instances where diagnosis is required. Unfortunately, papillomaviruses cannot be grown in cultured mammalian cells. Therefore, other methods such as immunohistochemistry, DNA hybridization and the polymerase chain reaction (PCR) need to be used to detect viral capsid protein or viral DNA, methods that are both expensive and specialized (Grayson et al., 2002; Ha et al., 2002; Kenny et al., 2002; Yamaguchi et al., 2002). The treatment of papillomas is not usually required except for cosmetic reasons or if the papilloma is malignant. Also, papillomas often regress spontaneously, although sometimes they may persist for years. They may be removed using liquid nitrogen, electrodiathermy or laser evaporation. Additionally, an anti-mitotic agent called podophyllin can be used.

Due to the incidence of papillomavirus infection and its recent association with cancer, the requirement for a vaccine has become an important issue (Sisk and Robertson, 2002). Although most papillomavirus infections are benign, the true incidence of their oncogenic potential remains poorly understood and further research is warranted to establish such potential. To date, the level and importance of their association with cancer is great enough to justify a vaccination policy. Although there are numerous types of papillomavirus, they are highly conserved at the molecular level. To date, a suitable vaccine has not been produced, but animal studies suggest that both prophylactic and therapeutic vaccination may be possible.

REFERENCES

Bosch, F.X. and de Sanjose, S. (2002). Human papillomavirus in cervical cancer. *Curr Oncol Rep* 4, 175–83.

Bosch, F.X., Lorincz, A., Munoz, N., Meijer, C.J. and Shah, K.V. (2002). The causal relation between human papillomavirus and cervical cancer. *J Clin Pathol* 55, 244–65.

Furumoto, H. and Irahara, M. (2002). Human papilloma virus (HPV) and cervical cancer. *J Med Invest* 49, 124–33.

Grayson, W., Rhemtula, H.A., Taylor, L.F., Allard, U. and Tiltman, A.J. (2002). Detection of human papillomavirus in large cell neuroendocrine carcinoma of the uterine cervix: a study of 12 cases. *J Clin Pathol* 55, 108–14.

Ha, P.K., Pai, S.I., Westra, W.H., *et al.* (2002). Real-time quantitative PCR demonstrates low prevalence of human papillomavirus type 16 in premalignant and malignant lesions of the oral cavity. *Clin Cancer Res* 8, 1203–9.

Kenny, D., Shen, L.P. and Kolberg, J.A. (2002). Detection of viral infection and gene expression in clinical tissue specimens using branched DNA (bDNA) in situ hybridization. *J Histochem Cytochem* 50, 1219–27.

Munger, K. (2002). The role of human papillomaviruses in human cancers. *Front Biosci* 7, d641–9.

Schneede, P. (2002). Genital human papillomavirus infections. *Curr Opin Urol* 12, 57–61.

Sisk, E.A. and Robertson, E.S. (2002). Clinical implications of human papillomavirus infection. *Front Biosci* 7, e77–84.

Wiley, D.J., Douglas, J., Beutner, K., *et al.* (2002). External genital warts: diagnosis, treatment, and prevention. *Clin Infect Dis* 35, S210–24.

Woodworth, C.D. (2002). HPV innate immunity. *Front Biosci* 7, d2058–71.

Yamaguchi, A., Hashimoto, N., Tsutae, W., *et al.* (2002). Detection of human papillomavirus DNA by PCR/microfluorometry for screening of cervical cancer. *Clin Chim Acta* 318, 41–9.

57

Polio

Polio is one of the few diseases that has affected humankind for as long as history can tell. It dates back over 3000 years to Egyptian stone engraving in the year 1500 BC, although it was not well recognized in Europe and North America until the late nineteenth century. Successful research into the disease began early in the twentieth century. Polio virus was transmitted to monkeys in 1909, but it was not until 1949 that it was possible to grow the virus in tissue culture cells of non-neuronal origin.

Polio is a member of the Picornaviridae family; it is an icosahedral virus. Each virion consists of a protein shell made of 60 copies of four proteins, named VP1–VP4, which encase the single-stranded RNA genome of 7.5 kb. There are three distinct serotypes of polio, named 1–3. Strains are named according to their serotype, name, country of isolation and year of isolation. Such strains may be indigenous, imported or derived from the live attenuated vaccine. Genotypic analysis of serotypes has indicated that there is usually less than 15% difference at the nucleotide level, and a single genotype is well conserved over time, making outbreak and epidemic tracing possible. During epidemics, point mutations occur infrequently, and generally deletions and insertions are uncommon. The virus follows a typical viral lifecycle (Figure 57.1). After ingestion, the virus binds to a host cell receptor, enters the cell, and then loses its viral envelope. Protein synthesis and RNA replication are then initiated, followed by RNA packaging and virus assembly.

Polio is primarily a disease of humans and primates. The normal route of infection is the oral route, although nasopharyngeal transmission may also occur. The virus initially replicates in the ton-

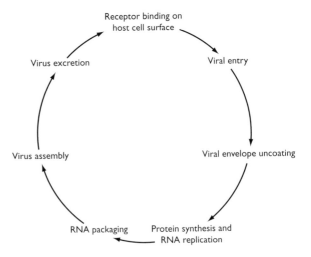

Figure 57.1   Schematic representation of the lifecycle of the polio virus.

sils, lymph nodes, Peyer's patches and small intestine. The incubation period before the onset of symptoms is between four and 35 days. Host restriction is due to the presence of a specific receptor on human and primate cells. However, certain strains of the virus, especially type 2, can cause paralytic disease in mice if the virus is inoculated artificially. After the transmission of polio to a susceptible individual, the virus continues to replicate in the intestine, where it persists; the basis of such tissue tropism is poorly understood. The initial symptoms of infection, which do not occur in all those infected, are fever, sore throat and flu-like illness. The patient usually recovers uneventfully after a few days. Circulating antibody normally restricts access of the virus to the central nervous system (CNS), but in unprotected individuals the virus circulates in the bloodstream before invading the CNS (Dalakas and Illa, 1991; Dalakas, 1995). Direct invasion of the CNS can also occur through the nerve fibres; the virus is then able to replicate in the motor neurones, which leads to cellular damage. Paralytic poliomyelitis occurs in less than 1% of cases 7–30 days after initial infection, affecting the limbs (spinal poliomyelitis), the respiratory muscles (bulbar poliomyelitis), or both (bulbospinal poliomyelitis). About 10% of paralysed individuals recover to a significant degree, 10% of cases are fatal, and 80% have significant residual paralysis. In the most severe cases, paralysis can lead to death by asphyxiation. As over 50% of polio cases occur in children under the age of three years, the disease burden on this age group in developing countries is enormous, with large numbers being permanently disabled. In some cases, the CNS may be infected without resulting paralysis, such as in aseptic meningitis.

Polio once had a worldwide distribution, but it is now most common is developing countries due to poor hygiene in such countries and the vaccination programmes that exist in developed countries. In the 1940s and 1950s, polio epidemics occurred each summer in developed countries, but the virus has now been eradicated from such countries. Improvements in hygiene reduce the incidence of the disease but also create a population of susceptible adults. The disease is also more common in areas where inactivated rather than live attenuated vaccines have been used. Prevalence of the virus is high in temperate countries during late summer and autumn, while in tropical countries it is endemic. Young children are the main reservoir of infection. A dramatic reduction in the incidence of polio has occurred due to global immunization programmes.

Various samples may be used for the laboratory diagnosis of polio, including faeces, throat swab, blood and post-mortem tissue. A throat swab is particularly useful for virus isolation at the onset of infection but may be positive up to 10 days after initial infection, while faeces should be tested as soon as possible after the onset of symptoms. Blood should be taken for antibody testing in both the acute and convalescent phases of infection,

although the polymerase chain reaction (PCR) may also be used (Chernesky, 1984; Corless et al., 2002). Post-mortem samples may include any tissue from the CNS for virus isolation or electron microscopy. Polio may be isolated on a number of cell lines. A cytopathic effect typical of the enterovirus group occurs 10–14 days after incubation and confirmation of identity and type may be achieved using polyclonal sera (Di Lonardo et al., 2002).

Immunity against polio infection may be gained following natural infection. Polio virus possesses two main antigens: the H antigen is associated with denatured virus and the N antigen is associated with infectious virus. In healthy individuals, the humoral immune response is directed at the viral H antigen during the acute phase of infection. During the convalescent phase, the humoral response develops after one to two weeks and is directed against the viral N antigen. However, virus excretion occurs for five weeks. A mucosal immunoglobulin A (IgA) response also develops after natural infection or after vaccination with the live attenuated virus. Patients with a humoral immunodeficiency are prone to polio infection. Immune serum containing anti-N antibodies is protective against infection.

There is no antiviral chemotherapy available against polio. In addition, each serotype is antigenically distinct, and therefore immunity to one serotype does not confer immunity to other serotypes. However, partial denaturation of virions exposes antigens that are cross-reactive between all three serotypes and may therefore provide cross-protection. The first polio vaccine was developed by Salk in 1955 and consisted of a formalin-inactivated formulation (Blume and Geesink, 2000). One major problem with this vaccine is that it requires injection by a trained worker and elicits only an immunoglobulin G (IgG) response; therefore, it prevents spread to the CNS but provides very little protection in the gut, so it is not useful for controlling transmission. A live attenuated vaccine was later developed by Sabin in 1961; this can be given orally and does not require administration by a trained worker. It stimulates IgA and IgG responses to protect against mucous membrane and bloodstream infection. The stimulation of an IgA response prevents person-to-person transmission in the early stages of infection. In addition, attenuated virus is excreted for a short time in the stools of vaccinated individuals and may therefore lead to passive immunization of close contacts in areas where hygiene is poor. The Sabin vaccine is relatively inexpensive, costing only eight US cents for each dose. Such vaccines have enabled the virus to be controlled in the developed world, and the vaccine strains developed in the 1950s still provide protective immunity today. The Sabin vaccine is produced by passage of the virus through various in vitro and in vivo systems, resulting in attenuation of virulence. The vaccine is composed of three strains to provide maximum immunity. It is very safe and results in vaccine-associated poliomyelitis in only one per 530 000 vaccinees. A comparison of the two vaccines is shown in Table 57.1.

Smallpox was made famous by its global eradication, and the World Health Organization (WHO) aims to repeat this with polio. At a meeting in 1988, the World Health Assembly (the governing body of the WHO) aimed to globally eradicate polio by 2000. However, although polio has declined by over 95%, eradication has not yet been attained (Hull and Aylward, 2001). The basis for polio eradication is its limited host range (humans), the availability of an effective and inexpensive vaccine that provides lifelong immunity, the absence of long-term carriers, and the virus's inability to survive in the environment. Such an eradication strategy is very similar to that of smallpox. Routine polio vaccination was introduced in many developing countries in the 1970s, when it was recognized that the disease was frequent and a major cause of morbidity in children in such countries. Wild polio virus has now been eradicated completely, and the disease is virtually controlled in the Western hemisphere and some developing countries. In the UK, for example, between one and four cases were reported each year between 1991 and 1998; none have been reported since (source: HPA CDSC). South Asia and sub-Saharan Africa remain the areas where eradication has not yet been achieved. However, due to the fact that polio is excreted in the faeces of immunized individuals, its existence in the environment after human eradication will complicate the issue (Horie et al., 2002; Yoshida et al., 2002). Other concerns have been raised regarding the accidental or deliberate release of the virus after polio eradication (Caceres and Sutter, 2001; Henderson, 2002; Minor, 2002), concerns that have been voiced with smallpox.

REFERENCES

Blume, S. and Geesink, I. (2000). A brief history of polio vaccines. *Science* 288, 1593–4.

Table 57.1 Comparison of the two available polio vaccines

Salk inactivated polio vaccine	Sabin oral polio vaccine
Given by injection: requirement for trained personnel	Given orally: no requirement for trained personnel
Long-term immunity but individual can remain a virus carrier	Long-term immunity and no possibility of virus carriage
No risk of vaccine-associated paralysis due to use of inactivated virus	Slight risk of vaccine-associated paralysis due to use of live attenuated virus
Vaccinee vaccinated: no close-contact passive vaccination	Vaccinee vaccinated and possibility of close contacts being vaccinated passively

Caceres, V.M. and Sutter, R.W. (2001). Sabin monovalent oral polio vaccines: review of past experiences and their potential use after polio eradication. *Clin Infect Dis* **33**, 531–41.

Chernesky, M.A. (1984). Current advances in viral diagnostic technology applicable to polio vaccination and diagnosis. *Rev Infect Dis* **6** (suppl 2), S525–7.

Corless, C.E., Guiver, M., Borrow, R., *et al.* (2002). Development and evaluation of a 'real-time' RT-PCR for the detection of enterovirus and parechovirus RNA in CSF and throat swab samples. *J Med Virol* **67**, 555–62.

Dalakas, M.C. (1995). The post-polio syndrome as an evolved clinical entity. Definition and clinical description. *Ann N Y Acad Sci* **753**, 68–80.

Dalakas, M. and Illa, I. (1991). Post-polio syndrome: concepts in clinical diagnosis, pathogenesis, and etiology. *Adv Neurol* **56**, 495–511.

Di Lonardo, A., Buttinelli, G., Amato, C., Novello, F., Ridolfi, B. and Fiore, L. (2002). Rapid methods for identification of poliovirus isolates and determination of polio neutralizing antibody titers in human sera. *J Virol Methods* **101**, 189–96.

Henderson, D.A. (2002). Countering the posteradication threat of smallpox and polio. *Clin Infect Dis* **34**, 79–83.

Horie, H., Yoshida, H., Matsuura, K., *et al.* (2002). Neurovirulence of type 1 polioviruses isolated from sewage in Japan. *Appl Environ Microbiol* **68**, 138–42.

Hull, H.F. and Aylward, R.B. (2001). Progress towards global polio eradication. *Vaccine* **19**, 4378–84.

Minor, P. (2002). Emerging/disappearing viruses future issues concerning polio eradication. *Virus Res* **82**, 33–7.

Yoshida, H., Horie, H., Matsuura, K., Kitamura, T., Hashizume, S. and Miyamura, T. (2002). Prevalence of vaccine-derived polioviruses in the environment. *J Gen Virol* **83**, 1107–11.

58

Parvovirus infection

Parvoviruses are members of the Parvoviridae family. Some have a small single-stranded DNA genome that can replicate independently, while others are 'defective' and require a helper virus for replication. Only parvovirus B-19 is pathogenic in humans (Anderson and Pattison, 1984), although other parvoviruses affect animals such as dogs (Bastianello, 1981). The virus was first isolated in the mid-1970s, but it was not until the early 1980s that its association with disease was understood (Thurn, 1988). The virus targets early erythroid progenitor cells, and therefore anaemia is a common clinical feature of infection. In order for the virus to survive, it must infect rapidly dividing cells. The cellular receptor for the virus is the P antigen, which is expressed in most individuals on mature erythrocytes and erythroid progenitors. However, the P antigen may also be expressed on megakaryocytes, endothelial cells, placenta cells, fetal liver cells and heart cells. Individuals who lack the P antigen are not susceptible to parvovirus B-19 infection.

Parvovirus B-19 infection, otherwise known as Fifth's disease or erythema infectiosum, is a common, endemic viral infection, and occurs most frequently among preschool and school-age children. Most cases occur sporadically. The virus may be spread from person to person by aerosols or by the exchange of body fluids. The latent period of the viral infection is between one and two days, and is followed by an erythematous malar rash, which is the classic feature of the infection. Infections among healthy children are short, lasting only one to two days, with low-grade fever and rash as the primary clinical manifestations (Anderson and Torok, 1991; Harnden, 1999). Fever, headache, malaise, myalgia and respiratory symptoms may also occur, sometimes accompanied by nausea, vomiting and abdominal pain. In adults, parvovirus B-19 infection is usually characterized by arthralgia and low-grade fever. The rash is less prominent in adults than in children, and may take a reticulated form over the face, trunk and extremities. Arthralgia or arthritis may accompany the initial symptoms, although many adults may have arthritis or arthralgia alone, without other preceding or concurrent symptoms (Balkhy et al., 1998; Gran et al., 1995). Other syndromes occur rarely, including vasculitis, encephalitis, meningitis, neuropathy, pneumonitis, glomerulonephritis, hepatitis and myocarditis. Parvovirus B-19 infection is of particular concern in anaemic and immunosuppressed patients. Studies have shown that between a quarter and a half of adults are immune to parvovirus B-19 infection due to childhood exposure to the virus.

Parvovirus B-19 infection has gained importance as a congenital infection of the unborn fetus (Brown, 1989). Serological studies among pregnant women during epidemics of parvovirus B-19 infection have suggested that between 3 and 19% of pregnant women will convert serologically to an immunoglobulin M (IgM) status. The vertical transmission rate for parvovirus B-19 is estimated to be 33% of those patients who show serological conversion. Serious fetal morbidity and mortality from parvovirus B-19 infection occurs in up to a fifth of patients who contract the virus during pregnancy. The second trimester of pregnancy appears to be the period of highest risk for fetal loss. Viral studies performed on spontaneous abortions in the first trimester have shown a 2–3% incidence of parvovirus B-19. Case reports of twin pregnancies discordant for congenital parvovirus B-19 infection suggest that vertical transmission is dependent on both maternal and fetal factors. Because parvovirus B-19 is a DNA virus, chronic recurrent infection in infants who have survived congenital parvovirus infection has been reported. Therefore, confirmed cases of congenital parvovirus infection should be reported to the paediatrician following delivery to allow for paediatric monitoring of potential chronic infection. There are isolated case reports of congenital deformities among infants with congenital parvovirus infection, but the pattern of abnormalities does not suggest a syndrome.

Some of the symptoms of parvovirus infection can resemble those of some other viral and bacterial infections, such as rubella, infectious mononucleosis, Lyme disease and meningococcal septicaemia (Table 58.1). Maternal diagnosis is difficult to make on clinical features alone because of the similarities between adult parvovirus B-19 infection and other viral syndromes. Serological testing with IgM and immunoglobulin G (IgG) shortly after exposure can confirm maternal immunity and relieve anxiety about potential vertical transmission (Chen *et al.*, 2000; Cubel *et al.*, 1996; Dieck *et al.*, 1999; Jones *et al.*, 1993). An alternative method of diagnosis is detection of the parvovirus B-19 DNA in maternal serum using the polymerase chain reaction (PCR) (Anderson *et al.*, 1985; Arnauld *et al.*, 1998; Cassinotti *et al.*, 1993; Clewley, 1989). The PCR test is also useful in immunocompromised individuals, who may not develop an immune response.

In most individuals, parvovirus infection is self-limiting. Unfortunately, there is no prophylaxis, treatment or vaccine available for maternal parvovirus B-19 infection, or indeed parvovirus B-19 infection in general (Harnden, 1999). For mothers and pregnant women, therefore, hand-washing is recommended in order to limit the spread of parvovirus infection. As individuals who develop parvovirus infection are contagious before symptoms appear, avoiding those who are infected will not limit the spread of infection. Treatment options for a fetus with suspected congenital parvovirus B-19 infection are limited but include high-dose IgG therapy and intrauterine fetal transfusion. In immunocompromised individuals, intravenous immunoglobulin may be useful.

REFERENCES

Anderson, M.J. and Pattison, J.R. (1984). The human parvovirus. Brief review. *Arch Virol* **82**, 137–48.

Anderson, L.J. and Torok, T.J. (1991). The clinical spectrum of human parvovirus B19 infections. *Curr Clin Top Infect Dis* **11**, 267–80.

Anderson, M.J., Jones, S.E. and Minson, A.C. (1985). Diagnosis of human parvovirus infection by dot-blot hybridization using cloned viral DNA. *J Med Virol* **15**, 163–72.

Arnauld, C., Legeay, O., Laurian, Y., *et al.* (1998). Development of a PCR-based method coupled with a microplate colorimetric assay for the detection of porcine parvovirus and application to diagnosis in

Table 58.1 Clinical symptoms of parvovirus infection

Erythema infectiosum	Most common in children
	Endemic or epidemic
	Self-limiting
Arthritis	Most common in adults
	May be protracted
Chronic anaemia	Occurs in immunocompromised patients

piglet tissues and human plasma. *Mol Cell Probes* **12**, 407–16.

Balkhy, H.H., Sabella, C. and Goldfarb, J. (1998). Parvovirus: a review. *Bull Rheum Dis* **47**, 4–9.

Bastianello, S.S. (1981). Canine parvovirus myocarditis: clinical signs and pathological lesions encountered in natural cases. *J S Afr Vet Assoc* **52**, 105–8.

Brown, K.E. (1989). What threat is human parvovirus B19 to the fetus? A review. *Br J Obstet Gynaecol* **96**, 764–7.

Cassinotti, P., Weitz, M. and Siegl, G. (1993). Human parvovirus B19 infections: routine diagnosis by a new nested polymerase chain reaction assay. *J Med Virol* **40**, 228–34.

Chen, M.Y., Lee, K.L. and Hung, C.C. (2000). Immunoglobulin M and G immunoblots in the diagnosis of parvovirus B19 infection. *J Formos Med Assoc* **99**, 24–32.

Clewley, J.P. (1989). Polymerase chain reaction assay of parvovirus B19 DNA in clinical specimens. *J Clin Microbiol* **27**, 2647–51.

Cubel, R.C., Oliveira, S.A., Brown, D.W., Cohen, B.J. and Nascimento, J.P. (1996). Diagnosis of parvovirus B19 infection by detection of specific immunoglobulin M antibody in saliva. *J Clin Microbiol* **34**, 205–7.

Dieck, D., Schild, R.L., Hansmann, M. and Eis-Hubinger, A.M. (1999). Prenatal diagnosis of congenital parvovirus B19 infection: value of serological and PCR techniques in maternal and fetal serum. *Prenat Diagn* **19**, 1119–23.

Gran, J.T., Johnsen, V., Myklebust, G. and Nordbo, S.A. (1995). The variable clinical picture of arthritis induced by human parvovirus B19. Report of seven adult cases and review of the literature. *Scand J Rheumatol* **24**, 174–9.

Harnden, A. (1999). Diagnosis and treatment of parvovirus B19. *Practitioner* **243**, 672–4.

Jones, M.F., Wold, A.D., Espy, M.J. and Smith, T.F. (1993). Serologic diagnosis of parvovirus B19 infections. *Mayo Clin Proc* **68**, 1107–8.

Thurn, J. (1988). Human parvovirus B19: historical and clinical review. *Rev Infect Dis* **10**, 1005–11.

59

Chickenpox and shingles

The virus varicella zoster is responsible for two diseases, chickenpox and shingles. Chickenpox is the primary illness caused by the virus and usually occurs during childhood. Shingles is a reactivation of infection with varicella zoster and occurs most often in later adulthood.

CHICKENPOX

Chickenpox is a highly contagious disease with a worldwide distribution (Arvin, 1996). It causes approximately 4 million cases of infection in the USA each year. The virus spreads from person to person by direct contact with the upper respiratory tract or symptomatic skin lesions, or through particle inhalation from the air. It is because of this that around 90% of individuals in a household who have not had chickenpox will become infected if exposed to the virus via another family member. Most cases of chickenpox occur in the late winter and spring. More than 95% of individuals have chickenpox during their childhood, and at this age the infection is usually mild. Infection in infants and immunocompromised individuals can be severe (Balfour, 1988; Chen *et al.*, 2002). Occasionally, the infection is not acquired until adulthood; at this time, the infection is usually more severe, often including major organ involvement, which may lead to hospitalization. Complications such as pneumonia can develop, which may have serious consequences if not treated rapidly.

After infection with varicella zoster, the characteristic symptoms of chickenpox develop. These consist of an itchy rash, which then forms blisters that dry and become scabs after about four days (Weller, 1996). The rash may be the first sign of infection, and sometimes may be accompanied by fever and general malaise. The number of lesions on the body of an infected person ranges from only a few to more than 500. The infection is contagious one to two days before the rash appears and until all blisters have turned into scabs. However, the symptoms of chickenpox infection take between 10 and 21 days to develop after contact with an infected person. There are around 7000 hospitalizations and 100 deaths in the USA annually due to chickenpox.

The diagnosis of chickenpox can be confirmed by laboratory testing, although this is not usually necessary in routine childhood cases. Serological tests, such as the complement fixation test (CFT), may be performed to detect antibody titres during chickenpox infection. Alternatively, the virus may be demonstrated in lesion fluid by electron microscopy, isolated in cell culture, or detected using the polymerase chain reaction (PCR) (Bergstrom, 1996; Burke *et al.*, 1997; Dlugosch *et al.*, 1991; Drew and Mintz, 1980; Espy *et al.*, 2000).

Varicella zoster immunoglobulin prevents or modifies clinical illness in susceptible individuals who have been exposed to varicella. The immunoglobulin is prepared from plasma obtained from healthy volunteer blood donors with high antibody titres. It is most beneficial when given as soon as possible after exposure; protection lasts about three weeks. Individuals who may be considered for varicella zoster immunoglobulin include immunocompromised patients, pregnant women, neonates and susceptible health workers.

A live attenuated varicella virus vaccine has been marketed since 1994 and was licensed for use in 1995 in the USA. The virus strain used in the vaccine was isolated in the 1970s from a Japanese child, and virus was subsequently attenuated through passage in human embryonic lung cells, embryonic guinea pig cells, and human diploid cells (Kamiya and Ihara, 1989; Kamiya *et al.*, 1988). The vaccine is approved in the USA for use in healthy children aged 12 months or older, in adolescents and adults. It is safe and has been documented to induce a lasting and protective immune response (Arbeter, 1996; Gershon *et al.*, 1996). The seroconversion rate of varicella vaccine among susceptible children aged between 12 months and 12 years is 97%. In older children, 78% seroconvert after the first dose and 99% seroconvert after a second dose. Breakthrough infection has been reported, but these cases are usually mild. The vaccine is not licensed in the UK and therefore is not part of the UK childhood immunization programme. However, it is available for people at particularly high risk of infection, such as immunocompromised patients.

SHINGLES

Following childhood chickenpox infection, the varicella zoster virus is not eliminated from the body. The virus remains dormant in sensory ganglia and may reactivate decades later to produce shingles, otherwise known as zoster or herpes zoster. The incidence of herpes zoster in the USA is estimated to be between 600 000 and 1 million cases per year. During adulthood, the virus is usually held at bay by cell-mediated immunity, but when this immunity declines, such as in advanced age, lymphoma or AIDS, the virus is able to revert to its infectious state and cause shingles.

The first symptom associated with shingles is pain near the site of reactivation, where nerve damage has occurred in latently infected ganglia (Arvin, 1996). The pain may range from mild itching or tingling to severe pain. This is sometimes accompanied by flu-like symptoms. Within five days of reactivation, a rash and clusters of clear vesicles develop, which soon develop into blisters. Shingles is unilateral and does not cross the midline. The most common regions affected are those supplied by the trigeminal nerve and thoracic ganglia, which include the chest and abdomen and the eyes (ophthalmic zoster). Normally, new zoster lesions continue to appear for two to three days, and within 14 days the lesions become pustular and crusty. At this point, they no longer contain the virus. As with chickenpox, complications can occur, one of the most common being bacterial infection. This can cause severe complications because of the possibility of superficial gangrene and subsequent scarring. In the case of ophthalmic zoster, severe infection can cause corneal opacification or secondary bacterial infection. It is estimated that between 10 and 20% of the adult population develop shingles. However, shingles is more common in immunocompromised individuals; since immunocompetence declines with age, around 50% of those aged 80 years and over may develop shingles.

Shingles is diagnosed by clinical presentation and laboratory confirmation (Morgan and King, 1998). The clinical diagnosis of shingles is fairly straightforward, and laboratory diagnosis can be achieved by rising antibody titres as for chickenpox. The treatment of shingles may be important in hospitalized cases to reduce the occurrence of complications. Aciclovir is used widely for the treatment of shingles because it reduces the appearance of new vesicles, the duration of pain, and the duration of viral shedding. Aciclovir variants may also be used. As for chickenpox, varicella zoster immunoglobulin may be given to infected or susceptible individuals.

REFERENCES

Arbeter, A.M. (1996). Clinical trials of varicella vaccine in healthy adolescents and adults. *Infect Dis Clin North Am* **10**, 609–15.

Arvin, A.M. (1996). Varicella-zoster virus: overview and clinical manifestations. *Semin Dermatol* **15**, 4–7.

Balfour, H.H., Jr (1988). Varicella zoster virus infections in immunocompromised hosts. A review of the natural history and management. *Am J Med* **85**, 68–73.

Bergstrom, T. (1996). Polymerase chain reaction for diagnosis of varicella zoster virus central nervous system infections without skin manifestations. *Scand J Infect Dis Suppl* **100**, 41–5.

Burke, D.G., Kalayjian, R.C., Vann, V.R., Madreperla, S.A., Shick, H.E. and Leonard, D.G. (1997). Polymerase chain reaction detection and clinical significance of varicella-zoster virus in cerebrospinal fluid from human immunodeficiency virus-infected patients. *J Infect Dis* **176**, 1080–84.

Chen, T.M., George, S., Woodruff, C.A. and Hsu, S. (2002). Clinical manifestations of varicella-zoster virus infection. *Dermatol Clin* **20**, 267–82.

Dlugosch, D., Eis-Hubinger, A.M., Kleim, J.P., Kaiser, R., Bierhoff, E. and Schneweis, K.E. (1991). Diagnosis of acute and latent varicella-zoster virus infections using the polymerase chain reaction. *J Med Virol* **35**, 136–41.

Drew, W.L. and Mintz, L. (1980). Rapid diagnosis of varicella-zoster virus infection by direct immunofluorescence. *Am J Clin Pathol* **73**, 699–701.

Espy, M.J., Teo, R., Ross, T.K., *et al.* (2000). Diagnosis of varicella-zoster virus infections in the clinical laboratory by LightCycler PCR. *J Clin Microbiol* **38**, 3187–9.

Gershon, A.A., LaRussa, P. and Steinberg, S. (1996). The varicella vaccine. Clinical trials in immunocompromised individuals. *Infect Dis Clin North Am* **10**, 583–94.

Kamiya, H. and Ihara, T. (1989). Clinical experience of Oka-strain live varicella vaccine. *Indian J Pediatr* **56**, 568–70.

Kamiya, H., Sakurai, M., Ihara, T., *et al.* (1988). Clinical use of Oka live varicella vaccine. *Acta Paediatr Jpn* **30**, 594–600.

Morgan, R. and King, D. (1998). Shingles: a review of diagnosis and management. *Hosp Med* **59**, 770–76.

Weller, T.H. (1996). Varicella: historical perspective and clinical overview. *J Infect Dis* **174** (suppl 3), S306–9.

PART IV

Parasitology

60

Toxoplasma

Toxoplasma gondii, the causative organism of toxoplasmosis, is an obligate, intracellular coccidian protozoan that was first isolated in 1908. It has been found as a parasite of many warm-blooded animals, but members of the cat family appear to be the only definitive hosts for the parasite's sexual stages. It is estimated that one-third of the global population has been exposed to the parasite (Hill and Dubey, 2002). Infection is acquired by ingestion of the oocyst stage after exposure to the faeces of infected cats, contaminated soil or undercooked meat. It can also be acquired transplacentally, by organ transplantation and from blood transfusion. After ingestion, the outer walls of the parasite oocysts are disrupted by enzymatic degradation in the stomach. The infective stages – bradyzoites and sporozoites – are liberated into the intestinal lumen, where they invade and multiply within the surrounding tissue (Bonhomme *et al.*, 1992). They are released from disrupted cells as tachyzoites, which subsequently invade the neighbouring cells and the blood. There is therefore widespread dissemination of the parasite. The host develops an immune response, and any free tachyzoites are killed. At this stage, tissue cysts are formed in various organs in which the parasite continues to multiply at a slow rate. After infection, mild symptoms may include lymphadenopathy or a syndrome similar to that of glandular fever, although most infected people do not show clinical signs of disease. Like a few other human pathogens, infection lasts for life because the cysts are able to persist in a dormant state in the host tissues. Toxoplasmosis in immunocompromised individuals may lead to severe or life-threatening disease. It is usually due to the secondary reactivation of cysts formed after

dissemination of the parasite in normal infection. Frequent complications include fever, persistent headache, rapid mental deterioration and focal neurological signs.

The most recognized complication of infection with *T. gondii* is congenital infection (Guerina, 1994). If infection is acquired during pregnancy, then 40% of women transmit the infection to the fetus (Cook *et al.*, 2000). However, about 90% of acute *Toxoplasma* infections in pregnant women go unrecognized due to subclinical infection. Some countries screen for *Toxoplasma* in pregnancy, but there is insufficient evidence to suggest the need for this in the UK (Gilbert and Peckham, 2002). It is during the parasitaemic stage of maternal infection that placental infection occurs. Fetal infection may occur depending on the stage of pregnancy at which the woman acquired the infection. About 10–15% of infections acquired in the first trimester of pregnancy result in fetal infection. This increases to 30% for infections acquired in the second trimester and to 60% for those acquired in the third trimester. Although the incidence of fetal infection is lowest in the first trimester, it is at this time that the effects on the fetus are most severe and may result in spontaneous abortion. Congenitally infected infants born to mothers who acquired the infection in the third trimester usually have no obvious signs of infection at birth. However, subsequent loss of vision and mental retardation may occur. An immunocompromised mother may transmit *Toxoplasma* to the fetus even if acquisition of the parasite was years before conception. A number of cases of toxoplasmosis have also been described in patients with acquired immunodeficiency syndrome (AIDS), systemic lupus erythematosus (SLE), Hodgkin's lymphoma and splenectomy (Filice *et al.*, 1993; Peacock *et al.*, 1983). In human immunodeficiency virus (HIV)-infected women, fetal transmission of *Toxoplasma* may occur due to recurrent parasitaemia throughout pregnancy.

The main method of preventing toxoplasmosis in pregnancy is by education. Exposure to the parasite can be prevented or at least reduced by following simple hygiene measures. A number of tests have been developed for the diagnosis of toxoplasmosis (Montoya, 2002); these may be divided into two main groups. The first group includes tests that use whole intact trophozoites as an antigen source; such tests include the dye test, direct agglutination and the fluorescent antibody test (Desmonts and Remington, 1980; Desmonts and Thulliez, 1985; Evans and Ho-Yen, 2000). The second group includes tests that use disrupted parasites as an antigen source, such as enzyme-linked immunosorbent assay (ELISA), latex agglutination, indirect haemagglutination and complement fixation (Desmonts *et al.*, 1981). The dye test is the accepted reference test for the detection of *Toxoplasma*-specific antibody. The test is a complement-mediated neutralizing antigen–antibody reaction, which is quantitative mainly for immunoglobulin G (IgG), although immunoglobulin M (IgM) is also fixed. Reactivity occurs within two weeks of infection, with titres peaking at >1000 IU/ml after six to eight weeks. The use of the dye test in conjunction with other appropriate tests can determine whether an individual has been exposed to *Toxoplasma* and whether the infection is acute or chronic. Serological diagnosis of congenital infection is more difficult. *Toxoplasma*-specific IgM may be detected in only half of those infected, and therefore IgG testing is necessary (Desmonts *et al.*, 1981). However, this cannot be performed accurately until the child is free of maternal IgG. Other non-specific laboratory findings in toxoplasmosis include elevated gamma-glutamyltransferase concentrations, total IgM concentrations, leukocyte counts and eosinophil counts. Thrombocytopenia also occurs. Poly-merase chain reaction (PCR) assays have also been developed for the diagnosis of toxoplasmosis (Cingolani *et al.*, 1996; Contini *et al.*, 1998; Costa *et al.*, 2000), which can be designed to detect specific stages of the parasite (Contini *et al.*, 1999; Contini *et al.*, 2002).

Spiramycin is commonly used for the treatment of toxoplasmosis and has been recommended for use in reducing the frequency of maternal transmission to the fetus. Such treatment should be continued throughout pregnancy. Studies have shown that pyrimethamine/sulfadiazine is more effective than spiramycin in altering the severity of fetal infection, although it should be noted that pyrimethamine is potentially teratogenic and should not be used during the first trimester.

Toxoplasma is a parasite that does not cause clinical disease in most individuals. However, it is of importance in pregnant women and immunocompromised patients. Upon reflection of the results of diagnostic tests, these individuals should be educated and, if necessary, appropriate therapy given.

REFERENCES

Bonhomme, A., Pingret, L. and Pinon, J.M. (1992). Review: *Toxoplasma gondii* cellular invasion. *Parassitologia* **34**, 31–43.

Cingolani, A., De Luca, A., Ammassari, A., *et al.* (1996). PCR detection of *Toxoplasma gondii* DNA in CSF for the differential diagnosis of AIDS-related focal brain lesions. *J Med Microbiol* **45**, 472–6.

Contini, C., Fainardi, E., Cultrera, R., *et al.* (1998). Advanced laboratory techniques for diagnosing *Toxoplasma gondii* encephalitis in AIDS patients: significance of intrathecal production and comparison with PCR and ECL-western blotting. *J Neuroimmunol* **92**, 29–37.

Contini, C., Seraceni, S. and Cultrera, R. (1999). Different PCR systems to detect *Toxoplasma gondii* tachyzoites or bradyzoites in clinical specimens from patients with and without overt disease. *J Eukaryot Microbiol* **46**, 77–8S.

Contini, C., Cultrera, R., Seraceni, S., *et al.* (2002). The role of stage-specific oligonucleotide primers in providing effective laboratory support for the molecular diagnosis of reactivated *Toxoplasma gondii* encephalitis in patients with AIDS. *J Med Microbiol* **51**, 879–90.

Cook, A.J., Gilbert, R.E., Buffolano, W., *et al.* (2000). Sources of toxoplasma infection in pregnant women: European multicentre case-control study. European Research Network on Congenital Toxoplasmosis. *Br Med J* **321**, 142–7.

Costa, J.M., Pautas, C., Ernault, P., Foulet, F., Cordonnier, C. and Bretagne, S. (2000). Real-time PCR for diagnosis and follow-up of *Toxoplasma* reactivation after allogeneic stem cell transplantation using fluorescence resonance energy transfer hybridization probes. *J Clin Microbiol* **38**, 2929–32.

Desmonts, G. and Remington, J.S. (1980). Direct agglutination test for diagnosis of *Toxoplasma* infection: method for increasing sensitivity and specificity. *J Clin Microbiol* **11**, 562–8.

Desmonts, G. and Thulliez, P. (1985). The toxoplasma agglutination antigen as a tool for routine screening and diagnosis of toxoplasma infection in the mother and infant. *Dev Biol Stand* **62**, 31–5.

Desmonts, G., Naot, Y. and Remington, J.S. (1981). Immunoglobulin M-immunosorbent agglutination assay for diagnosis of infectious diseases: diagnosis of acute congenital and acquired *Toxoplasma* infections. *J Clin Microbiol* **14**, 486–91.

Evans, R. and Ho-Yen, D.O. (2000). Evidence-based diagnosis of toxoplasma infection. *Eur J Clin Microbiol Infect Dis* **19**, 829–33.

Filice, G.A., Hitt, J.A., Mitchell, C.D., Blackstad, M. and Sorensen, S.W. (1993). Diagnosis of *Toxoplasma* parasitemia in patients with AIDS by gene detection after amplification with polymerase chain reaction. *J Clin Microbiol* **31**, 2327–31.

Gilbert, R.E. and Peckham, C.S. (2002). Congenital toxoplasmosis in the United Kingdom: to screen or not to screen? *J Med Screen* **9**, 135–41.

Guerina, N.G. (1994). Congenital infection with *Toxoplasma gondii*. *Pediatr Ann* **23**, 138–42, 147–51.

Hill, D. and Dubey, J.P. (2002). *Toxoplasma gondii*: transmission, diagnosis and prevention. *Clin Microbiol Infect* **8**, 634–40.

Montoya, J. G. (2002). Laboratory diagnosis of *Toxoplasma gondii* infection and toxoplasmosis. *J Infect Dis* **185** (suppl 1), S73–82.

Peacock, J.E., Jr, Folds, J., Orringer, E., Luft, B. and Cohen, M.S. (1983). *Toxoplasma gondii* and the compromised host. Antibody response in the absence of clinical manifestations of disease. *Arch Intern Med* **143**, 1235–7.

61

Malaria

Malaria occurs in both the Old and the New Worlds between the latitudes of 40 degrees north and 30 degrees south. It is a major cause of mortality in tropical regions. The disease kills 1 million children in Africa each year, and there are an estimated 300–500 million cases of malaria worldwide. *Plasmodium*, of which there are four species, is the parasite responsible for the disease. *P. falciparum* is the species responsible for the majority of fatalities due to malaria. The other species, *P. vivax*, *P. ovale* and *P. malariae*, cause febrile illnesses but are rarely fatal (Oh *et al.*, 2001). The incidence of imported malaria cases seen in the UK has increased over the past 20 years. This is due in part to the increase in foreign travel, as many more business and tourism visits to tropical regions now occur. Another reason is the increasing resistance of *P. falciparum* to anti-malarial drugs. Laboratories have therefore needed to be more aware of the requirements for the laboratory diagnosis of malaria (Anon, 1997).

The lifecycles and transmission of the four species of *Plasmodium* are very similar (Bray and Garnham, 1982; Florens *et al.*, 2002). Human infection results from the inoculation of sporozoites into the bloodstream after a bite from an infected *Anopheles* mosquito. The sporozoites invade the parenchyma cells of the liver, where they develop into exo-erythrocytic schizonts in one to two weeks. Each schizont ruptures, releasing thousands of merozoites into the bloodstream. These merozoites enter erythrocytes, where they undergo further development. They first become vacuolated as trophozoites and then enlarge to become erythrocytic schizonts, after which the nuclear material divides to form numerous merozoites.

Merozoite-containing erythrocytes rupture, releasing their contents into the bloodstream. These merozoites are able to infect other erythrocytes, leading to further infection cycles. Some merozoites form gametocytes, which develop further only if they are ingested by an *Anopheles* mosquito; further development occurs within the mosquito to eventually form sporozoites, which pass to the salivary glands and can therefore infect another host. The developmental stages in the *Anopheles* mosquito take approximately two weeks for *P. vivax*, 22 days for *P. falciparum* and one month for *P. malariae*. The epidemiology of malaria is complex because of the many factors relating to vector and human interactions.

The symptoms of falciparum malaria include fever and flu-like illness, with shaking, chills, headache, muscle aches and tiredness (O'Holohan, 1976; Ryan, 2001). Nausea, vomiting and diarrhoea may also occur. Malaria may also lead to anaemia and jaundice due to the loss of red blood cells. If falciparum malaria is not treated promptly, it may cause kidney failure, seizures, mental confusion, coma and eventually death. Non-falciparum malaria results in a febrile illness (Oh *et al.*, 2001). It rarely causes organ complications, and resistance to chloroquine is unusual. Falciparum malaria is a more serious illness. The symptoms are due solely to the erythrocyte stage of infection; there are no symptoms related to the liver stage. The incubation period is between one week and one month. The clinical features may include pyrexia, impaired consciousness, prostration and jaundice. Further, complications may follow, such as renal failure, respiratory distress syndrome, haemorrhage and coma.

The diagnosis of malaria relies on the detection of organisms in the peripheral blood (Avila and Ferreira, 1996; Bailey, 1998). Blood smears stained by the Giemsa method are used for examination under oil immersion. Thick and thin smears are made, the former being used for screening and the latter for detailed morphological examination. Peripheral blood used for the smears is best taken during a pyrexial period before any treatment is given. Malaria parasites are identified as bodies whose nuclear material stains red whilst the cytoplasm stains blue; dark pigmentation may be seen in later stages of development. Diagnosis may also be made by the indirect fluorescent antibody test (IFAT), the indirect haemagglutination test (IHAT), enzyme-linked immunosorbent assay (ELISA) and the polymerase chain reaction (PCR) (Avila and Ferreira, 1996; Becker et al., 1999; Ferrer-Rodriguez et al., 1999; Hanscheid, 1999; Lee et al., 2002). However, these tests are restricted to specialist laboratories and do not replace microscopic diagnosis.

Various types of therapy may be used for the prevention or treatment of malaria. Primary exo-erythrocytic schizonticides are used as a preventive therapy; these act by killing sporozoites after they are inoculated into the bloodstream or by killing schizonts occurring in the liver. Erythrocytic schizonticides are used to treat developed disease by killing erythrocytic schizonts. Secondary exo-erythrocytic schizonticides are used to prevent relapse of malarial infection. Finally, gametocytocides are used in late malaria to affect gametocytes so that they are unable to develop once ingested by the *Anopheles* mosquito. Many of the therapies have been available for a number of years, but drug resistance has been developing steadily (Price and Nosten, 2001). For example, chloroquine is still effective, although resistance to the drug is patchy but widespread (Adubofour, 1992). Resistance to other anti-malarials has also been reported and is therefore becoming a problem. In vitro resistance to mefloquine has even been reported in areas where the drug has not yet been introduced, but mefloquine may be useful in areas where chloroquine resistance exists (Croft and Garner, 1997).

Vaccine development is difficult due to the complex lifecycle of *P. falciparum* (Facer and Tanner, 1997). The possibility of developing a vaccine became a reality due to monoclonal antibody technology and the possibility of continuous in vitro culture of the parasite. Vaccines have included a recombinant DNA *P. falciparum* sporozoite vaccine, a synthetic circumsporozoite peptide vaccine and a polymeric synthetic hybrid vaccine. A recently developed vaccine called SPf66 has shown some promise in initial trials; this consists of three asexual blood-stage antigens (Genton and Corradin, 2002). Clinical trials of these vaccines have shown them to have varying efficacies. However, the prospect of a vaccine that reduces the burden of disease is getting closer. It therefore remains to be seen whether any of these vaccines will reach widespread use. As well as therapeutic measures, strategies such as vector control and bite prevention may be used to limit the spread of malaria. The genome of *P. falciparum* has now been sequenced, and it is hoped that this will lead to new therapies and a vaccine (Florens et al., 2002).

REFERENCES

Adubofour, K.O. (1992). Drug resistance in malaria: a review of the west African situation. *J Natl Med Assoc* **84**, 1025–9.

Anon (1997). The laboratory diagnosis of malaria. The Malaria Working Party of the General Haematology Task Force of the British Committee for Standards in Haematology. *Clin Lab Haematol* **19**, 165–70.

Avila, S.L. and Ferreira, A.W. (1996). Malaria diagnosis: a review. *Braz J Med Biol Res* **29**, 431–43.

Bailey, W. (1998). Latest developments in the laboratory diagnosis of malaria. *Afr Health* **20**, 16, 18.

Becker, K., Ortmann, C., Bajanowski, T., Brinkmann, B. and Peters, G. (1999). Use of polymerase chain reaction for postmortem diagnosis of malaria. *Diagn Mol Pathol* **8**, 211–15.

Bray, R.S. and Garnham, P.C. (1982). The life-cycle of primate malaria parasites. *Br Med Bull* **38**, 117–22.

Croft, A. and Garner, P. (1997). Mefloquine to prevent malaria: a systematic review of trials. *Br Med J* **315**, 1412–16.

Facer, C.A. and Tanner, M. (1997). Clinical trials of malaria vaccines: progress and prospects. *Adv Parasitol* **39**, 1–68.

Ferrer-Rodriguez, I., Vazquez, G.J., Cordova, G.J. and Serrano, A. E. (1999). Diagnosis of malaria by polymerase chain reaction. *P R Health Sci J* **18**, 99–103.

Florens, L., Washburn, M.P., Raine, J.D., *et al.* (2002). A proteomic view of the *Plasmodium falciparum* life cycle. *Nature* **419**, 520–26.

Genton, B. and Corradin, G. (2002). Malaria vaccines: from the laboratory to the field. *Curr Drug Targets Immune Endocr Metabol Disord* **2**, 255–67.

Hanscheid, T. (1999). Diagnosis of malaria: a review of alternatives to conventional microscopy. *Clin Lab Haematol* **21**, 235–45.

Lee, S.H., Kara, U.A., Koay, E., Lee, M.A., Lam, S. and Teo, D. (2002). New strategies for the diagnosis and screening of malaria. *Int J Hematol* **76** (suppl 1), 291–3.

Oh, M.D., Shin, H., Shin, D., *et al.* (2001). Clinical features of vivax malaria. *Am J Trop Med Hyg* **65**, 143–6.

O'Holohan, D.R. (1976). Clinical and laboratory presentation of malaria: an analysis of one thousand subjects with malaria parasitaemia. *J Trop Med Hyg* **79**, 191–6.

Price, R.N. and Nosten, F. (2001). Drug resistant falciparum malaria: clinical consequences and strategies for prevention. *Drug Resist Update* **4**, 187–96.

Ryan, E.T. (2001). Malaria: epidemiology, pathogenesis, diagnosis, prevention, and treatment – an update. *Curr Clin Top Infect Dis* **21**, 83–113.

62

Cyclosporiasis

Cyclospora cayetanensis was first described as a possible cause of gastrointestinal illness by Ashford (1979). The presence of similar organisms was noted in faeces during the 1980s, when screening for cryptosporidia became routine practice. It was also described as *Blastocystis hominis*, a coccidian, a flagellate, a mould spore and a cyanobacterium-like body (blue–green alga) (Babcock *et al.*, 1985; Bendall *et al.*, 1993; Long *et al.*, 1991; Shlim *et al.*, 1991). The latter description was due to conclusions drawn from its appearance under transmission electron microscopy. An increase in reports of the parasite from around the world developed from 1990 onwards, and it was not until this time that it was acknowledged as a novel cause of diarrhoea and was named *C. cayetanensis* (Ortega *et al.*, 1994).

The current taxonomic position of *C. cayetanensis* is based on the organism's maturation and sporulation characteristics (Ortega *et al.*, 1994). When species of *Cyclospora* mature, they possess two sporocysts per oocyst; upon excystation, two sporozoites are released from each sporocyst (a total of four sporozoites). Such characteristics are typical of *C. cayetanensis*. Its species name is derived from the name of the institution, Cayetano Heredia University, Peru, where much of the initial research was performed (Ortega *et al.*, 1993; Ortega *et al.*, 1994). Although the maturation and sporulation characteristics of *C. cayetanensis* are the same as those of other species of *Cyclospora*, the oocyst morphology is quite different. They are uniformly circular and between 8 and 10 μm in diameter, and an internal morula of 6–7 μm in diameter can usually be seen under light microscopy (Ortega *et al.*, 1994). Oocysts are excreted in human faeces in the oocyst form; they are undifferentiated and require envi-ronmental exposure to develop fully (Figure 62.1). However, sporulation of the oocysts may occur under laboratory conditions in potassium dichromate or water (Smith *et al.*, 1997). *C. cayetanensis* appears to infect the duodenum and small bowel; the organism has either been isolated from these organs or pathological changes have been seen. Oocysts are excreted in the faeces of infected individuals throughout the illness.

The distribution of *C. cayetanensis* appears to be worldwide. Cases of infection have been reported in individuals who live in or have visited the USA, Caribbean islands, Central and South America, southern Asia, South-East Asia and Eastern Europe (Clarke and McIntyre, 1994). A few sporadic cases have arisen outside these areas in individuals with no history of foreign travel, but it is not known how these people acquired the infection. Results of faecal screening studies in the UK indicate that the incidence of *C. cayetanensis* infection in travellers is low (Clarke and McIntyre, 1996). *C. cayetanensis* infection may be seen in individuals of all ages. The Health Protection

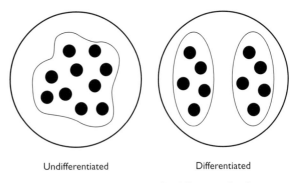

Undifferentiated   Differentiated

Figure 62.1 Schematic diagram of undifferentiated and differentiated *Cyclospora* oocysts.

Agency (HPA) Communicable Disease Surveillance Centre (CDSC) started receiving reports of *C. cayetanensis* infection in 1993 from laboratories in England and Wales. The low number of cases seen in the UK is probably due to the fact that the annual increase in cases in endemic areas is between April and August, and the height of the tourist season in these areas is not until later in the year. The source of *C. cayetanensis* infection is not known, although outbreaks in Chicago and Nepal have suggested that *C. cayetanensis* may be water-borne (Huang *et al.*, 1995; Rabold *et al.*, 1994; Wright and Collins, 1997). Humans are probably not the definitive hosts of *C. cayetanensis*; however, many animal species have been screened, without success, for the carriage of *C. cayetanensis*.

Patients infected with *C. cayetanensis* suffer from a number of symptoms, including diarrhoea, nausea, vomiting, anorexia, weight loss and abdominal pain (Clarke and McIntyre, 1994; Shlim *et al.*, 1991). Fever may also be present. These symptoms vary considerably between patients. Symptoms may last for two to three weeks. In an outbreak in Nepal in 1989, the duration of illness ranged from four to 107 days. The incubation period of *C. cayetanensis* infection is not known, although patients have developed symptoms soon after arriving in an endemic country, one patient within two days. Symptom-free carriage of the organism is rare.

The laboratory diagnosis of *C. cayetanensis* may be achieved with a number of techniques (Clarke and McIntyre, 1994). The oocysts may be concentrated using the formol-ether technique or Sheather's sucrose flotation method, or they can be stained using the modified Ziehl–Neelsen method. In the latter, oocysts are differentiated easily from the background faecal material because they stain variably: some stain dark red, while others do not stain at all and appear as non-refractile glassy spheres. Although their appearance by this method is similar to that of *Cryptosporidium* spp., they can be differentiated easily by their size: oocysts of *C. cayetanensis* measure 8–10 μm while those of *Cryptosporidium* spp. measure about 4 μm. Oocysts of *C. cayetanensis* also autofluoresce

under ultraviolet (UV) light (Berlin *et al.*, 1994; Long *et al.*, 1990). The outer wall of the oocysts fluoresces green if exposed to UV light using at a wavelength of 365 nm.

Little work has been published on the human immune response to infection with *C. cayetanensis*. One report has described the demonstration of antibody production in 12 patients with cyclosporiasis by an indirect immunofluorescence technique using thin sections of *C. cayetanensis* in epoxy resin, but in another study using a similar technique no serological response was detected (Clarke and McIntyre, 1997; Long *et al.*, 1991). Infection with *C. cayetanensis* may not confer immunity because patients have been identified in which successive infections have occurred in consecutive years.

A number of antimicrobial agents have been used in individuals infected with *C. cayetanensis*. Some of these have been used blindly to treat suspected bacterial or parasitic infection, while others have been used specifically to treat *C. cayetanensis*. Most of these antimicrobial agents have proven to be ineffective because they have not reduced the duration or severity of symptoms. However, co-trimoxazole has been used successfully for the treatment of *C. cayetanensis* infection (Hoge *et al.*, 1995). Eradication of *C. cayetanensis*, as determined by the analysis of stool samples, has correlated with clinical recovery in those treated with co-trimoxazole, and relapse of infection has not been noted.

In conclusion, *C. cayetanensis* is a novel gastrointestinal pathogen that causes a prolonged diarrhoeal syndrome. It should be considered in all patients, irrespective of age, who have returned from Central and South America, southern Asia or South-East Asia. It may be diagnosed in the clinical laboratory using wet-mount preparations or Ziehl–Neelsen stained faecal preparations.

REFERENCES

Ashford, R.W. (1979). Occurrence of an undescribed coccidian in man in Papua New Guinea. *Ann Trop Med Parasitol* **73**, 497–500.

Babcock, D., Houston, R., Kumaki, D. and Shlim, D. (1985). *Blastocystis hominis* in Kathmandu, Nepal. *N Engl J Med* **313**, 1419.

Bendall, R.P., Lucas, S., Moody, A., Tovey, G. and Chiodini, P.L. (1993). Diarrhoea associated with cyanobacterium-like bodies: a new coccidian enteritis of man. *Lancet* **341**, 590–92.

Berlin, O.G., Novak, S.M., Porschen, R.K., Long, E.G., Stelma, G.N. and Schaeffer, F.W., 3rd (1994). Recovery of *Cyclospora* organisms from patients with prolonged diarrhea. *Clin Infect Dis* **18**, 606–9.

Clarke, S.C. and McIntyre, M. (1994). Human infection with *Cyclospora*. *J Infect* **29**, 112–13.

Clarke, S.C. and McIntyre, M. (1996). The incidence of *Cyclospora cayetanensis* in stool samples submitted to a district general hospital. *Epidemiol Infect* **117**, 189–93.

Clarke, S.C. and McIntyre, M. (1997). An attempt to demonstrate a serological immune response in patients infected with *Cyclospora cayetanensis*. *Br J Biomed Sci* **54**, 73–4.

Hoge, C.W., Shlim, D.R., Ghimire, M., *et al.* (1995). Placebo-controlled trial of co-trimoxazole for *Cyclospora* infections among travellers and foreign residents in Nepal. *Lancet* **345**, 691–3.

Huang, P., Weber, J.T., Sosin, D.M., *et al.* (1995). The first reported outbreak of diarrheal illness associated with *Cyclospora* in the United States. *Ann Intern Med* **123**, 409–14.

Long, E.G., Ebrahimzadeh, A., White, E.H., Swisher, B. and Callaway, C.S. (1990). Alga associated with diarrhea in patients with acquired immunodeficiency syndrome and in travelers. *J Clin Microbiol* **28**, 1101–4.

Long, E.G., White, E.H., Carmichael, W.W., *et al.* (1991). Morphologic and staining characteristics of a cyanobacterium-like organism associated with diarrhea. *J Infect Dis* **164**, 199–202.

Ortega, Y.R., Sterling, C.R., Gilman, R.H., Cama, V.A. and Diaz, F. (1993). Cyclospora species – a new protozoan pathogen of humans. *N Engl J Med* **328**, 1308–12.

Ortega, Y.R., Gilman, R.H. and Sterling, C.R. (1994). A new coccidian parasite (Apicomplexa: Eimeriidae) from humans. *J Parasitol* **80**, 625–9.

Rabold, J.G., Hoge, C.W., Shlim, D.R., Kefford, C., Rajah, R. and Echeverria, P. (1994). Cyclospora outbreak associated with chlorinated drinking water. *Lancet* **344**, 1360–1361.

Shlim, D.R., Cohen, M.T., Eaton, M., Rajah, R., Long, E.G. and Ungar, B.L. (1991). An alga-like organism associated with an outbreak of prolonged diarrhea among foreigners in Nepal. *Am J Trop Med Hyg* **45**, 383–9.

Smith, H.V., Paton, C.A., Mitambo, M.M. and Girdwood, R.W. (1997). Sporulation of *Cyclospora* sp. oocysts. *Appl Environ Microbiol* **63**, 1631–2.

Wright, M.S. and Collins, P.A. (1997). Waterborne transmission of *Cryptosporidium*, *Cyclospora* and *Giardia*. *Clin Lab Sci* **10**, 287–90.

63

Cryptosporidiosis

Cryptosporidia continue to be a significant cause of gastrointestinal illness in the UK and the rest of the world. The parasite was first described in 1907 by Tyzzer, who found it in the peptic glands of laboratory mice. From the first description through to 1971, cryptosporidia were described in a number of mammals, birds and reptiles (Table 63.1) (de Graaf *et al.*, 1999; Sreter and Varga, 2000; Taylor *et al.*, 1999). These cryptosporidia were speciated according to the host in which they were found, but it was suggested later that there may be only one species with a wide host range. Others suggest that

Table 63.1 Animals in which cryptosporidia have been found

Calves
Cats
Chickens
Clams
Fish
Geese
Horses
Humans
Lambs
Lizards
Mice
Monkeys
Rabbits
Snakes
Tortoises
Turkeys

the species *C. baileyi* and *C. meleagridis* are specific to birds, while *C. parvum* and *C. muris* infect mammals. Other species have been described, and genetic data are informing scientists of the relationship between different species.

Cryptosporidium is an obligate parasite related to *Plasmodium* and *Toxoplasma*. Its taxonomy is shown in Table 63.2. It has a complex lifecycle involving sexual and asexual stages, which are completed within a single host. *Cryptosporidium* oocysts are stable in the environment and are resistant to many chemical agents. The oocysts are quite resistant to chlorine and therefore filtration during water treatment is important both at large treatment plants and at other facilities, such as swimming pools. Antibiotics are largely ineffective, and those that do have an effect on the organism are toxic to humans.

Although *Cryptosporidium* has long been known as a cause of diarrhoea in animals, it was not until 1976 that the organism was first recognized in humans. The first report of diarrhoea was in a girl in the USA. A number of reports came later from acquired immunodeficiency syndrome (AIDS)

Table 63.2 Simplified taxonomy of *Cryptosporidium*

Phylum	Apicomplexa
Class	Sporozoea
Subclass	Coccidia
Order	Eucoccidiida
Suborder	Eimeriina
Family	Cryptosporiidae
Genus	*Cryptosporidium*

patients, but it is now recognized as an important cause of diarrhoea in both immunocompromised and healthy individuals around the world. Infection with *Cryptosporidium* may be acquired from a number of sources, including contaminated food and water, animals and person-to-person contact (Franzen and Muller, 1999; Griffiths, 1998; Rose and Slifko, 1999). The infectious dose is thought to be small, although the actual number of oocysts that must be ingested to result in infection is not known; some researchers suggest that 10 or fewer oocysts may be sufficient. After ingestion of *Cryptosporidium* oocysts, there is an incubation period of five days to two weeks. The clinical features of cryptosporidiosis that follow are a flu-like illness, with watery diarrhoea, cramps, fever, malaise and nausea (Farthing, 2000). These symptoms are similar to many other gastrointestinal infections, and therefore laboratory diagnosis is important for public health reasons. The illness is self-limiting and, like the incubation period, lasts between five days and two weeks in immunocompetent individuals. However, in immunocompromised patients, the symptoms of cryptosporidiosis may be severe, protracted and life-threatening.

Outbreaks of cryptosporidiosis have been reported due to contaminated domestic water supplies, milk and swimming pools (Anon, 1996; Cicirello *et al.*, 1997; Duke *et al.*, 1996; Frisby *et al.*, 1997; Harper *et al.*, 2002; Howe *et al.*, 2002; Patel *et al.*, 1998). A number of waterborne outbreaks were reported in the 1980s and 1990s in the UK and the USA:

- Texas, USA, 1984: 49 of 79 individuals tested positive.
- Georgia, USA, 1987: approximately 13 000 cases.
- Ayrshire, UK, 1988: 27 cases.
- Swindon, Oxfordshire, UK, 1989: 500 laboratory-confirmed but up to 5000 cases.
- Milwaukee, USA, 1993: more than 400 000 cases.

Further outbreaks occurred in the UK between 1989 and 1990, all thought to be due to contaminated water supplies. Outbreaks associated with contaminated swimming pool water have also occurred in the UK. The peak incidence of cryptosporidiosis occurs during the spring and during outbreaks. Laboratory surveys have shown that the parasite is found in approximately 2% of all faecal specimens examined in the laboratory, although in children the incidence is usually higher, at about 4% (Thomas *et al.*, 1990). It may also be the third most frequently identified enteric pathogen after *Campylobacter* and rotavirus.

Due to the potential public health implications resulting from cryptosporidiosis, laboratory diagnosis is extremely important. The usual size range of *Cryptosporidia* oocysts is 3–6 μm. Measurement of oocysts and the use of positive controls in the diagnosis of cryptosporidiosis is important. Oocysts may be confused with fungal spores or *Cyclospora cayetanensis*. *C. cayetanensis* is treatable with co-trimoxazole, but there is currently no suitable therapy for cryptosporidiosis. A number of methods are available for the diagnosis of cryptosporidiosis, that used most often being the cold Ziehl–Neelsen test, which was introduced by Henrikson and Pohlenz in 1981. With this method, the oocyst stains red and the background stains green. Another, more sensitive method is the auramine-phenol stain. Oocysts hold the auramine and fluoresce when viewed under a suitable light source. This method is particularly useful for screening large numbers of specimens. Immunofluorescence methods that employ an antibody stage and are therefore more specific are also available commercially. Finally, a safranin-methylene blue method has been described in which the oocysts stain pink. However, this method does not work well in all hands, and therefore the former methods are those of choice. Furthermore, unstained methods for the diagnosis of cryptosporidiosis are unreliable due to the parasite's similarity in size and morphology to other artefacts and faecal organisms. Although concentration methods are available, these are not usually required for the diagnosis of acute infections. Polymerase chain reaction (PCR) methods are now also becoming available, although these are currently limited to reference laboratories (Morgan *et al.*, 1998).

Cryptosporidium remains an important pathogen worldwide. Although the number of reports does not appear to be increasing in the UK, outbreaks are often large and can have serious public health consequences. Treatment does not seem to be a possible option because antibiotics are largely useless. As with many diseases, prevention is therefore the obvious method of reducing the incidence of cryptosporidiosis. It is essential that water supplies are clean and that recreational water facilities, such as swimming pools, are maintained. Finally, the public must be educated so that the spread of the organism via foods and animals can be reduced.

REFERENCES

Anon (1996). Foodborne outbreak of diarrheal illness associated with *Cryptosporidium parvum* – Minnesota, 1995. *MMWR Morb Mortal Wkly Rep* **45**, 783–4.

Cicirello, H.G., Kehl, K.S., Addiss, D.G., *et al.* (1997). Cryptosporidiosis in children during a massive waterborne outbreak in Milwaukee, Wisconsin: clinical, laboratory and epidemiologic findings. *Epidemiol Infect* **119**, 53–60.

De Graaf, D.C., Vanopdenbosch, E., Ortega-Mora, L.M., Abbassi, H. and Peeters, J.E. (1999). A review of the importance of cryptosporidiosis in farm animals. *Int J Parasitol* **29**, 1269–87.

Duke, L.A., Breathnach, A.S., Jenkins, D.R., Harkis, B.A. and Codd, A.W. (1996). A mixed outbreak of cryptosporidium and campylobacter infection associated with a private water supply. *Epidemiol Infect* **116**, 303–8.

Farthing, M.J. (2000). Clinical aspects of human cryptosporidiosis. *Contrib Microbiol* **6**, 50–74.

Franzen, C. and Muller, A. (1999). Cryptosporidia and microsporidia – waterborne diseases in the immunocompromised host. *Diagn Microbiol Infect Dis* **34**, 245–62.

Frisby, H.R., Addiss, D.G., Reiser, W.J., *et al.* (1997). Clinical and epidemiologic features of a massive waterborne outbreak of cryptosporidiosis in persons with HIV infection. *J Acquir Immune Defic Syndr Hum Retrovirol* **16**, 367–73.

Griffiths, J.K. (1998). Human cryptosporidiosis: epidemiology, transmission, clinical disease, treatment, and diagnosis. *Adv Parasitol* **40**, 37–85.

Harper, C.M., Cowell, N.A., Adams, B.C., Langley, A.J. and Wohlsen, T.D. (2002). Outbreak of *Cryptosporidium* linked to drinking unpasteurised milk. *Commun Dis Intell* **26**, 449–50.

Howe, A.D., Forster, S., Morton, S., *et al.* (2002). Cryptosporidium oocysts in a water supply associated with a cryptosporidiosis outbreak. *Emerg Infect Dis* **8**, 619–24.

Morgan, U.M., Pallant, L., Dwyer, B.W., Forbes, D.A., Rich, G. and Thompson, R.C. (1998). Comparison of PCR and microscopy for detection of *Cryptosporidium parvum* in human fecal specimens: clinical trial. *J Clin Microbiol* **36**, 995–8.

Patel, S., Pedraza-Diaz, S., McLauchlin, J. and Casemore, D.P. (1998). Molecular characterisation of *Cryptosporidium parvum* from two large suspected waterborne outbreaks. Outbreak Control Team South and West Devon 1995, Incident Management Team and Further Epidemiological and Microbiological Studies Subgroup North Thames 1997. *Commun Dis Public Health* **1**, 231–3.

Rose, J.B. and Slifko, T.R. (1999). *Giardia*, *Cryptosporidium*, and *Cyclospora* and their impact on foods: a review. *J Food Prot* **62**, 1059–70.

Sreter, T. and Varga, I. (2000). Cryptosporidiosis in birds – a review. *Vet Parasitol* **87**, 261–79.

Taylor, M.A., Geach, M.R. and Cooley, W.A. (1999). Clinical and pathological observations on natural infections of cryptosporidiosis and flagellate protozoa in leopard geckos (*Eublepharis macularius*). *Vet Rec* **145**, 695–9.

Thomas, A.G., Phillips, A.D. and Walker-Smith, J.A. (1990). Cryptosporidiosis in England and Wales: prevalence and clinical and epidemiological features. Public Health Laboratory Service Study Group. *Br Med J* **300**, 774–7.

64

Microsporidiosis

The range of parasites now known to infect humans is growing as foreign travel increases, infections are imported, and techniques for their detection develop. During the past two decades, three 'new' parasites that infect humans have been described: *Cryptosporidia*, *Cyclospora* and microsporidia. The former two parasites have been described in previous chapters. Microsporidia are poorly understood compared with *Cryptosporidium* and *Cyclospora*, even though they were first discovered over 100 years ago (Weiss, 2001). Their disease potential and the number of species causing human disease continue to be researched.

Microsporidia are obligate, intracellular protozoan parasites (Weiss, 2001). They have a proliferative tissue phase and a spore-forming phase during host infection. 'Microsporidia' is the term given to a number of genera, partly because classification of these organisms has proven difficult. However, they are sufficiently different to other intracellular parasites, in terms of the diseases they cause and their morphology, to be contained within their own phylum. Although microsporidia may be waterborne, other sources of infection are poorly understood (Franzen and Muller, 1999a). However, person-to-person spread is a possibility once initial human infection has occurred, and individuals who have visited or lived in the tropics, and those with other major parasitic diseases, are more likely to be infected. Insect vectors may be responsible for disease transmission in such areas. A number of risk factors have been determined for the acquisition of microsporidia in human immunodeficiency virus (HIV)-infected patients, including drinking unfiltered tap water, swimming in rivers,

and close contact with other infected individuals. Microsporidia are considered to be emerging pathogens, and the number of reported cases of disease is still relatively small. However, in the USA, hundreds of cases of gastrointestinal disease in immunocompromised patients are known to have been due to microsporidia. Since far fewer cases have occurred in immunocompetent individuals. Microsporidia have therefore been largely overlooked, except in immunocompromised patients.

A number of genera of microsporidia have been associated with human disease. They affect many sites of the body, resulting in a wide range of clinical symptoms (Shadduck and Greeley, 1989; Weber *et al.*, 2000). In HIV-positive individuals, intestinal microsporidiosis is thought to result in diarrhoea and weight loss (Bryan *et al.*, 1991). In other types of microsporidiosis, the symptoms depend on the site of infection:

- *Nosema*: disease at multiple body sites.
- *Encephalitozoon*: disease of the gastrointestinal tract, respiratory tract and eyes.
- *Enterocytozoon*: disease of the gastrointestinal tract.
- *Septata*: disease of the gastrointestinal tract.
- *Pleistophora*: disease of muscle tissue.
- *Microsporidium*: disease of the eye.

The term 'microsporidia' is also a catch-all term for those microsporidia not yet fully characterized and speciated. *Enterocytozoon* is the genus of Microspora most commonly associated with human disease. There is currently no standard antimicrobial treatment for microsporidial infection, although a number of therapies are available for HIV-positive individuals on a case-by-case basis (Conteas *et al.*, 2000).

Microsporidia infection is not limited to humans; they also cause disease in a number of other animals, including birds, rabbits, foxes and rats (Deplazes *et al.*, 2000; Wasson and Peper, 2000). Some species are also commercially useful for pest control purposes. *Nosema locustae* is available for controlling grasshoppers and crickets. *Nosema pyrausta* infects several insect species, including the European corn borer, for which it can be an important natural control, and is being developed for commercial use. *Vairimorpha necatrix* is another microsporidium with a wide host range that is also being developed for commercial use.

Microsporidia multiply extensively within the host cell cytoplasm. The general cycle of division includes a phase of repeated divisions by binary fission (merogeny) or multiple fission (schizogony) and a phase resulting in spore production (sporogony). Spores are used as the basis for the characterization of microsporidia. The spores possess a complex tubular extrusion mechanism for injecting the infective material, known as the sporoplasm, into the host cell. This mechanism is activated by environmental stimuli, whereby the polar vacuole distends and the subsequent intracellular pressure everts the polar tubule with its attached sporoplasm. The force of the eversion is enough to inject the sporoplasm into the host cell.

The laboratory diagnosis of microsporidiosis is based on the detection of spores from infected patient material (Garcia, 2002; Weber *et al.*, 2000). The spores are between 1 and 4 μm in diameter and are difficult to visualize without the use of electron microscopy. However, histological sections stained with periodic acid Schiff (PAS) and methenamine silver can be used, as a PAS-positive granule and the spore outline can be seen, respectively. In the case of intestinal microsporidial infection, diagnosis is difficult because few spores are present. As microsporidiosis can also be a disseminated disease, diagnosis may be achieved using stool, urine or nasal washings. To identify microsporidia to species level, the spore size, the nucleus configuration and the host–parasite relationship must all be determined (Franzen and Muller, 1999b). All microsporidia possess common morphological characteristics; for example, a polar tubule is present in all microsporidia and is one of the main features used to distinguish them from other protozoa. Furthermore, the number of coils of the polar tubule may also be used to differentiate microsporidia genera. The polymerase chain reaction (PCR) can now also be used for the detection and possible speciation of microsporidia (da Silva *et al.*, 1996; da Silva *et al.*, 1997; Franzen *et al.*, 1998; Muller *et al.*, 1999).

Microsporidia are emerging human pathogens with a wide host range for potential transmission of disease to humans. Although at present they are mainly a cause of disease in immunocompromised patients, the true incidence of infection in immunocompetent individuals is not known due to the lack of laboratories testing for the organisms and a general lack of understanding of the parasite's biology and epidemiology. As more laboratories look for microsporidia, the true importance will become better understood and more genera or species will most likely be found.

REFERENCES

Bryan, R.T., Cali, A., Owen, R.L. and Spencer, H.C. (1991). Microsporidia: opportunistic pathogens in patients with AIDS. *Prog Clin Parasitol* **2**, 1–26.

Conteas, C.N., Berlin, O.G., Ash, L.R. and Pruthi, J.S. (2000). Therapy for human gastrointestinal microsporidiosis. *Am J Trop Med Hyg* **63**, 121–7.

Da Silva, A.J., Schwartz, D.A., Visvesvara, G.S., de Moura, H., Slemenda, S.B. and Pieniazek, N.J. (1996). Sensitive PCR diagnosis of infections by *Enterocytozoon bieneusi* (microsporidia) using primers based on the region coding for small-subunit rRNA. *J Clin Microbiol* **34**, 986–87.

Da Silva, A.J., Bornay-Llinares, F.J., del Aguila de la Puente Cdel, A., *et al.* (1997). Diagnosis of *Enterocytozoon bieneusi* (microsporidia) infections by polymerase chain reaction in stool samples using primers based on the region coding for small-subunit ribosomal RNA. *Arch Pathol Lab Med* **121**, 874–9.

Deplazes, P., Mathis, A. and Weber, R. (2000). Epidemiology and zoonotic aspects of microsporidia of mammals and birds. *Contrib Microbiol* **6**, 236–60.

Franzen, C. and Muller, A. (1999a). Cryptosporidia and microsporidia – waterborne diseases in the immunocompromised host. *Diagn Microbiol Infect Dis* **34**, 245–62.

Franzen, C. and Muller, A. (1999b). Molecular techniques for detection, species differentiation, and phylogenetic analysis of microsporidia. *Clin Microbiol Rev* **12**, 243–85.

Franzen, C., Muller, A., Hartmann, P., *et al.* (1998). Polymerase chain reaction for diagnosis and species differentiation of microsporidia. *Folia Parasitol (Praha)* **45**, 140–48.

Garcia, L.S. (2002). Laboratory identification of the microsporidia. *J Clin Microbiol* **40**, 1892–1901.

Muller, A., Stellermann, K., Hartmann, P., *et al.* (1999). A powerful DNA extraction method and PCR for detection of microsporidia in clinical stool specimens. *Clin Diagn Lab Immunol* **6**, 243–6.

Shadduck, J.A. and Greeley, E. (1989). Microsporidia and human infections. *Clin Microbiol Rev* **2**, 158–65.

Wasson, K. and Peper, R.L. (2000). Mammalian microsporidiosis. *Vet Pathol* **37**, 113–28.

Weber, R., Deplazes, P. and Schwartz, D. (2000). Diagnosis and clinical aspects of human microsporidiosis. *Contrib Microbiol* **6**, 166–92.

Weiss, L.M. (2001). Microsporidia: emerging pathogenic protists. *Acta Trop* **78**, 89–102.

65

Schistosomiasis

Schistosomiasis, otherwise known as bilharziasis, is a parasitic disease that is endemic in many developing countries and is the second most prevalent tropical disease. The World Health Organization (WHO) estimates that 800 million individuals are at risk of infection and that around 200 million people are infected (Capron *et al.*, 2002). The disease, like many other infectious diseases, is associated with poverty, inadequate sanitation and poor living conditions. It is caused by one of five species of schistosome (also known as blood fluke) in humans. The three most important species to infect humans are *Schistosoma mansoni*, *S. haematobium* and *S. japonicum*; the other two are *S. intercalatum* and *S. mekongi*.

S. mansoni is the cause of intestinal schistosomiasis. It is found in 52 countries in Africa, the Caribbean, the eastern Mediterranean and South America (Chitsulo *et al.*, 2000; Ruppel *et al.*, 2002; Urbani *et al.*, 2002). *S. japonicum* and *S. mekongi* are present in seven Asian countries and the Pacific region. *S. intercalatum* is prevalent in 10 African countries. *S. haematobium* is found in 54 African countries and in the eastern Mediterranean; it is responsible for urinary schistosomiasis. Schistosome infection arises after contact with infected water. A lack of health education is responsible for further spread of the organism. Schistosome eggs are released in human excreta. When they are in contact with water, the eggs open to release the young form, known as the miracidium, which must infect a freshwater snail in order to complete its lifecycle. Once the miracidium has found its snail host, it divides to produce thousands of cercariae, which are then excreted by the snail into the surrounding water, where they can survive

for about 48 hours. It is the cercariae that are able to penetrate human skin and find their way into the bloodstream, where they develop into adult worms. This development takes between 30 and 45 days. Female worms lay between 200 and 2000 eggs per day over an average period of five years. In intestinal schistosomiasis and urinary schistosomiasis, the adult worms remain in the blood vessels surrounding the intestine and urinary tract, respectively. Only about half of the eggs are excreted in the faeces or urine; it is the remaining eggs rather than the adult worm that cause damage to other organs.

Initial symptoms of schistosomiasis are a rash and itchy skin around the area at which the cercariae penetrated the skin. Within one to two months, symptoms of infection, such as fever, chills, cough and muscle aches, may develop, although most individuals do not succumb to symptoms at this stage. This stage is known as Katayama fever, and its symptoms and severity may vary according to the infecting species. Schistosome eggs may travel to the liver, spleen, intestine or bladder, where they may cause symptoms and damage, resulting in cirrhosis or cancer (De Cock, 1986; Elliott, 1996). If eggs are present in the intestine or bladder, then blood may be seen in the faeces or urine, respectively. Most of the symptoms are due to the immune reactions mounted by the patient against the parasite. Complications may arise in some cases. For example, infection with *S. japonicum* can lead to cerebral involvement, such as epilepsy, hemiplegia and blindness.

Laboratory diagnosis of schistosomiasis is based on microscopy of terminal urine or faeces, depending on the symptoms and therefore the species of schistosome implicated. The schistosome ova are either elongated ellipsoid or roughly circular in shape, and are typically large (up to 170 μm in length and 70 μm in width). The presence and location of a spine can often be used to differentiate between species. In addition to microscopy, various serological tests, such as enzyme-linked immunosorbent assay (ELISA), are available (Hamilton *et al.*, 1998; Tarp *et al.*, 2000; Zhu *et al.*, 2002). For travellers returning home from an endemic area, serology should be performed at least three months after return. Safe and effective drugs are available for the treatment of schistosomiasis; these are effective against all species of schistosome (Elliott, 1996). As the dosage varies according to the infecting species, accurate diagnosis is important. Successful treatment cannot be confirmed by serology because antibodies persist after infection. Therefore, clearance of schistosome eggs as determined by microscopy is the chosen method and must be performed six weeks to three months after treatment.

The control of schistosomiasis has been attempted in endemic areas by interrupting the three main conditions of the disease (WHO Expert Committee, 2002; Bergquist, 2002; Chitsulo *et al.*, 2000; Sturrock, 2001; Urbani *et al.*, 2002; Yuan *et al.*, 2002): the contamination of water by infected individuals, the existence of a snail population, and contact by uninfected individuals with infected water. The interruption of any one of these conditions breaks the schistosome lifecycle. To achieve this, the education of local communities is important. Schistosome control has succeeded partly, and in the past 50 years the global distribution has changed significantly. Successful control has occurred in Asia, the Americas, north Africa and the Middle East. Schistosomiasis has been eradicated from Japan and the Lesser Antilles islands, and transmission has been stopped in Tunisia and reduced in Morocco, the Philippines, Saudi Arabia and Venezuela. Such control has been due to political commitment and the allocation of an effective control strategy. The control of *S. japonicum* was the most difficult to attain due to its zoonotic nature (it may also be found in cattle), and it is now

endemic in China, Indonesia, the Philippines and Thailand. However, the control of some species has led to an increased incidence of other species. For example, *S. japonicum* and *S. haematobium*, previously the two main causes of schistosomiasis, have decreased in prevalence and distribution, and *S. mansoni* has now become the most prevalent and widespread of the three species. In addition, recent environmental changes have resulted in the spread of the disease to previously low or non-endemic areas. For example, the construction of dams in some countries has led to new reservoirs for schistosomiasis. It is hoped that the control strategies can continue to decrease the burden of schistosomiasis on people living in endemic areas. However, the task is large and will require full support of the associated governments along with health agencies such as the WHO.

REFERENCES

Bergquist, N.R. (2002). Schistosomiasis: from risk assessment to control. *Trends Parasitol* **18**, 309–14.

Capron, A., Capron, M. and Riveau, G. (2002). Vaccine development against schistosomiasis from concepts to clinical trials. *Br Med Bull* **62**, 139–48.

Chitsulo, L., Engels, D., Montresor, A. and Savioli, L. (2000). The global status of schistosomiasis and its control. *Acta Trop* **77**, 41–51.

De Cock, K.M. (1986). Hepatosplenic schistosomiasis: a clinical review. *Gut* **27**, 734–45.

Elliott, D.E. (1996). Schistosomiasis. Pathophysiology, diagnosis, and treatment. *Gastroenterol Clin North Am* **25**, 599–625.

Hamilton, J.V., Klinkert, M. and Doenhoff, M.J. (1998). Diagnosis of schistosomiasis: antibody detection, with notes on parasitological and antigen detection methods. *Parasitology* **117** (suppl), S41–57.

Ruppel, A., Kennedy, M.W. and Kusel, J.R. (2002). Schistosomiasis immunology, epidemiology and diagnosis. *Trends Parasitol* **18**, 50–52.

Sturrock, R.F. (2001). Schistosomiasis epidemiology and control: how did we get here and where should we go? *Mem Inst Oswaldo Cruz* **96** (suppl), 17–27.

Tarp, B., Black, F.T. and Petersen, E. (2000). The immunofluorescence antibody test (IFAT) for the diagnosis of schistosomiasis used in a non-endemic area. *Trop Med Int Health* 5, 185–91.

Urbani, C., Sinoun, M., Socheat, D., *et al.* (2002). Epidemiology and control of mekongi schistosomiasis. *Acta Trop* 82, 157–68.

WHO Expert Committee (2002). Prevention and control of schistosomiasis and soil-transmitted helminthiasis. *World Health Organ Tech Rep Ser* 912, i–vi, 1–57, back cover.

Yuan, H., Jiang, Q., Zhao, G. and He, N. (2002). Achievements of schistosomiasis control in China. *Mem Inst Oswaldo Cruz* 97 (suppl 1), 187–9.

Zhu, Y., He, W., Liang, Y., *et al.* (2002). Development of a rapid, simple dipstick dye immunoassay for schistosomiasis diagnosis. *J Immunol Methods* 266, 1–5.

66

Onchocerciasis

River blindness, or onchocerciasis, is the world's second leading cause of blindness. It affects people in over 30 countries in Africa, Latin America and the Arabian Peninsula (Hoerauf *et al.*, 2003). It is estimated that 120 million people are at risk and around 18 million people have the disease. Most of those infected live in Africa. The disease is caused by the parasite *Onchocerca volvulus*. It results in blindness or severe visual impairment, but it is a chronic systemic disease and may, therefore, also result in disfigurement, musculoskeletal complaints and weight loss (Murdoch *et al.*, 2002; Sabrosa and Zajdenweber, 2002). Sometimes, epilepsy and growth arrest occur. The disease is spread by its vector, the *Simulium* fly (*Simulium damnosum*).

The microfilariae of O. *volvulus* were first observed in 1875, and the adult worm was described 20 years later. Infection occurs after being bitten by an infected *Simulium* fly. These flies are crucial in the transmission of the disease; they lay their eggs in fast-flowing rivers, and the adults emerge 8–12 days later. Between one and three months after infection, the larvae have developed into adult worms. Adult worms are contained within nodules, which are usually located over prominent bones. Each nodule contains two to three adult female worms and one or two adult male worms. While the adult worms are within the nodules, they are recognized but not attacked seriously by the patient's immune system. The nodules also contain eosinophils and lymphocytes at their periphery, and macrophages are found within the nodules around the adult worms. The adult female worm releases hundreds of microfilariae each day for around a decade. Adult worms may live for up to 14 years. The microfilariae, which live for up to

two years, can move easily through skin and connective tissue and are therefore often found in the skin and eyes. They may be detected in blood, urine, cerebrospinal fluid and various internal organs. As many as 100 million microfilariae may be present in heavily infected individuals.

The clinical symptoms of onchocerciasis are due mostly to the immune responses to dying or dead microfilariae; these are mainly humoral responses, but there are also some cellular responses. Immune responses vary between individuals, and therefore the symptoms can be quite different. Eosinophils are the important cellular response of the immune system and cause the skin damage associated with the disease. The risk of visual impairment due to onchocerciasis increases as the prevalence of infection in a community rises. The microfilarial stage may enter the cornea from the surrounding conjunctiva, resulting in a punctate keratitis (Kale, 1998). After prolonged infection, sclerosing keratitis and indocyclitis develop, resulting in permanent visual impairment or even blindness. Symptoms associated with disease of the skin may be mild or very severe. In their mildest form, there is itching and a localized maculopapular rash, which may clear within a few months; in some cases, however, the lesions become chronic and generalized and the itching more severe. After years of infection, degenerative skin changes occur. Elastic fibres are destroyed, resulting in thinned skin, which begins to sag.

Onchocerciasis should be considered in those who live in, or have visited, areas endemic for the disease, particularly in people with itching. The clinical diagnosis of onchocerciasis is usually achieved by sampling a small amount of skin (Boatin *et al.*, 1998a). This skin is immersed in saline so that the microfilariae emerge into solution, where they can be counted. Alternatively, the Mazzotti test may be performed, whereby diethylcarbamazine is administered, resulting in itching and possibly intense inflammation at the site of microfilarial infection. Other laboratory tests based on the detection of microfilarial DNA, such as polymerase chain reaction (PCR) and enzyme-linked immunosorbent assay (ELISA), are also available (Vincent *et al.*, 2000; Zimmerman *et al.*, 1994). Onchocerciasis may be treated with ivermectin, a drug introduced in 1987 and that was considered to be a milestone for tropical disease treatments (Boatin *et al.*, 1998b; Kale, 1998). This drug is provided free by the manufacturer to people with the disease and who are living in areas where eradication programmes are in progress. It is given as a single dose of 150 µg/kg, which clears microfilariae from the skin for several months, although it does not kill the adult worms. Although diethylcarbamazine can be used for treatment, the side effects can be quite serious, as indicated by the Mazzotti test. Other drugs are needed, however, to control the disease effectively (Hoerauf *et al.*, 2002).

The control of onchocerciasis has been an ongoing effort. The World Health Organization (WHO) initiated the Onchocerciasis Control Programme in 1974, which initially encompassed seven west African countries but was later expanded to 11 countries to cover a total land area of 1.23 million km² and a population of 30 million people (Hougard *et al.*, 2002). The programme is supported by four agencies and has resulted in some remarkable achievements. Vector control has resulted in clearance of the disease in areas such as the Volta River Basin. The programme costs up to 2002 amounted to $550 million. Although this appears to be a huge sum of money, the actual cost for each protected person was less than $1. The programme has also opened up an estimated 25 million hectares of fertile land suitable for housing and cultivation and with a potential to feed 17 million people annually. This is important so that the local population is not only cleared of disease but is also able to live and farm. Hopefully, the control programme will be extended with further funding and agency support (Murdoch *et al.*, 2002; Seketeli

et al., 2002). If not, onchocerciasis may well return to cleared areas.

REFERENCES

Boatin, B.A., Toe, L., Alley, E.S., Dembele, N., Weiss, N. and Dadzie, K.Y. (1998a). Diagnostics in onchocerciasis: future challenges. *Ann Trop Med Parasitol* **92** (suppl 1), S41–5.

Boatin, B.A., Hougard, J.M., Alley, E.S., *et al.* (1998b). The impact of Mectizan on the transmission of onchocerciasis. *Ann Trop Med Parasitol* **92** (suppl 1), S46–60.

Hoerauf, A., Adjei, O. and Buttner, D.W. (2002). Antibiotics for the treatment of onchocerciasis and other filarial infections. *Curr Opin Investig Drugs* **3**, 533–7.

Hoerauf, A., Buttner, D.W., Adjei, O. and Pearlman, E. (2003). Onchocerciasis. *Br Med J* **326**, 207–10.

Hougard, J.M., Yameogo, L. and Philippon, B. (2002). Onchocerciasis in West Africa after 2002: a challenge to take up. *Parasite* **9**, 105–11.

Kale, O.O. (1998). Onchocerciasis: the burden of disease. *Ann Trop Med Parasitol* **92** (suppl 1), S101–15.

Murdoch, M.E., Asuzu, M.C., Hagan, M., *et al.* (2002). Onchocerciasis: the clinical and epidemiological burden of skin disease in Africa. *Ann Trop Med Parasitol* **96**, 283–96.

Sabrosa, N.A. and Zajdenweber, M. (2002). Nematode infections of the eye: toxocariasis, onchocerciasis, diffuse unilateral subacute neuroretinitis, and cysticercosis. *Ophthalmol Clin North Am* **15**, 351–6.

Seketeli, A., Adeoye, G., Eyamba, A., *et al.* (2002). The achievements and challenges of the African Programme for Onchocerciasis Control (APOC). *Ann Trop Med Parasitol* **96** (suppl 1), S15–28.

Vincent, J.A., Lustigman, S., Zhang, S. and Weil, G.J. (2000). A comparison of newer tests for the diagnosis of onchocerciasis. *Ann Trop Med Parasitol* **94**, 253–8.

Zimmerman, P.A., Guderian, R.H., Aruajo, E., *et al.* B. (1994). Polymerase chain reaction-based diagnosis of *Onchocerca volvulus* infection: improved detection of patients with onchocerciasis. *J Infect Dis* **169**, 686–9.

67

Acanthamoeba infection

Acanthamoeba infection is poorly publicized, yet it has devastating effects for infected individuals. The poor publicity is probably associated with the relatively small number of cases that occur each year. Furthermore, it cannot be found in many microbiological texts more than 10 years old. The genus *Acanthamoeba* was first described in the 1930s and now includes 18 species assigned to three groups I–III (Table 67.1) (Visvesvara, 1991). They are free-living amoebae and are ubiquitous in the environment. They have been found in many freshwater and seawater sources as well as swimming pools and air-conditioning units. They have also been isolated from fish, reptiles, birds and mammals, and have even been found as possible commensals in the upper respiratory tract and intestinal tract of humans. As amoebae, they exist in several stages of development: the trophozoite stage is irregularly shaped and between 15 and 45 μm in diameter, while the cyst stage is spherical and between 15 and 20 μm in diameter, and possesses a thick double wall that may be spherical or wrinkled. Both the trophozoite and cyst stages possess a single nucleus with a large, centrally located nucleolus.

The recent increase in interest in *Acanthamoeba* and its associated diseases has led to the requirement of a better method of classification. Several researchers are attempting to classify the organism based on its ribosomal RNA sequence (Chung *et al.*, 1998), and this follows the general trend of the application of genomic sequencing technology to the identification and classification of other microbes.

Early interest in the organisms was not because it caused human disease but because it was encoun-

Table 67.1 The 18 species of *Acanthamoeba*

Group I	Group II	Group III
A. astronyxis	A. castellanii	A. culbertsoni
A. comandoni	A. divionensis	A. lenticulata
A. echinulata	A. griffini	A. royeba
A. tabiashi	A. hatchetti	A. palestinensis
	A. lugdunensis	
	A. mauritaniensis	
	A. polyphaga	
	A. quina	
	A. rhysodes	
	A. triangularis	

tered as a culture contaminant. However, in the 1950s it was recognized that *Acanthamoeba* could cause disease after the organism was inoculated into animals who later died from encephalitis. The first confirmed case of fatal *Acanthamoeba* encephalitis was not reported until 1971 in the USA. In addition, interest in *Acanthamoeba* increased amongst ophthalmologists during the 1980s due to the occurrence of eye infections, and more research on the organism was performed.

Acanthamoeba causes two main diseases in humans: chronic granulomatous encephalitis and keratitis (Marciano-Cabral *et al.*, 2000). Granulomatous encephalitis due to *Acanthamoeba* is a disease that evolves slowly from a subacute condition to a chronic disease that results in granulomatous lesions within the brain (Sell *et al.*, 1997). The disease usually results in death following bronchopneumonia and coma. Keratitis is most common in contact-lens wearers; it has therefore gained more interest in the last decade due to the increase in the number of people who wear contact lenses (McCulley *et al.*, 2000; Sharma *et al.*, 2000). Disseminated disease may also occur in acquired immunodeficiency syndrome (AIDS) patients, other immunocompromised patients, and people with predisposing factors, such as liver disease, renal failure and splenectomy.

The diagnosis of *Acanthamoeba* infection is important. In cases of encephalitis, an early diagnosis is preferred, although there is currently no effective treatment. In cases of *Acanthamoeba* keratitis, delayed diagnosis or misdiagnosis may lead to extensive corneal inflammation and visual loss. Treatment usually consists of combination therapy with a number of biocides (Kumar and Lloyd, 2002; Lindquist, 1998). Corneal scrapings or contact-lens fluid may be used as samples for the identification of *Acanthamoeba* keratitis. Acridine orange has been used for the staining of corneal scrapings for the morphological identification of *Acanthamoeba* cysts (Hahn *et al.*, 1998; Kilvington *et al.*, 1990; Martinez and Visvesvara, 1991). The wrinkled appearance of cysts is a good preliminary identification trait of *Acanthamoeba*. Polymerase chain reaction (PCR) tests have also been devel-

oped that enable early and specific diagnosis of *Acanthamoeba* infection (Khan and Paget, 2002).

Much remains to be learnt about *Acanthamoeba* infection. The pathogenic mechanisms are currently poorly understood, and the reason for its relative rarity in causing human disease is unknown. It is not known whether some species or strains are more virulent than others, or whether all free-living *Acanthamoeba* are equally capable of causing disease in humans. The epidemiology of human disease has remained stable in recent years, suggesting that *Acanthamoeba* does not represent a threat as an emerging problem. However, since the disease is so severe in both its encephalitis and keratitis forms, further research on the organism is justified.

REFERENCES

Chung, D.I., Yu, H.S., Hwang, M.Y., *et al.* (1998). Subgenus classification of *Acanthamoeba* by riboprinting. *Korean J Parasitol* **36**, 69–80.

Hahn, T.W., O'Brien, T.P., Sah, W.J. and Kim, J.H. (1998). Acridine orange staining for rapid diagnosis of *Acanthamoeba* keratitis. *Jpn J Ophthalmol* **42**, 108–14.

Khan, N.A. and Paget, T.A. (2002). Molecular tools for speciation and epidemiological studies of *Acanthamoeba*. *Curr Microbiol* **44**, 444–9.

Kilvington, S., Larkin, D.F., White, D.G. and Beeching, J.R. (1990). Laboratory investigation of *Acanthamoeba* keratitis. *J Clin Microbiol* **28**, 2722–5.

Kumar, R. and Lloyd, D. (2002). Recent advances in the treatment of *Acanthamoeba* keratitis. *Clin Infect Dis* **35**, 434–41.

Lindquist, T.D. (1998). Treatment of *Acanthamoeba* keratitis. *Cornea* **17**, 11–16.

Marciano-Cabral, F., Puffenbarger, R. and Cabral, G.A. (2000). The increasing importance of *Acanthamoeba* infections. *J Eukaryot Microbiol* **47**, 29–36.

Martinez, A.J. and Visvesvara, G.S. (1991). Laboratory diagnosis of pathogenic free-living amoebas: *Naegleria*, *Acanthamoeba*, and *Leptomyxida*. *Clin Lab Med* **11**, 861–72.

McCulley, J.P., Alizadeh, H. and Niederkorn, J.Y. (2000). The diagnosis and management of *Acanthamoeba* keratitis. *Clao J* **26**, 47–51.

Sell, J.J., Rupp, F.W. and Orrison, W.W., Jr (1997). Granulomatous amebic encephalitis caused by acanthamoeba. *Neuroradiology* **39**, 434–6.

Sharma, S., Garg, P. and Rao, G.N. (2000). Patient characteristics, diagnosis, and treatment of non-contact lens related *Acanthamoeba* keratitis. *Br J Ophthalmol* **84**, 1103–8.

Visvesvara, G.S. (1991). Classification of *Acanthamoeba*. *Rev Infect Dis* **13** (suppl 5), S369–72.

68

Parasitic cestodes

Tapeworms are cestode parasites. There are numerous genera distributed throughout the world, although only a few are pathogenic to humans. Larval tapeworms are found in extraintestinal tissues and cause systemic infections, whereas adult tapeworms are found in the small intestine and are usually asymptomatic. Adult tapeworms are segmented; each segment possesses a complete male and female reproductive system. The lifecycle of most tapeworms involves a definitive host and an intermediate host, each cycle having particular larval forms. The pathology caused by tapeworm infection is due to the presence and activity of the worms themselves, by the erosive action caused by the scolex hooks possessed by some worms, or by the reduced host intake of vitamin B12. Allergic reactions may also occur. Most tapeworm infections cause a limited host immune response, apart from a moderate eosinophilia and an increase in immunoglobulin E (IgE) levels. *Hymenolepis nana*, however, causes a strong immune response when the host is infected by the eggs.

The beef tapeworm (*Taenia saginata* or *Taeniarhynchus saginatus*) and pork tapeworm (*Taenia solium*) are the most common cestode parasites of humans. They are estimated to cause infection in over 60 million people worldwide (Hoberg, 2002). They have a global distribution, but they are more common in poor areas, where there is a lot of contact with domestic animals and where food may often be undercooked. Other *Taenia* species infect cats and dogs, although these will not be described. Around 4 million people are infected with *T. solium*. The lifecycles of both tapeworms are similar, except for the stage that occurs in either cattle or pigs.

BEEF TAPEWORM (*T. SAGINATA*)

The adult beef tapeworm usually reaches a length of 5–10 m, but it may grow as long as 25 m (Fan and Chung, 1998; Hoberg, 2002). The adult tapeworm lives in the small intestine of the definitive host, where it attaches itself to the intestinal wall using its hooked scolex. Thousands of proglottids are produced, which mature, become gravid, and break off from the adult worm. The gravid proglottids migrate to the anus, during which time the eggs contained within them are released. Up to 100 000 eggs may be present inside each proglottid, and these are passed in the faeces. The eggs can survive in the environment for years, but to complete the lifecycle they must be ingested by an intermediate host. Alternatively, a complete proglottid may be released in the faeces and then be ingested by a new host, which results in the release of the eggs. Larvae (oncospheres) hatch from the eggs, and attach to and then penetrate the intestinal wall. They then enter the blood system to enable them to reach striated muscle tissue. The oncosphere fills with fluid and develops into the cysticercus (larval cyst), a small infective body about 8 mm in diameter. They survive here in the intermediate host for a number of years. If raw or improperly cooked infected beef is ingested by humans, then this cysticercus is digested and the scolex attaches to the wall of the small intestine. Gravid segments are released into the intestine, starting the lifecycle again. It takes between two and three months after initial attachment for the worm to reach its adult length of 4–5 m. Adult worms may live for 20 years or more. There are few pathogenic or immunogenic effects from infection, which accounts for the long lifespan of the worm.

PORK TAPEWORM (*T. SOLIUM*)

The lifecycle of *T. solium* is similar to that of *T. saginata*, except that the intermediate host is the pig (Garcia and Del Brutto, 2000; Sciutto *et al.*, 2000). There are usually fewer than 1000 proglottids, each of which is less active than those of *T. saginata*, although they often contain more than 50 000 eggs. The major difference is that the larval stage can also take place in humans, resulting in severe cysticercosis. The scolex is similar to that of *T. saginata*, apart from the arrangement of the hooks; however, this results in some pathogenicity and inflammation. *T. solium* can be a serious systemic infection, depending on the size of the cysticerci. The central nervous system is a common site of infection, and the larvae often develop in the brain; however, they can develop in all other organs. Human cysticercosis is a widespread disease in developing countries, particularly Latin America.

The clinical symptoms due to infection with either worm are usually limited to nausea, vomiting, loss of appetite and weight loss. An upsetting condition is the crawling of worm segments from the anus. However, if *T. solium* infection occurs in the brain or other major organs, then it is more serious and can result in major complications or death.

Table 68.1 shows the main features of *T. saginata* and *T. solium*.

LABORATORY DIAGNOSIS OF TAPEWORM INFECTION

The diagnosis of tapeworm infection still relies upon microscopy. *Taenia* infections are diagnosed by the presence of gravid segments or eggs in stool specimens by microscopy. The eggs of *T. saginata* and *T. solium* are very similar, so the species identification is by proglottid and scolex analysis. The diagnosis of the presence of tapeworm larvae is more difficult because these are present in tissues. Cysts may be identified in biopsies or by radiography, depending on the site of the larval cyst. Serological methods, such as enzyme-linked immunosorbent assay (ELISA) and indirect haemagglutination, may also be used, but often these are not diagnostic due to the lack of sensitivity and specificity (Fan and Chung, 1998).

HYDATID DISEASE

Hydatid disease (echinococcosis) is caused by the larval stages of the tapeworms *Echinococcus granulosus* and *Echinococcus multilocularis*. It is common in sheep-raising areas, such as Eastern Europe, the Mediterranean, Australia and New Zealand (Ammann and Eckert, 1996). The adult worms are small (less than 1 cm in length) and reside in the small intestine of carnivores such as dogs, foxes and

Table 68.1 Features of *Taenia saginata* and *Taenia solium*

Characteristic	*T. saginata*	*T. solium*
Definitive host	Humans	Humans
Intermediate host	Cattle	Pigs (or humans)
Mode of infection	Ingestion of cysticerci	Ingestion of cysticerci
Site of infection in intermediate host	Striated muscle	Any major organ

wolves. Several worms are usually present in the infected animal. Each worm consists of a scolex possessing four suckers. The mature terminal segment, known as the proglottid, ruptures to release thousands of ova. These ova, which are morphologically indistinguishable from those of *T. saginata* and *T. solium*, are voided in the faeces. The intermediate hosts, usually sheep and cattle, become infected after ingestion of contaminated pastures or, in the case of humans, contaminated vegetables. Once the animal or human is infected, the egg hatches in the duodenum to release the oncosphere, which penetrates the intestinal wall to enter the portal system, where the embryo can be distributed to any part of the body. One or more cysts (hydatids) may develop in any tissue, including all the major organs. The clinical symptoms vary according to the tissue involved and the size of the cyst. The hydatid of *E. granulosus* grows slowly but reaches a diameter of about 30 cm. It is filled with fluid and an inner lining, from which thousands of scoleces bud off into the surrounding lumen. The scoleces enlarge and develop into vesicular daughter hydatids, which may produce a third generation of hydatids. Symptoms may go unnoticed for many years but then, depending on the site, appear without warning. Such episodes may range from the development of deafness to anaphylactic shock.

Infection with *E. multilocularis* (the multiloculate or alveolar tapeworm) is rare. Although the appearance and lifecycle of this parasite is similar to that *of E. granulosus*, the cyst is much more invasive and does not remain confined. It develops a series of chambers and results in pathology resembling malignant growth. The primary cyst usually develops in the liver and, as it is usually diagnosed late, infection is often fatal.

DWARF TAPEWORM (HYMENOLEPIS NANA)

Infection with *H. nana* is common. It has a worldwide incidence, but it is particularly prevalent in crowded conditions, such as those that occur in some areas of India and China (Mirdha and Samantray, 2002; Sirivichayakul *et al.*, 2000). It is acquired after ingesting eggs contained within the faeces of another infected animal through contaminated food, water or direct contact. Infection with this tapeworm is usually asymptomatic, but heavy infection may cause nausea and vomiting, diarrhoea and general abdominal pain. Ingested eggs hatch in the duodenum, and the oncospheres penetrate into the villi, where they develop into cysticercoid larvae. They are then released into the gut lumen, they attach to the intestinal mucosa, and they develop into adult worms after 5–10 days. The worms are small (15–40 mm long), and they have a scolex possessing four suckers. Terminal gravid segments contain eggs, which are released within the faecal bolus. Most species of *Hymenolepis* larvae are found in insect or crustacean hosts, except for those of *H. nana*, which develop in insects or the human small intestine.

RAT TAPEWORM (HYMENOLEPIS DIMINUTA)

The rat tapeworm is larger than *H. nana* (up to 60 cm long). Its lifecycle involves grain insects. *H. diminuta* does not commonly cause human infection, but it can if an insect that carries cysticercoids of the worm is ingested. Young children are therefore most commonly infected. The symptoms are mild diarrhoea (Hamrick *et al.*, 1990).

DOUBLE-PORED TAPEWORM (DIPYLIDIUM CANINUM)

Otherwise known as the 'cucumber tapeworm', this worm causes infection in dogs and cats and is spread by fleas or lice, which are the intermediate hosts. The perineum of the animal becomes contaminated with eggs when they are passed in the faeces. The eggs may then be ingested by a flea or louse. Proglottids may also be released in the animal faeces; these resemble the shape of a cucumber or rice grain, hence the nickname. Dogs or cats become infected when they ingest an infected flea or louse. Children and others in close contact with pets may contract the infection after accidental ingestion of a flea containing cysticercoids, but such infection is usually asymptomatic (Raitiere, 1992).

BROAD FISH TAPEWORM (*DIPHYLLOBOTHRIUM LATUM*)

This parasite is common in temperate and sub-Arctic regions, such as Scandinavia, Japan and central Europe, and where freshwater fish are eaten raw (Lee *et al.*, 1994). It is the largest parasite to cause infection in humans: the adult worm may reach a length of 10 m, consisting of thousands of segments that produce around a million ova each day. The adult worm is identified by its scolex, which has a pair of linear sucking grooves instead of suckers and hooks, and also by its rosette-shaped uterus, which has a pore through which eggs are passed. Eggs are therefore shed into the surroundings rather than within a segment. Infection does not usually cause any pathology, although symptoms such as mild diarrhoea, vomiting and fatigue may occur occasionally. Megaloblastic anaemia may occur, but this is seen rarely due to improved diet and better treatment.

The parasite has an aquatic component to its lifecycle, unlike other cestode parasites that affect humans (von Bonsdorff and Bylund, 1982). To begin the lifecycle, fresh water must be contaminated with faeces containing parasite eggs from a human or wild animal. The eggs hatch, releasing the ciliated coracidium, which contains the oncosphere. This is then ingested by a water flea, where it develops into the second-stage embryo, the procercoid. If the infected water flea is ingested by a small fish, then the procercoid penetrates the gut within a few hours and develops into the third-stage larva, the plerocercoid. The infected small fish are consumed by larger fish, where the plerocercoid penetrates the muscle tissue. If these large fish are then eaten raw by humans, the plerocercoid is released, attaches to the gut wall, and starts in development as an adult worm.

COENURUS TAPEWORM (*TAENIA MULTICEPS*)

This worm is found in dogs and other wild canids. Sheep are the intermediate hosts. It has also been found in other wild animals and pets (Fountain, 2000; Huss *et al.*, 1994; Ing *et al.*, 1998). Human infection with the parasite is rare but may occur after accidental ingestion of dog faeces or food or water contaminated by dog faeces that contain eggs. In temperate areas, infection is usually confined to the brain, but in tropical areas infection affects the eye or subcutaneous tissue (Williams and Templeton, 1971). Treatment is usually by surgery, although some antiparasitic drugs may be beneficial.

REFERENCES

Ammann, R.W. and Eckert, J. (1996). Cestodes. Echinococcus. *Gastroenterol Clin North Am* **25**, 655–89.

Fan, P.C. and Chung, W.C. (1998). *Taenia saginata asiatica*: epidemiology, infection, immunological and molecular studies. *J Microbiol Immunol Infect* **31**, 84–9.

Fountain, K. (2000). *Coenurus serialis* in a pet rabbit. *Vet Rec* **147**, 340.

Garcia, H.H. and Del Brutto, O.H. (2000). *Taenia solium* cysticercosis. *Infect Dis Clin North Am* **14**, 97–119, ix.

Hamrick, H.J., Bowdre, J.H. and Church, S.M. (1990). Rat tapeworm (*Hymenolepis diminuta*) infection in a child. *Pediatr Infect Dis J* **9**, 216–19.

Hoberg, E.P. (2002). Taenia tapeworms: their biology, evolution and socioeconomic significance. *Microbes Infect* **4**, 859–66.

Huss, B.T., Miller, M.A., Corwin, R.M., Hoberg, E.P. and O'Brien, D.P. (1994). Fatal cerebral coenurosis in a cat. *J Am Vet Med Assoc* **205**, 69–71.

Ing, M.B., Schantz, P.M. and Turner, J. A. (1998). Human coenurosis in North America: case reports and review. *Clin Infect Dis* **27**, 519–23.

Lee, S.H., Chai, J.Y., Seo, M., *et al.* (1994). Two rare cases of *Diphyllobothrium latum parvum* type infection in Korea. *Kisaengchunghak Chapchi* **32**, 117–20.

Mirdha, B.R. and Samantray, J.C. (2002). *Hymenolepis nana*: a common cause of paediatric diarrhoea in urban slum dwellers in India. *J Trop Pediatr* **48**, 331–4.

Raitiere, C.R. (1992). Dog tapeworm (*Dipylidium caninum*) infestation in a 6-month-old infant. *J Fam Pract* **34**, 101–2.

Sciutto, E., Fragoso, G., Fleury, A., *et al.* (2000). *Taenia solium* disease in humans and pigs: an ancient parasitosis disease rooted in developing countries and emerging as a major health problem of global dimensions. *Microbes Infect* **2**, 1875–90.

Sirivichayakul, C., Radomyos, P., Praevanit, R., Pojjaroen-Anant, C. and Wisetsing, P. (2000). *Hymenolepis nana* infection in Thai children. *J Med Assoc Thai* **83**, 1035–8.

Von Bonsdorff, B. and Bylund, G. (1982). The ecology of *Diphyllobothrium latum*. *Ecol Dis* **1**, 21–6.

Williams, P.H. and Templeton, A.C. (1971). Infection of the eye by tapeworm coenurosis. *Br J Ophthalmol* **55**, 766–9.

PART V

Mycology

69

Candidiasis

Fungi and yeasts belong to the *Eumycetes*. They are eukaryotic organisms with a differentiated nucleus and a rigid cell wall. Originally described as plants without chlorophyll, they are now grouped with the protozoa. The growth requirements of fungi and yeasts are generally simple. They can survive in the environment and grow at temperatures between 28 and 37 °C, although this varies according to the individual fungus or yeast. Fungi grow slowly compared with yeasts.

Only a relatively small number of fungi and yeasts are human pathogens. Most infections, such as athlete's foot, are superficial but common. The rare infections tend to be invasive and are usually severe and often fatal. Almost 12 000 fungal isolates were reported in England and Wales between 1990 and 1999, accounted for by 73 different species (source: HPA CDSC).

Yeasts are fungi that grow as single cells and produce daughter cells by budding or by binary fission. They differ from most other fungi, which grow as thread-like hyphae. However, yeasts cannot be differentiated from other fungi on this distinction because some fungi can alternate between the yeast and hyphal phases. Yeasts are considered a universal model for the understanding of cell division, differentiation and other cell processes. Classical and molecular genetics have utilized the yeasts heavily over the past few decades and successfully improved our understanding of genes and proteins and their functions. Yeasts are mostly opportunistic pathogens, but they have also been used by humankind for the production of beer and bread as far back as Egyptian times in 2600 BC.

- *Saccharomyces cerevisiae* is the common baker's yeast used for breadmaking.
- *Candida albicans* is a common cause of minor infections in humans.
- *Cryptococcus neoformans* is a pathogen of humans.

Candida, when present in low numbers, is part of the normal mouth, intestinal and vaginal flora (Soll, 2002). It may also be found on the skin of healthy individuals. In most people, commensal bacteria control the quantity of *Candida* within the body. However, as an opportunistic pathogen, due to the administration of antibiotics, immunosuppression or the presence of an underlying medical condition, *Candida* can cause infection (candidiasis). Opportunistic infection may occur during pregnancy, after trauma, in diabetics and in alcoholics. Candidiasis results in a mild, superficial inflammatory reaction at the location of infection, occurring mostly on the mucosa, such as in the mouth and the vagina. Candidiasis of mucosal surfaces is generally known as thrush. Secondary infections may occur in the lower respiratory tract and urinary tract, although these are less common. Septicaemia is also possible in people with severe candidiasis. The majority of yeast infections are caused by *C. albicans*. However, there are six other species that may cause human infection, the sites of which are similar to those caused by *C. albicans*; these species are responsible for only about 10% of *Candida* infections (Gutierrez *et al.*, 2002; Krcmery and Barnes, 2002; Moosa and Sobel, 2002).

The most common infection is vaginal candidiasis (vaginal thrush) (Sobel, 2002). In the UK in 2000, there were over 68 000 cases of candidiasis in women, an increase from 51 000 in 1990 (source: HPA CDSC). A whitish discharge is seen, which contains pus cells and yeasts. Pregnant women are particularly susceptible to vaginal thrush due to hormonal imbalances and changes in the vaginal microbial flora. Oral candidiasis, which is also called thrush, is a fungal infection of the mouth and/or throat. Candidiasis of the throat is called oesopharyngeal candidiasis. While oral candidiasis can sometimes occur without symptoms, the most common symptoms are discomfort and burning of the mouth and throat, and an altered sense of taste. Creamy white or yellowish spots in the mouth and throat that can be removed by light scraping are also common. These may be accompanied by cracking, redness, soreness and swelling at the corners of the mouth. A bad case can include mouth sores. Oral candidiasis is rare if CD4-positive white cell counts are above 500. Infection is more common as the count drops to 100. Oral candidiasis may be more difficult to treat when CD4-positive cell counts fall below 50. Certain drugs can alter the ability of commensal organisms to survive in the mouth, which can then promote the growth of *Candida*. These include long-term antibiotics, steroids and oral contraceptives with a high oestrogen content.

Invasive candidiasis is a fungal infection that occurs when *Candida* enter the bloodstream (Spellberg and Edwards, 2002). Candidaemia is now one of the most common bloodstream infections in Western nations. Those at risk of candidaemia include prematurely born babies, surgical patients, and immunocompromised people (Blash, 2002). The symptoms of invasive candidiasis are not specific but include fever and chills, which do not improve after antibiotic therapy. Infection can spread to organs such as the kidneys, liver, bones, muscles, joints, spleen and eyes. Additional specific symptoms may develop, depending on the site of infection. If infection does not respond to antibiotic therapy, then this can lead to organ failure and death.

The laboratory diagnosis of candidiasis is usually straightforward (Richardson and Ellis, 2000). The yeast survives well in exudates and blood, as well as most laboratory media. Yeasts will also grow in standard blood culture systems, and therefore diagnosis in patients with candidaemia is straightforward. Yeast cells are seen easily under microscopy, with or without staining, although dark field or phase contrast microscopy is better. They are Gram-positive when stained. *Candida* grow well on blood or Sabouraud agar at temperatures between 20 and 37 °C. As most yeast infections are caused by *C. albicans*, speciation is not usually required, although more formal identification can be determined by sugar utilization and pseudomycelium production. Serology is not an established method of diagnosis, but the polymerase chain reaction (PCR) is being used more widely; its use is not required often as the yeast can usually be seen by microscopy or can be isolated rapidly from body fluids. Molecular methods can be employed to speciate or type *Candida* isolated during outbreaks in hospital wards and institutions such as nursing homes. Such methods include PCR, restriction enzyme electrophoresis and DNA probes. However, these are restricted to research and reference laboratories.

The treatment of candidiasis is two-fold. First, the underlying cause of infection must be determined; second, antifungal treatments such as nystatin, amphotericin B and clotrimazole may be given. Antifungal treatment depends on the site and seriousness of the infection, and care must be taken with the emergence of *Candida* that are resistant to antifungal drugs (Morschhauser, 2002; Sanglard and Odds, 2002).

REFERENCES

Blash, J.L. (2002). Systemic *Candida* infections in patients with leukemia: an overview of drug therapy. *Clin J Oncol Nurs* 6, 323–31.

Gutierrez, J., Morales, P., Gonzalez, M.A. and Quindos, G. (2002). *Candida dubliniensis*, a new fungal pathogen. *J Basic Microbiol* **42**, 207–27.

Krcmery, V. and Barnes, A.J. (2002). Non-albicans *Candida* spp. causing fungaemia: pathogenicity and antifungal resistance. *J Hosp Infect* **50**, 243–60.

Moosa, M.Y. and Sobel, J.D. (2002). Non-albicans *Candida* infections in patients with hematologic malignancies. *Semin Respir Infect* **17**, 91–8.

Morschhauser, J. (2002). The genetic basis of fluconazole resistance development in *Candida albicans*. *Biochim Biophys Acta* **1587**, 240–48.

Richardson, M. and Ellis, M. (2000). Clinical and laboratory diagnosis. *Hosp Med* **61**, 610–14.

Sanglard, D. and Odds, F.C. (2002). Resistance of *Candida* species to antifungal agents: molecular mechanisms and clinical consequences. *Lancet Infect Dis* **2**, 73–85.

Sobel, J.D. (2002). Treatment of vaginal *Candida* infections. *Expert Opin Pharmacother* **3**, 1059–65.

Soll, D.R. (2002). Candida commensalism and virulence: the evolution of phenotypic plasticity. *Acta Trop* **81**, 101–10.

Spellberg, B. and Edwards, J.E. (2002). The pathophysiology and treatment of *Candida* sepsis. *Curr Infect Dis Rep* **4**, 387–99.

70

Ringworm

Although most of the thousands of species of filamentous fungi are non-pathogenic, about 100 of them cause infection in humans (Yates and Concannon, 2002). They are responsible for infections of the nail, hair, skin, respiratory tract, gastrointestinal tract, eye and deep tissues. They can also be responsible for sensitization and poisoning. Worldwide, between 0.5 and 10% of the population has a ringworm infection, depending on the country, climate and age group (Aste *et al.*, 2003; Ayaya *et al.*, 2001; Devliotou-Panagliotidou *et al.*, 2001; Silverberg *et al.*, 2002). One-third of all ringworm infections involve the nails.

Ringworm, or tinea, is a very common infection of the skin, hair and nails. It is caused by about 40 filamentous fungi; 90% of infections are caused by *Microsporum audouinii*, *M. canis*, *Trichophyton rubrum*, *T. mentagrophytes*, *T. verrucosum* and *Epidermophyton floccosum* (Hainer, 2003). These dermatophytes live only on keratinized surfaces and do not invade non-keratinized tissue. In the host, they exist as hyphae and arthrospores, but in vitro they also form asexual spores known as microconidia and macroconidia. Microconidia are small (2–5 μm), unicellular, and round or pear-shaped. Macroconidia are multicellular and differ in size, shape and morphology depending on the genus: in *Microsporum* they are spindle-shaped, rough-surfaced and 40–150 μm in length; in *Epidermophyton* they are pear-shaped, smooth-surfaced and 30–40 μm in size; and in *Trichophyton* they are smooth, cylindrical and 10–50 μm in length.

Infections are often named according to the site of infection (Pomeranz and Sabnis, 2002):

- Tinea capitis is infection of hair on the head.
- Tinea corporis is infection of the trunk and extremities.
- Tinea pedis is infection of the foot (also known as athlete's foot).
- Tinea cruris is infection of the groin.
- Tinea barbae is infection of the beard area and neck.
- Tinea faciale is infection of the face.
- Tinea unguium is infection of the nail.

Infection can spread rapidly in the dead keratinized layer in the hyphal form. Due to the infection taking place in dead matter, the inflammatory reaction is usually mild and restricted to dry scaling or hyperkeratosis. Irritation, erythema, oedema and vesiculation may occur. The irregular pink periphery at the infection site gives rise to the name 'ringworm'. Infection of the nails renders them irregular, discoloured and friable. Scalp infection is caused by epidermal and hair follicle infection, and results in hair loss and the formation of a black dot or spore-covered stump at the site of infection. Ringworm infection can be transmitted in a variety of ways:

- Direct skin-to-skin contact with an infected person.
- Contact with an infected pet or farm animal.
- Contact with an infected individual's clothing, shoes or personal items.
- Contact with a contaminated surface, such as in bathrooms and changing rooms.

Ringworm rarely results in serious infection. However, cellulitis can occur in the lower extremities, leading to the formation of broken skin, particularly between the toes. This can be followed by the entry of opportunistic bacteria and is a frequent complication, particularly in the elderly (Brook, 2002). Also, immunocompromised patients are susceptible to atypical and particularly aggressive ringworm infections, which lead to extensive skin disease, subcutaneous abscesses and dissemination.

Laboratory diagnosis of ringworm is usually by microscopy and culture of infected material (Elewski, 1996; Liu *et al.*, 1997; Weinstein and Berman, 2002), although the polymerase chain reaction (PCR) may now also be used (Liu *et al.*, 1997). Care must be taken in the quality and quantity of sample taken. For example, nail clippings rarely result in a positive diagnosis. However, good sampling often results in friable or minute samples, which are then difficult to use in the laboratory. If a good sample is collected, hyphae may be seen by microscopy. Culture, which takes at least three days but may take weeks, is followed by identification as described above. Dermatophytes may be isolated on Sabouraud agar at 26–28 °C. Identification of the fungus may be difficult, as the colonial appearance varies considerably between species and on different media. Identifying features include the rate of growth, folding and zoning of the colony itself, colony texture and pigmentation.

Treatment for ringworm may include griseofulvin, which must be given for two to three weeks for skin and hair infection and up to a year for nail infections (Anon, 1996; Hainer, 2003; Pomeranz and Sabnis, 2002; Weinstein and Berman, 2002). The new skin, hair or nail must grow back and be clean of infection before treatment can stop. Infection can be avoided by good hygiene practices and by avoiding the sharing of hats, socks and other clothes. However, swimming pools and changing rooms remain sources of infection.

REFERENCES

Anon (1996). Management of scalp ringworm. *Drug Ther Bull* **34**, 5–6.

Aste, N., Pau, M. and Biggio, P. (2003). Tinea pedis observed in Cagliari, Italy, between 1996 and 2000. *Mycoses* **46**, 38–41.

Ayaya, S.O., Kamar, K.K. and Kakai, R. (2001). Aetiology of tinea capitis in school children. *East Afr Med J* **78**, 531–5.

Brook, I. (2002). Secondary bacterial infections complicating skin lesions. *J Med Microbiol* **51**, 808–12.

Devliotou-Panagliotidou, D., Koussidou-Eremondi, T., Chaidemenos, G.C., Theodoridou, M. and Minas, A. (2001). Tinea capitis in adults during 1981-95 in northern Greece. *Mycoses* **44**, 398–400.

Elewski, B.E. (1996). Diagnostic techniques for confirming onychomycosis. *J Am Acad Dermatol* **35**, S6–9.

Hainer, B.L. (2003). Dermatophyte infections. *Am Fam Physician* **67**, 101–8.

Liu, D., Coloe, S., Baird, R. and Pedersen, J. (1997). PCR identification of *Trichophyton mentagrophytes* var. *interdigitale* and *T. mentagrophytes* var. *mentagrophytes* dermatophytes with a random primer. *J Med Microbiol* **46**, 1043–6.

Pomeranz, A.J. and Sabnis, S.S. (2002). Tinea capitis: epidemiology, diagnosis and management strategies. *Paediatr Drugs* **4**, 779–83.

Silverberg, N.B., Weinberg, J.M. and DeLeo, V.A. (2002). Tinea capitis: focus on African American women. *J Am Acad Dermatol* **46**, S120–24.

Weinstein, A. and Berman, B. (2002). Topical treatment of common superficial tinea infections. *Am Fam Physician* **65**, 2095–102.

Yates, Y.J. and Concannon, M.J. (2002). Fungal infections of the perionychium. *Hand Clin* **18**, 631–42, discussion 643–6.

71

Aspergillosis

Aspergillus, like many fungi, is an opportunistic pathogen. The fungus is widespread in nature and can be found in soil, water and decaying vegetation. Although spores may be inhaled frequently, infection is actually uncommon. The genus *Aspergillus* possesses septate hyphae and reproduces by asexual conidia, which are produced in chains from elongated cells called sterigmata. These are borne on the expanded end of a specialized hypha known as the conidiophore. The morphology of the sporing structures is used in species identification.

A. fumigatus and *A. flavus* are the most frequently isolated *Aspergillus* in patients with proven aspergillosis (Perea and Patterson, 2002; Walsh and Groll, 2001). Nosocomial aspergillosis has been recognized increasingly as a cause of severe illness and mortality in highly immunocompromised patients, in diabetics, and after trauma, medical intervention and antibiotic therapy (Marr *et al.*, 2002). The most important nosocomial infection due to *Aspergillus* is pneumonia. In contrast to most bacterial pneumonias, the primary route of acquiring *Aspergillus* infection is by inhalation of fungal spores. A role for nasopharyngeal colonization with *Aspergillus* as an intermediate step before invasive pulmonary disease has been proposed but remains to be elucidated. Colonization of the lower respiratory tract by *Aspergillus*, especially in patients with pre-existing lung disease such as chronic obstructive lung disease, cystic fibrosis or inactive tuberculosis, can predispose to invasive pulmonary or disseminated infection. Colonization and growth of *Aspergillus* in the lungs leads to the formation of a mycelial mass known as a 'fungus ball' or aspergilloma. This leads to a productive

cough but few other symptoms. Importantly, tissue invasion does not occur. In severely immunocompromised patients, primary *Aspergillus* pneumonia results from local lung tissue invasion. Subsequently, the fungus may disseminate via the bloodstream, leading to the formation of septic emboli, which may lodge in the brain, heart and kidneys. *Aspergillus* may also disseminate to deep organs. Individuals with or without invasive aspergillosis may also become sensitized to the spores, leading to asthmatic symptoms and a mucofibrinous sputum.

In the UK, there were 873 reports of *Aspergillus* infection between 1990 and 1999, but only 389 of these were considered invasive infections (Lamagni *et al.*, 2001). However, the diagnosis of aspergillosis remains important. The diagnosis of *Aspergillus* pneumonia is often difficult without the performing of invasive procedures. Bronchoalveolar lavage has been a useful screening test, but lung biopsy is still considered the most reliable technique. Histopathological demonstration of tissue invasion by fungal hyphae is usually required in addition to isolation of *Aspergillus* from respiratory tract secretions because the latter, by itself, may indicate colonization. However, *Aspergillus* grown from the sputum of a febrile, granulocytopoenic patient with a new pulmonary infiltrate is indicative of pulmonary aspergillosis. Routine blood cultures are insensitive for detecting *Aspergillus*, but serology and polymerase chain reaction (PCR) may be useful (Bialek *et al.*, 2002; Centeno-Lima *et al.*, 2002; Raad *et al.*, 2002). When isolated in the laboratory from clinical samples such as sputum, *A. fumigatus* grows as white, velvety colonies at first but then becomes green, yellow or black as the conidia are formed. The organism can grow at temperatures up to 50 °C. A number of traits may be used to speciate and characterize *A. fumigatus*:

- culture and morphology;
- use of secondary metabolites;
- DNA probing;
- microsatellite patterns;
- restriction fragment hybridization analysis.

The treatment of aspergillosis relies on amphotericin B and itraconazole. However, the efficacy of these drugs in vivo is low and therefore the mortality rate of invasive aspergillosis remains high. Effective means of avoiding exposure to *Aspergillus* are also important for at-risk individuals. Environmental disturbances due to construction or renovation activities in and around hospitals markedly raise the airborne spore counts and have been associated with nosocomial aspergillosis (Kistemann *et al.*, 2002). Outbreaks of invasive aspergillosis reinforce the importance of maintaining an environment as free as possible of *Aspergillus* spores for at-risk patients. To achieve this, specialized services, such as bone-marrow transplant services, can install protected environments for the care of such patients, as well as reduce the risk of environmental exposure during hospital construction and routine maintenance of hospital air-filtration and ventilation systems. Laminar airflow systems have been shown to decrease or eliminate the risk of nosocomial aspergillosis in at-risk patients. However, such systems are costly to install and maintain. Substances such as copper-8-quinolinolate have been used on environmental surfaces contaminated with *Aspergillus* spp. to control outbreaks. They have also been used, although not commonly, in building materials to decrease the environmental spore burden.

A single case of nosocomial *Aspergillus* pneumonia is often difficult to link to a specific environmental exposure. However, additional cases may remain undetected without an active search that includes an intensive retrospective review of microbiological, histopathological and post-mortem records. When additional cases are detected, the likelihood is increased that a hospital environmental source of *Aspergillus* spp. can be identified. New molecular typing techniques such as karyotyping and DNA endonuclease profiling may aid significantly in identifying the source of an outbreak (Chazalet *et al.*, 1998; Mondon *et al.*, 1997). The availability of the *Aspergillus* genome sequence will also increase our understanding of the fungus and how it causes disease and therefore may lead to improved therapies (Brakhage and Langfelder, 2002; Denning *et al.*, 2002).

REFERENCES

Bialek, R., Moshous, D., Casanova, J.L., Blanche, S. and Hennequin, C. (2002). Aspergillus antigen and PCR assays in bone marrow transplanted children. *Eur J Med Res* **7**, 177–80.

Brakhage, A.A. and Langfelder, K. (2002). Menacing mold: the molecular biology of *Aspergillus fumigatus*. *Annu Rev Microbiol* **56**, 433–55.

Centeno-Lima, S., de Lacerda, J.M., do Carmo, J.A., Abecasis, M., Casimiro, C. and Exposto, F. (2002). Follow-up of anti-Aspergillus IgG and IgA antibodies in bone marrow transplanted patients with invasive aspergillosis. *J Clin Lab Anal* **16**, 156–62.

Chazalet, V., Debeaupuis, J.P., Sarfati, J., *et al.* (1998). Molecular typing of environmental and patient isolates of *Aspergillus fumigatus* from various hospital settings. *J Clin Microbiol* **36**, 1494–500.

Denning, D.W., Anderson, M.J., Turner, G., Latge, J.P. and Bennett, J.W. (2002). Sequencing the *Aspergillus fumigatus* genome. *Lancet Infect Dis* **2**, 251–3.

Kistemann, T., Huneburg, H., Exner, M., Vacata, V. and Engelhart, S. (2002). Role of increased environmental Aspergillus exposure for patients with chronic obstructive pulmonary disease (COPD) treated with corticosteroids in an intensive care unit. *Int J Hyg Environ Health* **204**, 347–51.

Lamagni, T.L., Evans, B.G., Shigematsu, M. and Johnson, E.M. (2001). Emerging trends in the epidemiology of invasive mycoses in England and Wales (1990–9). *Epidemiol Infect* **126**, 397–414.

Marr, K.A., Patterson, T. and Denning, D. (2002). Aspergillosis. Pathogenesis, clinical manifestations, and therapy. *Infect Dis Clin North Am* **16**, 875–94, vi.

Mondon, P., Brenier, M.P., Symoens, F., *et al.* (1997). Molecular typing of *Aspergillus fumigatus* strains by sequence-specific DNA primer (SSDP) analysis. *FEMS Immunol Med Microbiol* **17**, 95–102.

Perea, S. and Patterson, T.F. (2002). Invasive Aspergillus infections in hematologic malignancy patients. *Semin Respir Infect* **17**, 99–105.

Raad, I., Hanna, H., Huaringa, A., Sumoza, D., Hachem, R. and Albitar, M. (2002). Diagnosis of invasive pulmonary aspergillosis using polymerase chain reaction-based detection of aspergillus in BAL. *Chest* **121**, 1171–6.

Walsh, T.J. and Groll, A.H. (2001). Overview: non-fumigatus species of Aspergillus: perspectives on emerging pathogens in immunocompromised hosts. *Curr Opin Investig Drugs* **2**, 1366–7.

72

Histoplasmosis

Histoplasmosis is a disease caused by the fungus *Histoplasma*. The genus has one species, *H. capsulatum*, although there are two varieties, *capsulatum* and *duboisii*. This dimorphic fungus is found in many parts of the world, but it is encountered most frequently in tropical regions. Histoplasmosis is the most common mycosis in North America, where it is found mainly in the Ohio and Mississippi River valleys. It is found in rich soils, such as those containing droppings from birds or animals. *H. capsulatum* grows in soil and material contaminated with bat or bird droppings. Spores become airborne when contaminated soil is disturbed. Inhaling the spores causes infection. The disease is not transmitted from an infected person to other people, although infection occurs naturally in rodents, dogs, cats, bats and humans. The fungus has been found in poultry house litter, caves, areas harbouring bats, and bird roosts.

In humans, the symptoms of histoplasmosis vary greatly, from an acute benign pulmonary infection to a chronic pulmonary or fatal disseminated disease (Woods *et al.*, 2001). This is mostly dependent on the intensity of exposure and the immunity of the exposed individual. Infants, young children and older people, particularly those with chronic lung disease, are at increased risk for severe disease. Disseminated disease is seen more frequently in people with cancer or acquired immunodeficiency syndrome (AIDS). Most exposed individuals have few or no symptoms. However, if symptoms do occur, they will start within 3–17 days (average 10 days) after exposure. The acute respiratory disease is characterized by respiratory symptoms, a general ill feeling, fever, chest pains and a dry or non-productive cough (Kauffman,

2001). Distinct patterns may be seen on chest X-ray. About 10–20% of cases will develop chronic disease, including progressive pulmonary disease and disseminated infection. Chronic lung disease resembles tuberculosis and can worsen over months or years; other organs can also be affected. The disseminated form is fatal unless treated.

The diagnosis of histoplasmosis is often by histological examination of skin biopsies. Smears can be stained with Giemsa to aid in recognition. Positive histoplasmin skin tests occur in as many as 80% of the people living in areas where *H. capsulatum* is endemic, such as the eastern and central USA. Antigen detection tests and the polymerase chain reaction (PCR) may also be used for diagnosis (Bialek *et al.*, 2002; Rickerts *et al.*, 2002; Wheat *et al.*, 2002). Being a dimorphic fungus, *Histoplasma* grow differently in different conditions, particularly different temperatures. In soil and in vitro culture at 25–28 °C, *Histoplasma* grow after two weeks as a white or slightly brown woolly mould. Septate mycelia bear microconidia, which are between 2 and 5 µm in width. In mammals and in vitro culture at 37 °C, *Histoplasma* grow as oval yeasts up to 4 µm in size and form moist, buff-coloured yeast-like colonies. Demonstration of conversion from yeast to mould is useful for identification purposes.

Antifungal medications are used to treat severe cases of acute histoplasmosis and all cases of chronic and disseminated disease (Mocherla and Wheat, 2001). Mild disease usually resolves without treatment, and past infection results in partial protection against ill effects if reinfection occurs. For example, during a large outbreak in Ohio, USA, all patients recovered within three weeks without any treatment. Therefore, the actual treatment of histoplasmosis depends on the severity of the disease and the immune competency of the patient. Many patients, including those with pericardial and rheumatic manifestations, can be observed without treatment. For severe disease where treatment is indicated and where mortality may reach 80% without treatment, amphotericin B, itraconazole and fluconazole are used. With treatment, mortality can be as low as 25%, although relapse of infection may occur.

REFERENCES

Bialek, R., Feucht, A., Aepinus, C., *et al.* (2002). Evaluation of two nested PCR assays for detection of *Histoplasma capsulatum* DNA in human tissue. *J Clin Microbiol* **40**, 1644–7.

Kauffman, C.A. (2001). Pulmonary histoplasmosis. *Curr Infect Dis Rep* **3**, 279–85.

Mocherla, S. and Wheat, L.J. (2001). Treatment of histoplasmosis. *Semin Respir Infect* **16**, 141–8.

Rickerts, V., Bialek, R., Tintelnot, K., Jacobi, V. and Just-Nubling, G. (2002). Rapid PCR-based diagnosis of disseminated histoplasmosis in an AIDS patient. *Eur J Clin Microbiol Infect Dis* **21**, 821–3.

Wheat, L.J., Garringer, T., Brizendine, E. and Connolly, P. (2002). Diagnosis of histoplasmosis by antigen detection based upon experience at the histoplasmosis reference laboratory. *Diagn Microbiol Infect Dis* **43**, 29–37.

Woods, J.P., Heinecke, E.L., Luecke, J.W., *et al.* (2001). Pathogenesis of *Histoplasma capsulatum*. *Semin Respir Infect* **16**, 91–101.

Appendix: useful websites

CHARITIES AND FUNDING AGENCIES

Leverhulme Trust, UK: www.leverhulme.org.uk/
Meningitis Research Foundation, UK:
    www.meningitis.org/
National Meningitis Trust, UK:
    www.meningitis-trust.org.uk/
Wellcome Trust, UK: www.wellcome.ac.uk/
Medical Research Council: www.mrc.ac.uk/

SOCIETIES AND PROFESSIONAL BODIES

Institute of Biomedical Science, UK:
    www.ibms.org/
American Society for Microbiology:
    www.asm.org/
Society for General Microbiology, UK:
    www.socgenmicrobiol.org.uk/
British Society for Antimicrobial Chemotherapy:
    www.bsac.org.uk/
Society for Applied Microbiology, UK:
    www.sfam.org.uk/
Royal College of Pathologists, UK:
    www.rcpath.org/
Hospital Infection Society, UK: www.his.org.uk/
The Royal Society, UK: www.royalsoc.ac.uk/
International Society of Infectious Diseases:
    www.isid.org/
World Health Organization: www.who.int/en/

GOVERNMENT BODIES

Health Protection Agency, UK: www.hpa.org.uk/
Medical Devices Agency, UK:
    www.medical-devices.gov.uk
Health and Safety Executive, UK:
    www.hse.gov.uk/index.htm
Scottish Centre for Infection and Environmental
    Health: www.show.scot.nhs.uk/scieh/
Scottish Health on the Web:
    www.show.scot.nhs.uk/
UK Department of Health:
    www.doh.gov.uk/index.htm
National Institutes of Health, USA: www.nih.gov/
Centers for Disease Control and Prevention, USA:
    www.cdc.gov/

ACCREDITATION BODIES

Clinical Pathology Accreditation:
    www.cpa-uk.co.uk/
UK Accreditation Service: www.ukas.com/

SEQUENCING AND GENOMICS

Multilocus sequence typing: www.mlst.net/
Institute for Genome Research, USA:
    www.tigr.org
Sanger Centre, UK: www.sanger.ac.uk/
National Centre for Biotechnology and
    Information: www.ncbi.nlm.nih.gov/
Lab on a Chip: www.lab-on-a-chip.com/home/
    index.asp
Nanoapex: http://news.nanoapex.com/

Index

Page numbers in bold type refer to tables